". . . this book is essential reading. Drs. Brown, Gerbarg, and Muskin have written a text that has the potential to revolutionize mainstream mental health care, and provide practitioners and consumers alike the confidence to seek out alternative treatments."

—**Amy Weintraub**,
Founder and Director of LifeForce Yoga®
Healing Institute and author of
Yoga for Depression

"[A]n excellent reference . . . that will appeal to CAM consumers and practitioners as well as conventional physicians. All will find a thoughtful review of practical guidelines for the application of CAM treatments for neurology and psychiatry. I give it a thumbs up!"

— *HerbalGram Magazine*

"[I]nvaluable for practicing physicians and those in the mental health industry."

—*Midwest Book Review*

"[A] powerful book . . . has the potential to blow a gaping hole in the current wall of psychiatric ignorance of natural therapies."

— **Chris Kilham**,
founder, Medicine Hunter Inc.

"Well organized and clearly written, this valuable guide emphasizes the evidence for yoga, herbals, and other natural therapies in the management of common mental and emotional disorders . . . a comprehensive yet accessible book for clinicians and consumers seeking to understand and apply basic principles of integrative care in ways that are effective *and* safe."

—**James Lake MD**,
Chair, APA Caucus on Complementary,
Alternative and Integrative Medicine, author of
Integrative Mental Health Care

"This book is for everyone . . . an invaluable resource for practitioners and consumers alike."

—*Townsend Letter*

W9-BHG-693

"Brown, Gerbarg, and Muskin have distilled an otherwise daunting field of treatment down to its basics: their overriding approach is to present the CAM methods that are most practical in a clinical setting, easy to administer, and low in side effects."
—*Current Psychiatry* **Online**

"[T]he best book on this difficult topic that I have come across."
—**Martin Guha,** *Journal of Mental Health*

"Using wonderfully written and helpful clinical vignettes, these experienced clinicians provide us with a roadmap to understanding the options and challenges that both practitioners and patients need to navigate. For mental health professionals and consumers alike, this is a must-have book!"
—**Michelle Riba, MD,**
   Professor of Psychiatry, Associate Chair for
   Integrated Medicine and Psychiatric Services,
   Department of Psychiatry, University of Michigan

"A truly impressive compilation of the latest research in the field of integrative mental health care. Optimal treatment of our patients demands that we challenge our biases about healing and that we educate ourselves about the latest in integrative technologies. This book, with its rich clinical examples and informative treatment guidelines, is an excellent resource for doing just that."
—**Erin L. Olivo, PhD, MPH,**
   Assistant Clinical Professor of Medical Psychology,
   Director, Integrative Medicine Program,
   Columbia University, College of
   Physicians and Surgeons

How to Use
HERBS, NUTRIENTS & YOGA
in Mental Health

How to Use
HERBS, NUTRIENTS & YOGA
in Mental Health

Richard P. Brown, MD
Patricia L. Gerbarg, MD
Philip R. Muskin, MD

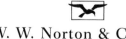

W. W. Norton & Company
New York • London

For informtion about special discounts for bulk purchases, please contact
W. W. Norton Special Sales at specialsales@wwnorton.com or 800-233-4830

Manufacturing by Courier Westford
Book design by Molly Heron
Production manager: Leeann Graham
Digital production: Joe Lops

Library of Congress Cataloging-in-Publication Data

Brown, Richard P.
How to use herbs, nutrients, & yoga in mental health /
Richard P. Brown, Patricia L. Gerbarg, Philip R. Muskin.
p. cm.
Originally published: How to use herbs, nutrients & yoga in mental
health care / Richard P. Brown, Patricia L. Gerbarg, Philip R. Muskin.
Includes bibliographical references and index.
ISBN 978-0-393-70744-1 (pbk.)
1. Mental illness—Alternative treatment. 2. Alternative medicine.
I. Gerbarg, Patricia L. II. Muskin, Philip R. III. Brown, Richard P. How
to use herbs, nutrients & yoga in mental health care. IV. Title. V.
Title: How to use herbs, nutrients and yoga in mental health.
RC480.5.B762 2012
616.89'1—dc23
2011017280

W. W. Norton & Company, Inc., 500 Fifth Avenue, New York, NY. 10110
www.wwnorton.com

W. W. Norton & Company Ltd.,
Castle House, 75/76 Wells Street,
London W1T 3QT

1 3 5 7 9 0 8 6 4 2

For their love,
patience, and support,
we dedicate this book
to our families.

Contents

Expanded Contents

CHAPTER 4

DISORDERS OF COGNITION AND MEMORY

CHAPTER 5

ATTENTION-DEFICIT DISORDER AND LEARNING DISABILITIES

CHAPTER 10

CAM to Counteract Medication Side Effects

Acknowledgments

We wish to thank the friends and colleagues who read and critiqued our manuscript. Our deepest appreciation goes to Dr. Sharon Sageman for her extraordinarily insightful comments on every chapter. She shared her clinical expertise, contributed several cases from her practice, and authored several of the important studies cited in the sections on post-traumatic stress disorder and bipolar disorder. We could not have found a more supportive, conscientious reader. She dedicated her time and attention to this book as though it were her own. We cannot thank her enough. She is our pearl of wisdom.

We would also like to thank Dr. Charles Silberstein, who provided many practical suggestions to improve the clarity and accessibility of the material in this book. For those readers who notice that some of the scientific material is intelligible, you have Charlie to thank. He brought to our attention the kinds of questions that would be of interest to practitioners and let us know which sections needed more explanation and which approaches were most effective.

We also must thank Naomi Gerbarg, BSW, MA, who shared her perspective as a nonmedical reader seeking health care information. Her skills as a reader and as a writer helped our book relate better to its audience. On behalf of our book, we thank Naomi for her time and her sensitivity to the needs of readers.

Many colleagues, teachers, and mentors contributed generously by sharing their expertise and the fruits of their research with us. Dr. Zakir Ramazanov taught us about *Rhodiola rosea* and gave us his extensive translations of Russian research on adaptogens. Dr.

Teodoro Bottiglieri guided us through the metabolic mysteries of S-adenosylmethionine, homocysteine, and methylfolate. Dr. Stephen Porges and Dr. Teodoro Beauchaine have enhanced our understanding of the role of the autonomic nervous system in mental health.

We also want to express our deep appreciation to Dr. Beth Adelson, Dr. Lorenzo Bernardi, Mark Blumenthal, Laura Braslow, Joshua Braslow, Dr. Gerard Byrne, Dr. Janis Carter, Dr. Bud Craig, Dr. R. Damodoran, Teresa Descilo, MSW, CTS, Dr. Patricia Eagon, Dr. Julia Eilenberg, Stephen Elliot, Dr. Jim Farrow, Dr. B. N. G. Gangadhar, Dr. Liselotte Gootjes, Dr. A-Min Huang, Dr. Martin Katzman, Dr. Vinod Kochupillai, Dr. James Lake, Dr. Stephen Larsen, Robin Larsen, Dr. Elena Lilioukina, Shad Meshad, MSW, Dr. Elizabeth Schauer, Dr. Leslie Sherlin, Dr. Shirley Telles, Dr. Irena Strigo, Dr. A. Vedamurthachar, Dr. Arielle Warner, and Aimee Weintraub. Our knowledge and experience of mind–body practices derive from the wisdom and training of Sri Sri Ravi Shankar, creator of Sudarshan Kriya Yoga, Aikido Master Sensei Imaizumi, Qigong Master Robert Peng, Zen from Sensei Tadashi Nakamura, Tai Chi from Master Tsu Kuo Shih, and Dr. Lester Fehmi, originator of the Open Focus technique.

The editors and staff of Norton Professional Books deserve our thanks for their understanding and enthusiastic support in bringing this book to publication. They gave priority to the needs of clinicians for practical training in complementary and alternative medicine.

Most of all, we wish to thank our patients who had the courage to keep trying new and alternative approaches to overcome their difficulties, and who trusted us to guide them toward recovery. Their unwillingness to give up when standard treatments failed gave us the opportunity to develop the approaches presented in the chapters ahead. In addition, several of the treatments were brought to us by patients who had come across them in their own searches, proving that one can learn a great deal from listening to patients. Our knowledge base could only have been built with their collaboration.

Preface

Complementary treatments are being used by the majority of consumers, with or without the advice of their health care practitioners. Although many physicians and therapists believe that herbs
and mind–body practices enhance health, they hesitate to integrate
such approaches into their clinical work. This is understandable considering that few had access to courses in complementary and alternative medicine (CAM) during their training. Once in practice, it is
difficult to find time to master the use of hundreds of herbs or to
connect with an experienced clinician for supervision, an essential
part of mental health training. By focusing on evidence-based treatments that have significant benefits and minimal side effects, clinicians can develop enough expertise to give their clients the best that
CAM has to offer while protecting them from unnecessary risks.

Some consumers pursue CAM because they want to enhance
health, prevent illness, slow aging processes, or feel more in control
of their health care choices. Others are dissatisfied with the effects
of prescription medications, cannot tolerate the side effects from
drugs, or fear long-term adverse effects. Unfortunately, without the
guidance of knowledgeable health care providers, many become
casualties of the misinformation superhighway or practitioners who
profit financially from the sale of products they recommend.

In this book we concentrate on CAM treatments that we find
most helpful in clinical practice, relatively easy to administer, and low
in side effects. With this knowledge, health care professionals will be
able to respond to the concerns of their clients and develop integrated

treatment plans leading to health enhancement, disease prevention, and optimal symptom resolution with minimal side effects.

A tiered decision-making approach to common problems encountered in the office will show which treatments to consider first and how to add complementary layers for more and more improvements. For each condition, we present our best picks from the herb garden and the most effective, least time-consuming mind–body techniques. Chapters will begin with the most useful CAM treatments followed by those with more circumscribed benefits.

This book may be used by clinicians interested in broadening their knowledge of CAM and in learning practical methods to safely introduce new treatments into their work. As a study guide, this book provides material and case examples for teaching courses on CAM for students in any mental health or medical field. Major areas of mental health are covered, including mood disorders, anxiety disorders, disorders of cognition and memory, hormone-related problems and life stage issues, psychological aspects of medical illnesses, schizophrenia, and substance abuse.

Consumers and clinicians will find here a resource of practical information for many of the health issues they and their families are facing. For example, the chapter on attention-deficit disorders and learning disabilities will prove helpful for families looking for alternatives to medication for their children. Women will find new approaches to premenstrual syndrome, infertility, mood disorders during and after pregnancy, physical and cognitive changes of menopause, and sexual enhancement. The chapter on disorders of cognition and memory introduces ways to improve mental function and quality of life for people with age-associated memory decline, poststroke, traumatic brain injury, Alzheimer's disease, and Parkinson's disease. Information on improving mental and emotional well-being in patients with medical conditions, such as cancer and HIV, is offered in the chapter on medical illnesses.

Whether you devour this book from cover to cover or just nibble on the topics that satisfy your particular needs, we hope that you will be inspired to continue learning about the ongoing discoveries in complementary and mind–body medicine. Each chapter covers a major diagnostic category in the broad field of mental health. Complementary and alternative treatments that the authors have found to be beneficial for the conditions within those categories are presented. For each treatment, the research evidence, clinical experience, risks, and benefits are discussed. Case examples are used to illustrate practical ways to apply and combine complementary treatments with standard treatments, such as medications and psychotherapies, to bring each patient as close to full remission as possible. Clinical pearls highlight important knowledge points. Summary lists, charts, and appendixes are included. References and other resources are given to assist readers in pursuing more information in the areas of greatest interest to them.

This book is intended as a guide to integrating complementary and alternative practices into standard mental health care. Rather than an encyclopedic review of all CAM modalities, the focus is on treatments that are of practical use to most clinicians. Treatment recommendations should be considered in the context of the individual patient's needs, medical conditions, physical state, and use of other medications. The patient's physician should always be informed on all CAM treatments and the regimen checked for possible adverse interactions. The tables at the end of each chapter outline common adverse reactions, but do not cover all possible side effects and medication interactions. Clinical judgment and further checking of the resources (see Appendix B) regarding specific treatments is advised in order to obtain all the available information to ensure the safe use of CAM. As with most prescription medications, the safety of most CAM treatments in children, pregnancy, and breast-feeding has not been established.

How to Use

HERBS, NUTRIENTS & YOGA

in Mental Health

CHAPTER 1

Basic Principles of Integrative Mental Health Care

Integrative mental health care encompasses the whole person (body, mind, and spirit), including all aspects of lifestyle. It emphasizes the therapeutic relationship and makes use of all appropriate therapies, including conventional, alternative, and complementary.

—Adapted from the definition of *integrative medicine* by
The Program in Integrative Medicine, University of Arizona

Whether you are a general practitioner, psychiatrist, neurologist, internist, or other medical specialist, a psychologist, nurse, social worker, counselor, physician's assistant, chiropractor, physical therapist, acupuncturist, mind–body therapist, nutritionist, homeopathic practitioner, dentist, or other health care provider, you already know the basic principles of good clinical practice in your field. We offer a few suggestions regarding how to apply what you know to improve your practice of complementary and alternative medicine (CAM) and to seamlessly integrate it into your work.

A study of information-seeking behavior among the health sciences faculty at the University of California, San Francisco concluded that the majority of health professionals are unable to locate the CAM information they need for research, teaching, and practice (Owen & Fang, 2003). While 41% of respondents got useful information from the Web and 40% from journals, 46% relied on their colleagues for advice. Reliable information is the foundation of clinical work. In Appendix B you will find useful resources for CAM information. In each chapter you will find treatments that we have found beneficial in clinical practice and in Appendix A information on where to obtain products of good quality.

The quality and quantity of scientific information on CAM treatments varies greatly. This can add to the clinician's uncertainty about using such treatments. In addition to indicating the extent and validity of the scientific research for each treatment, we will put this information in the context of clinical decision making. Keep in mind that a lack of research often has little to do with the potential benefits of an herb and more to do with whether a company would profit enough from sales to offset the costs of doing a double-blind, placebo-controlled study (approximately $500,000 to $2,000,000). Unlike synthetic drugs, patents usually cannot protect the sale of natural herbs, so no single company would profit enough from exclusive sales to pay the cost of research. Many companies obtain patents for herbal combinations with "proprietary blends." While we prefer to see large-scale controlled studies, these are available for only a few CAM treatments. In most cases, there is preliminary or pilot data. Each clinician must decide how long to wait for positive preliminary results to be validated by further studies before using these treatments.

While most health care professionals agree that double-blind randomized placebo-controlled trials are the gold standard of research, in many cases such studies are no guarantee of efficacy or safety. Numerous drugs have been pulled from the market due to serious adverse effects or lack of efficacy after initial positive results in such studies. This may be due to the fact that most studies use carefully selected subjects without comorbid conditions who do not represent the range of patients in clinical practice. Furthermore, few studies run for more than six weeks and therefore yield little information on long-term effects.

We have a lower threshold for trying CAM treatments based on preliminary data than for synthetic drugs for several reasons. First, synthetic pharmaceuticals are new to biological systems. Because most CAM treatments have been used by large groups of people of all ages and stages of health for hundreds if not thousands of years, we have much more information about their safety and potential side effects than we could possibly have for drugs that are often tested for six weeks in a carefully selected group of physically healthy subjects.

Second, in general, CAM treatments have far fewer and far milder side effects than prescription medications or surgery. The relatively high safety profile of most CAM treatments weighs in favor of trying them even if the scientific research is limited.

The context and options are also important in deciding whether to offer complementary treatments. If a patient is suffering and has not responded to standard treatments or cannot tolerate side effects, then it makes sense to offer low-risk alternatives with few adverse effects. The level of evidence for medical treatments is an assessment of the amount and the quality of research available to support the use of each treatment. For example, if there are six well-documented double-blind randomized placebo-controlled studies of a substantial number of patients that all report significant positive benefits, the level of evidence is rated as high. In contrast, if there is only one study or if there are only a few small open, uncontrolled studies, then the level is lower. Rather than dismissing all but those treatments with the highest levels of evidence, we suggest that different clinical situations warrant different levels of evidence for treatment. Here are several scenarios in which the clinician might accept a lower level of evidence in recommending CAM treatments:

1. The patient has tried and failed to respond to standard treatments.
2. The patient is unable to tolerate side effects of standard treatments.
3. The patient has a condition for which there is no effective standard treatment.
4. Standard treatments and augmentation strategies partially relieve symptoms, but the patient is still symptomatic.
5. The patient is taking necessary medications and those medications are causing side effects that could be alleviated by CAM treatments.
6. The patient wants to reduce or mitigate the effects of risk factors, for example, a family history of Alzheimer's disease, a personal history of cigarette smoking, or head trauma.
7. The patient wants to explore the full range of preventive, antiaging, or function-enhancing (e.g., cognitive or sexual) options.
8. The patient is in a situation in which there is no access to standard treatments, for example, a mass disaster or war zone.

9. The patient is uncomfortable with traditional pharmaceuticals and is more comfortable starting with CAM.
10. The patient cannot afford traditional pharmaceuticals and wants to start with lower cost alternatives.

It is best to start by focusing on a small number of CAM treatments to develop in-depth knowledge as you gain experience. Clinicians add to their repertoire of CAM treatments over time. As is true in all areas of health care, it is important to know one's limits and when to refer to other providers in order to do no harm. The same principles of good clinical judgment used in standard practice apply to CAM, including objectively weighing risks versus benefits, evaluating the evidence base for each treatment, flexibility in adapting treatments to the individual patient's needs, and risk reduction. Along the way you will discover through clinical work which experts provide information that really helps your patients do well. Once you identify such experts, you can attend their lectures or contact them for advice or supervision if needed. Reading their articles can offer an opportunity to dig for diamonds in their reference lists.

It is essential to learn how each CAM treatment works. Simplistic tables that say use herb X for symptom Y are of limited use. Knowledge of the underlying mechanisms of action for each treatment allows better understanding of all the ways it may affect the patient, including interactions with medications. Look for CAM lectures and courses sponsored by reputable organizations such as professional societies and academic institutions.

The quality of products used in CAM varies greatly. Not knowing which brands are of high quality is a major obstacle for practitioners. Stable supplements that are easy to produce, such as vitamin C, can be purchased from any large reliable company. However, the purity and potency of herbal preparations may depend on where they were grown, when they were harvested, and the specific extraction techniques. Certain nutrients, such as S-adenosylmethionine, are highly unstable and require great care not only in production, but also in the manufacturing and packaging of the tablet. For those supplements that require special attention for processing and manufacturing, we provide a list of products believed to be of good quality in the tables in Appendix A. The intention is to help practitioners identify reliable products that they can begin to use while gaining experience. These lists do not cover all available products. Exclusion from a list does not mean that we have assessed other products to be inferior. In developing the list of quality herbal products, we took into consideration the following sources of information:

1. Some companies were asked to supply detailed information about the source of their materials, the methods of extraction and manufacture, documents such as high-pressure liquid chromatography as proof of purity, reports of all tests and clinical studies done on their products, and evidence of testing for shelf life (how long the product retains full potency while sitting on the shelf). If a company was unable or unwilling to supply adequate documentation, they were not included on our list.
2. Specific products that demonstrated efficacy in controlled studies published in peer-reviewed journals were considered of high quality.
3. Information gathered from independent testers such as ConsumerLab and SupplementWatch was also used.
4. Observations over many years of clinical practice provided us with valuable information about the efficacy and tolerability of products.

The information about quality products is not intended to promote any company. We have attempted to provide several options in each category. Some companies specialize in combination products tailored to specific clinical problems. In such cases, the choices may be limited to one or two product lines.

ETHICAL PRACTICES

We recommend avoiding the temptation to profit from the sale of CAM products. Practitioners are often approached by herbal companies offering financial incentives to prescribe or sell their products. One can promote ethical practices by just saying no. Even if you believe that a product is of good quality, as soon as you start to sell it in your office, you are on the slippery slope of allowing money to influence clinical judgment. Although many CAM experts believe in the quality of their name brand products, they have opened the door for conflict of interest to erode trust. However, there are exceptions. For example, some CAM products and medications used in other countries can only be purchased by a licensed physician. In such cases, the physician may have to purchase and resell the product to patients. To prevent any compromise of ethics, we advise selling such products at cost without profit. This may seem a bit austere, but the unconscious is a greedy beast that can subvert clinical judgment. Even when the practitioner's decision to prescribe a CAM product is not influenced by profit, if the practitioner benefits financially from the sale of that product, the patient's trust may be undermined by the appearance of a conflict of interest. Accepting customary lecture fees is also within the bounds of ethical practice. It is best to apply the same ethical standards to CAM that you would use with prescription medications.

LIABILITY ISSUES

Fear of malpractice liability prevents many practitioners from integrating CAM into their work. Many are uncertain about how to handle liability issues. In discussing legal and regulatory issues, malpractice experts Michael Cohen and Ronald Schouten (2007) suggest that the following categories of malpractice could be applied to CAM: misdiagnosis, failure to treat, failure of informed consent, fraud and misrepresentation, abandonment, vicarious liability, and breach of privacy and confidentiality. Obviously, patients who request CAM treatments are entitled to the same level of diagnostic evaluation as those who seek conventional treatments.

While, in general, the same approach used to address liability issues in standard practice is applicable to all categories of liability in integrative mental health care, in using CAM treatments, the issue of failure to treat raises several potential scenarios worth noting:

1. If scientific evidence supports the safety and efficacy of a CAM treatment, then it is not likely to lead to a liability. There could be cases in which a patient who is unable to tolerate or respond to conventional treatments could be treated with a reasonably safe and effective CAM therapy. In such cases, one could argue that it would be negligent not to inform the patient of the CAM treatment and offer the option to try it.

2. If scientific evidence indicates that a particular CAM treatment is ineffective or is likely to cause harm, then the practitioner should try to dissuade the patient.
3. If the evidence for the safety or efficacy of a CAM treatment is equivocal, then the practitioner should discuss with the patient all of the known potential risks as well as the quality of the evidence both in favor of and against the treatment. If the patient decides to try the treatment after this discussion (which has been documented in the chart), then the practitioner should monitor the patient during the trial and intervene if any adverse reactions occur.
4. If the patient has a condition that can be easily or rapidly cured by standard treatment, and if the use of CAM delays effective treatment such that the patient suffers harm or the illness progresses, this could be considered malpractice, negligence, or substandard care.

The same principles that govern informed consent in conventional treatments can be applied to CAM. Practitioners should consult their individual state regulations governing the practice of CAM. The Federation of State Medical Boards (FSMB; 2002) of the United States approved model guidelines for the use of CAM therapies in medical practice (http://www.fsmb.org/pdf/2002_grpol_complementary_alternative_therapies.pdf). They recommend that before offering any recommendation for treatment, the physician should conduct an appropriate medical history and physical examination of the patient as well as a review of the patient's medical records. The FSMB (2002) guidelines note:

> The evaluation shall include, but not be limited to, conventional methods of diagnosis and may include other methods of diagnosis as long as the methodology utilized for diagnosis is based upon the same standards of safety and reliability as conventional methods, and shall be documented in the patient's medical record. The medical record shall also document:
>
> • what medical options have been discussed, offered or tried, and if so, to what effect, or a statement as to whether or not

certain options have been refused by the patient or guardian; that proper referral has been offered for appropriate treatment;
• that the risks and benefits of the use of the recommended treatment to the extent known have been appropriately discussed with the patient or guardian;
• that the physician has determined the extent to which the treatment could interfere with any other recommended or ongoing treatment.

Sidebar 1.1 shows an example of how to write a note to document the decision to treat a depressed patient with S-adenosylmethionine, an alternative antidepressant described in Chapter 2. Including a direct quote from the patient adds credibility to the record.

Written informed consent forms for CAM can be created by adapting language found on conventional forms and including space to fill in the potential risks, drug interactions, and benefits. However, clinicians will find that it is cumbersome and time consuming to ask the patient to sign a form every time a treatment is initiated. Moreover, this does not obviate the need for full documentation of the decision-making process and discussion in the patient record.

In general, referral to a CAM therapist should not engender liability for the referring conventional practitioner. However, the practitioner may be considered liable if the referral delays medical care and leads to harm for the patient, if the conventional practitioner knows or should know that the CAM therapist is incompetent, or if there is a joint treatment (Cohen & Schouten, 2007).

Practitioners of conventional medicine, CAM, and integrative medicine can minimize liability risks by becoming well-informed about the treatments they recommend, completing a thorough diagnostic workup, fully informing the patient of treatment options (both conventional and CAM), clearly documenting treatment discussions in the medical record, monitoring the patient for progress as well as adverse reactions, engaging the patient in treatment decisions, and communicating clearly with the patient about treatment issues. Ultimately, the single most effective way to prevent liability problems is to maintain a caring and responsive professional relationship with the patient.

SIDEBAR 1.1 **SAMPLE NOTE FOR DOCUMENTATION OF CAM**

Impressions and Recommendations:

1. The patient has major depression, recurrent moderate causing significant difficulties functioning at work and at home. Previous trials of 8 prescription antidepressants, including 2 TCAs, 3 SSRIs, venlafaxine, bupropion, mirtazepine, and 2 mood stabilizers have been unsuccessful because of intolerable side effects (sedation, weight gain, cognitive impairment, elevated liver enzymes, and sexual dysfunction).

2. The patient has been informed of the risks and benefits of further medication trials including MAOIs and mood stabilizers. I also discussed the potential risks and benfits of an alternative antidepressant, S-adenosylmethionine (SAMe), including nausea, diarrhea, headache, palpitations, insomnia, anxiety, agitation, and mania in bipolar patients. I informed the patient that SAMe has been approved by the FDA for over-the-counter sale in the United States as a nutraceutical.

3. I recommended SAMe because it does not cause any sedation, weight gain, cognitive impairment, liver enzyme elevations, or sexual dysfunction. SAMe has no adverse interactions with any of the medications the patient is taking.

4. The patient chose to begin a trial of SAMe because she prefers to avoid medication side effects if possible. The patient states, "I've suffered enough from the prescriptions I've already tried. I want to try some alternative treatments."

BEGIN AT THE BEGINNING: DIFFERENTIAL DIAGNOSIS

The differential diagnosis is a working list of the possible diagnoses that could account for the patient's symptoms. Sometimes the diagnosis is evident in the first encounter, but usually it unfolds over time. Diagnosis and treatment can be like a game of chess in that as it evolves, only certain moves are possible at each moment in time. Every therapy opens with the building of trust based on understanding and compassion. As you elicit the clinical history, inquire respectfully about the patient's attitudes toward and experiences with CAM as well as standard treatments. Has the patient benefited from complementary approaches? What products is the patient using? Does the patient engage in mind–body practices? Often patients will tell you that years ago they did yoga or meditation or Tai Chi, but that they had forgotten how good it made them feel. Others will say that they tried meditation but never could do it because they were thinking too much. In Chapter 3 we show how useful these nuggets of information can be as you formulate a treatment plan.

> If you drink too much from a bottle marked "poison," it is almost certain to disagree with you, sooner or later.
> —*Alice's Adventures in Wonderland* by Lewis Carroll

Alice remembered to read the label before following the directions "Drink Me" on the bottle she found on a glass table. Clinicians also need to read the labels on bottles of herbs while keeping in mind that labels do not tell all that you might wish to know. As Alice discovered, the absence of a "poison" label is no assurance of safety. We ask patients to bring to the office all of the vitamins and supplements they are taking and we keep a magnifying glass handy for reading the fine print. Obtaining previous treatment records and knowing what substances your patient has been ingesting are essential in working through the differential diagnosis.

INTRODUCING CAM

The patient's level of interest in or resistance to CAM is an important consideration in the treatment plan. Take time to explain the pros and cons of standard and alternative treatments pertinent to the symptoms. When the client absolutely favors prescription medication and maintains a completely negative attitude toward CAM, it makes sense to start with prescription drugs if they are appropriate. If the response to medication is robust with few side effects, then

CAM may not be necessary. However, if after doing appropriate medication trials the patient is only 50% or 75% improved or if there are troublesome side effects, it may be time to reopen the CAM discussion. By this time, the patient has learned from experience the limitations of prescription medication and is probably more willing to try alternative approaches. You can share what you know with the patient by discussing CAM options, explaining how each one works and the potential benefits and risks. When you record this discussion in the chart along with your reasons for recommending CAM, you will also be reducing the liability risks.

Conversely, if patients come to you strongly favoring CAM, then you first need to understand the reasons for their interest and make certain that you fully inform them of both standard and alternative treatment options. The history may show that the patient has already run the gamut of medication trials without satisfactory results. Again, be sure to document in the chart that you have fully informed the patient about standard and CAM treatments.

CAM is not a panacea, but it can contribute to recovery and well-being. Enabling the patient to participate in the decision-making process strengthens the therapeutic relationship. Many come from backgrounds in which they had no choice but to obey what others imposed upon them. Approaching the integration of CAM as an exploratory collaboration supports the therapeutic process.

Many of the case examples used in this book involve assessing, augmenting, or changing prescription medications. Practitioners and students who are not licensed to prescribe medication will find a guide to medications in Appendix C. Even if you cannot write prescriptions, you may still contribute to an integrative treatment plan through team discussions and by providing clients and other practitioners with current information on CAM treatments. Those who offer CAM treatments need to be aware that patients who have medical conditions and those taking prescription medications should be advised to consult their physician before adding or substituting herbs or supplements.

Focus on Stress

The most useful concept in complementary medicine is stress—psychological, environmental, and physical. Directly and indirectly,

CAM works by reducing stress, enhancing stress resistance, or ameliorating the adverse effects of stress.

We can consider stress to be any condition in which the demands for activity exceed the supply of energy. This applies at the cellular level as well as to the organism as a whole. Energy is generated in mitochondria and stored in energy molecules such as adenosine triphosphate and creatine phosphate. This energy fuels all functions of life including cellular repair. Cells are subject to constant damage from free radicals, radiation, inflammation, infections, toxins, and aging. Oxygen, nutrients, and energy are required to continuously repair the damage inflicted on cell membranes, mitochondria, DNA, and other cellular components.

Prescription antidepressants target specific neurotransmitters involved in mood regulation. Alternative approaches support the optimal functioning of all neurons by ensuring a rich supply of vitamins and nutrients known to support cellular energy production and metabolic pathways, prevent damage to cellular components, reduce excess inflammation and lipid peroxidation, and enhance cellular repair. Furthermore, through mind–body practices it is possible to increase oxygenation and to shift the chemical and electrical activity of the nervous system toward more integrated, synchronous, and effective functioning with a reduction in energy expenditure.

Under conditions of emotional or physical stress, cells burn energy at a higher rate while generating more free radicals as by-products. The main components of the stress response system are the sympathetic nervous system (SNS) and the hypothalamic-pituitary-adrenal axis (HPA). When we perceive danger, the SNS prepares the body for fight or flight by releasing neurotransmitters that accelerate the heart rate and respiration, increase blood flow to muscles, and reduce blood flow to the digestive tract. The HPA contributes hormones such as adrenaline to stimulate the heart and nervous system. Cortisol is released to mobilize glucose stores. The human stress response system is designed for short periods of intense activity to be followed by long periods of rest and recovery. Once the immediate danger has passed, the parasympathetic nervous system (PNS) is supposed to become more active to slow the heart and respiration, relax the gastrointestinal tract, restore energy reserves, and enhance cellular repair. Failure of the PNS to counterbalance the SNS is critical in the pathogenesis of anxiety, depression, and stress-related conditions including heart disease, diabetes, irritable bowel disease, cancer, and diseases of aging.

Stress is a major factor in most illnesses of the mind, body, and spirit. It is well known that prolonged emotional stress can lead to chronic overactivation of the SNS. Common symptoms of elevated SNS activity include anxiety, agitation, insomnia, excess worry, overreactivity, rapid or irregular heartbeat, elevated blood pressure, abdominal pain (e.g., a knot in the stomach), and weight gain. In more extreme cases, all of the symptoms of panic, post-traumatic stress disorder, or chronic fatigue syndrome can appear. Pharmacological interventions for stress symptoms have targeted the SNS. Anxiolytics and many antidepressants dampen SNS responses. However, more recent studies are showing that underactivity of the PNS is an important feature of anxiety disorders and many other conditions including panic, PTSD, depression, ADHD, aggression, sociopathy, and autism. Medications have not been shown to boost the activity of the PNS even though it is critical for restoring balance within the stress response system (Glassman, Bigger, Gaffney, & Van Zyl, 2007). Adaptogenic herbs such as *Rhodiola rosea* may boost PNS activity (Baranov, 1994). The importance of autonomic nervous system function and methods to enhance PNS activity using certain mind–body techniques are discussed in Chapter 3.

Go for the Gold: Optimal Health

The goal of treatment is remission, the complete relief of symptoms and resumption of full functioning in all areas of life. While 100% remission is not possible in all cases, it is well worth exploring complementary treatments to increase the patient's progress toward this goal. Integrative mental health care broadens the focus from reducing the burden of disease to attaining optimal health. Clients who have struggled with mental health issues for many years may not know what level of function they might attain. While a past history of limited treatment response is important, the clinician should leave no stone unturned in questioning previous diagnoses and treatments while searching for opportunities to help the patient go for the gold.

CHAPTER 2 OUTLINE

1. **Nutraceuticals**: S-adenosylmethionine for depression, antidepressant augmentation, arthritis, fibromyalgia, liver disease, Parkinson's disease, HIV/AIDS

2. **Herbs**: St. John's Wort, *Rhodiola rosea*

3. **Vitamins**: B vitamins, L-methylfolate, and vitamin D

4. **Nutrients**: choline, inositol, omega-3 fatty acids, 5-hydroxy-L-tryptophan (5-HTP), N-acetylcysteine

5. **Hormones**: dehydroepiandrosterone (DHEA) and 7-Keto DHEA

6. **Mind–Body Practices**: yoga—Iyengar, Shavasana, Hatha, Qigong, Sudarshan kriya

7. **Complex Cases**: multilayered approaches for integrative treatments in depression and bipolar disorder

CHAPTER 2

Mood Disorders

This chapter explores nutraceuticals, herbs, vitamins, nutrients, hormones, mind–body practices, and multi-layered approaches for the treatment of depression and bipolar disorder. Although the signs and symptoms of depression are well known, it is one of the most undertreated illnesses today. The general consensus has been that combining verbal psychotherapy with medication has been more effective than either treatment alone in the long-term management of depression (Pampallona, Bollini, Tibaldi, Kupelnick, & Munizza, 2004). Prescription antidepressants have become the mainstay of treatment despite the expense, the risks, the side effects, and the limited benefits associated with their use. Studies of antidepressant medications show that fewer than one third of all patients achieve full remission within eight weeks (Thase, 2003). Approximately 30% are partial responders and about 30% are non-responders (Baghai, Moller, & Rupprecht, 2006).

Knowing the method of patient selection and the definition of *outcome* in antidepressant treatment studies is crucial to understanding why we do not see many patients being "cured" of depression despite so many reports from double-blind, placebo-controlled studies claiming response rates above 60%. The results of many clinical trials cannot be generalized to the population of patients seen in most practice settings because the commonly used exclusion criteria preselect patients with uncomplicated depression. Recognizing this problem, the National Institute of Mental Health funded Sequenced Treatment Alternatives to Relieve Depression (STAR*D), a more naturalistic study of 4,000 patients including those with chronic depression and comorbid psychiatric and medical conditions (Trivedi, Rush, Wisniewski, Nierenberg, Warden et al., 2006). To simulate the most widely used approaches in psychiatric and primary care settings, patients were initially treated with a selective serotonin reuptake inhibitor (SSRI), in this study citalopram (Celexa) in doses up to 60 mg/day. The remission rate was only 27% (response rate 47%). Nonresponders were augmented or switched to other antidepressants with about a 30% remission rate (Trivedi et al., 2006). Most studies of antidepressants exclude patients with anxiety disorder, personality disorder, suicide attempts, long duration of illness, substance abuse, and medical disorders or those who were previously unresponsive to treatment. This means that 60–80% of your patients would not qualify for an antidepressant study. While the results of such studies have some relevance, understanding that most of your patients differ clinically from those selected for medication studies puts the benefit of standard psychotropic treatment into a more realistic perspective and highlights the need for multiple augmentation strategies.

In most studies, a responder is any subject whose scores on measures of depression decrease by 50% or more. This means that those who start with high depression scores may be called responders even if they are left with significant residual symptoms of depression. We do recognize the substantial benefits of antidepressants. For example, giving a patient 50% improvement in symptoms of depression can mean the difference between hope and despair. It can enable a dysfunctional individual to return to work. However, an optimal state of well-being would be 100% remission of symptoms. Residual symptoms of depression take the joy out of life. Moreover, they put the patient at higher risk for relapse, according to the Depression Clinical and Research Program at Massachusetts General Hospital (Fava, 2006; Petersen, 2006).

We suggest one way to make a simple assessment of the degree of improvement in depression among your patients. Just ask them to roughly estimate the percentage improvement in depression that they have noticed since starting antidepressant medication. Most will report 30–70%. Additional improvements using complementary and alternative medicine (CAM) can bring them closer to total remission. Prescription medications are necessary for recovery from depression in many cases. However, if we rely solely on prescriptions, we will not be giving our patients the opportunity for more complete and lasting recovery.

Nonadherence to medication protocols is a common cause of treatment failure. A three-year study of members of the Harvard Pilgrim Health Care managed care plan found an average noncompliance rate of 75% among patients on antidepressant medications (Bambauer, Adams, Zhang, Minkoff, Grande et al., 2006). Although laziness and disorganization may be factors, we believe that people vote with their feet. Most people stop taking their medication because they feel that what they get out of their pill is not worth putting up with the side effects and costs. If a treatment regimen really makes people feel good, they tend to continue it.

Assessing the efficacy of CAM treatments in depression is challenging. Few large-scale randomized, controlled studies have been done. Furthermore, it is difficult in general to obtain clear positive results in depression studies, particularly in outpatients with mild to moderate depression. Approximately 50% of well-controlled studies of prescription antidepressants submitted for U.S. regulatory approval failed to show positive results. These same antidepressants were later approved for use by the Food and Drug Administration (FDA) based on other positive studies. In other words, a negative outcome in a depression study does not necessarily mean that a drug lacks antidepressant efficacy (Khan, Khan, Walens, Kolts, & Giller, 2003).

Evaluating the quality of evidence for CAM is complex because most rating systems and meta-analyses are limited to substances used as solo treatments and tend to exclude studies of adjunctive treatments. While CAM can be used as a monotherapy, it is often combined with other treatments. Moreover, researchers find it easier to get permission for studies of CAM as an adjunctive rather than as a solo treatment. This chapter discusses methods for understanding and using nutraceuticals, herbs, nutrients, mind–body practices, and exercise in the treatment of mood disorders. It includes major depression, dysthymia, depression in patients with medical illnesses, bipolar disorder, and bipolar disorder associated with post-traumatic stress disorder.

NUTRACEUTICALS

Nutraceuticals are a special class of supplements that have been found by the FDA to be safe enough for sale over the counter in the United States without a prescription.

S-adenosylmethionine, Ademetionine

SAMe (S-adenosylmethionine) has been a first-line, mainstream antidepressant in many European countries for over 20 years. It is still considered an alternative treatment in the United States where the FDA approved its use as an over-the-counter nutraceutical in 1998.

SAMe is an essential molecule that participates in hundreds of biochemical reactions within the cells of all living organisms (see Figure 2.1). Cells produce SAMe through the condensation of methionine and adenosine triphosphate. SAMe donates essential molecules (methyl groups) for the production of DNA, proteins, phospholipids, neurotransmitters (serotonin, norepinephrine, and dopamine), and many other important building blocks. It also

---

CLINICAL PEARL

Neutraceuticals, herbs, and nutrients can be used as first-line treatments for mild to moderate depressions. Although most severe depressions require antidepressant medication for optimal response during the acute response phase (first 2 weeks) and for remission (8 weeks), CAM can also help by improving the initial response, increasing the rate and degree of remission, supporting long-term remission, and reducing side effects.

donates sulfate groups, for example in the synthesis of the major antioxidant glutathione (Bottiglieri, 2002).

SAMe was shown to be safe and effective for the treatment of major depression in 16 open trials, 13 double-blind placebo-controlled studies, and 19 double-blind controlled trials in comparison to standard antidepressants. For a detailed review of SAMe metabolism and a critique of the research studies, see Brown, Gerbarg, and Bottiglieri (2002). Because SAMe is a natural metabolite

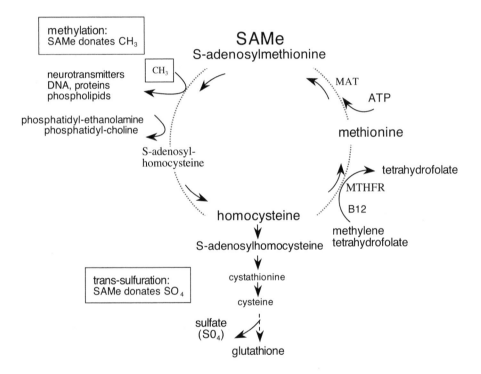

Figure 2.1 S-adenosylmethionine (SAMe) metabolic pathways build essential molecules. Methionine + ATP $\rightarrow$ SAMe. Methionine adenosyltransferase (MAT) enzyme converts methionine and adenosine triphosphate (ATP) into S-adenosylmethionine (SAMe). SAMe donates methyl groups (CH3) for synthesis of neurotransmitters, proteins, and other essential molecules. SAMe pathway leads to production of glutathione (major antioxidant). Methylene-tetrahydrofolate reductase (MTHFR) enzyme and B12 cofactor regenerate methionine (needed to maintain SAMe synthesis) and convert methylene tetrahydrofolate to tetrahydrofolate.

(more like a vitamin), it is very low in side effects when compared with prescription antidepressants and it has a more rapid onset of action. There are no reported adverse interactions with other medications. In fact, SAMe protects the liver from the toxic effects of other medications. SAMe can augment the action of standard antidepressants and restore efficacy when they have lost it. SAMe is the only antidepressant that has been studied in combination with monoamine oxidase inhibitors with good results (Torta et al., 1988). In addition to its antidepressant effects, SAMe has numerous long-term health benefits and advantages for patients with a wide range of serious medical conditions.

The electroencephalogram profile of SAMe is similar to that of tricyclic antidepressants (TCAs), while the profile of St. John's Wort is like that of SSRIs. The effects of SAMe on cortical nerve cell metabolism also overlap with those of TCAs. A review of SAMe noted three controlled studies showing that it enhances the action of TCAs (Brown, Gerbarg, & Bottiglieri, 2000). SAMe is more like a TCA, but with minimal side effects, rendering it more tolerable.

Side Effects

The most common side effect of SAMe is mild nausea. This can usually be relieved by eating a light snack before taking SAMe, taking ginger capsules or tea, or by reducing the SAMe dose. Loose bowels, flatulence, and abdominal pain can also occur. For patients who tend to be constipated, this is a boon. However, those who are prone to nausea, gastric irritation, or irritable bowel symptoms may not do well. Rarely, the nausea or diarrhea can become too problematic, requiring discontinuation of SAMe. Occasionally patients complain of headache. Because SAMe is activating, it can occasionally exacerbate anxiety, panic, or agitation, as can any activating antidepressant (see below). Antidepressants, including SAMe, can trigger hypomania or mania in patients with bipolar disorder (manic-depressive). A diagnosis of bipolar disorder is a strong contraindication against the use of SAMe. There have been rare cases in which patients with palpitations have complained of an increase in these irregular heartbeats when given SAMe, although it is generally well tolerated by individuals with cardiovascular disease. However, if it exacerbates symptoms, it should be discontinued.

SAMe does not cause sexual side effects, sedation, weight gain, or cognitive interference. The absence of these troubling side effects makes SAMe readily acceptable to many clients.

How to Use SAMe in the Treatment of Depression

SAMe tends to be an activating antidepressant. It helps to energize patients whose depression is characterized by low energy, tiredness, low motivation, and hypersomnia. It works best when taken at least 20 to 30 minutes before breakfast and lunch on an empty stomach for maximal absorption. If the patient forgets to take it before meals, it can be taken two hours after a meal when the stomach has emptied. If taken later in the day, there may be interference with sleep.

For patients whose depression includes significant symptoms of anxiety and agitation, it is often necessary to use a benzodiazepine or buspirone during the first few weeks because the stimulating effects of SAMe can exacerbate anxiety (as also occurs with stimulating antidepressants such as SSRIs). However, within two or three weeks, as the antidepressant action is established, it is usually possible to taper off anxiolytics.

Case 1—SAMe for Depression

Jim, a 50-year-old business consultant, was having his fourth episode of depression. Normally an outgoing, dynamic self-starter, he was feeling insecure, indecisive, and afraid. His mind was filled with worries about a business slowdown. Usually, a business slump would motivate him to aggressively find new clients, but instead he felt paralyzed. Unable to sleep at night, he spent hours on the phone seeking reassurance from family and friends, all to no avail. Jim's depressions had always responded to sertraline (Zoloft) or fluoxetine (Prozac). He had been well for two years off medication. Jim was reluctant to resume prescription SSRIs because they destroyed his libido and caused erectile dysfunction. He asked about alternatives and chose a trial of SAMe, starting with 400 mg in the morning. At 1,200 mg/day, he began to feel less anxious and less depressed. On 800 mg twice a day he had complete remission of depression.

After he had been asymptomatic for three months, SAMe was gradually reduced. Jim experienced no adverse effects and was comfortable staying on a maintenance dose of SAMe 400 mg twice a day.

SAMe Dosages

In patients who are elderly or who have medication sensitivities, significant anxiety, gastrointestinal problems, or serious medical conditions, one can start with a test dose of 200 mg SAMe 20 minutes before breakfast for a few days. It this is well tolerated, increase to 400 mg 20 minutes before breakfast for 3–7 days. The rate of increase in SAMe doses depends on your clinical assessment of the patient. For elderly, frail, or unstable patients, allow more time for increases. If the patient reports side effects, then allow more time to adjust before the next increase. In general, the dose for mild depression is 400–600 mg/day; moderate depression, 600–1,200 mg/day; severe depression, 1,200–1,600 mg/day; very severe treatment-resistant depression, 1,600–2,400 mg/day. Before you exceed 1,600 mg/day (the maximum dose that has been used in clinical trials), consider augmenting SAMe with other CAM treatments and prescription antidepressants or obtaining a CAM consultation. Inform the patient that SAMe has been used safely in high doses, but that clinical trials have not exceeded 1,600 mg, and record this discussion in the patient's chart (see Chapter 1).

SAMe Augmentation With B Vitamins

The pathways by which SAMe donates methyl groups (methylation) for the production of the major neurotransmitters involved in mood regulation require the cofactors B_{12} (methylcobalamine) and folate (see Figure 2.1). Low levels of these cofactors have been found in association with severe depression. Adding 1,000 mcg/day B_{12}, 800 mcg folate, and 50–100 mg/day B_6 will often enhance the antidepressant effects of SAMe as well as other antidepressant medications (see below). B vitamins and folate should not be given to men with cardiac stents because they can accelerate restenosis in those whose baseline homocysteine is less than 15 μmol/liter.

Clinical Applications and Practical Considerations

SAMe is as effective as prescription antidepressants for mild to severe depression. If the patient is unable to afford SAMe, then St. John's Wort and *Rhodiola rosea* could be tried first in mild to moderate depression. When moderate to severe depression is the primary diagnosis, SAMe should be the first-line CAM treatment to consider. Although SAMe contributes to the production of serotonin, norepinephrine, and dopamine, its profile of pharmacological activity is similar to that of a noradrenergic agent. A history of good response to a noradrenergic antidepressant (e.g., tricyclic or tetracyclic) would weigh more heavily on the side of starting with SAMe. It has far fewer side effects than standard antidepressants and it works more rapidly. Patients who complain of sexual dysfunction or weight gain on prescription antidepressants may do well on SAMe because it does not cause either of these disturbing side effects. SAMe is quite useful in augmenting the effects of other antidepressants.

SAMe works well in the geriatric population and is often better tolerated than conventional antidepressants. It has unique benefits in treating depression in patients with arthritis, fibromyalgia, liver disease, and HIV/AIDS (see section below). It should also be seriously considered for patients who take medications that impair liver function such as statins (for hypercholesterolemia). Patients receiving statins in addition to prescription antidepressants are at increased risk for liver dysfunction. SAMe has no adverse hepatic effects and has been shown to protect against liver damage from numerous prescription medications.

Cost is a major drawback for SAMe because it is not yet covered by insurance companies in most countries. Prices vary from $20 to $60 for a package of 20 of the 400 mg tablets. Encourage your patient to comparison shop (among the listed quality brands) as large chain stores and online websites often have sales. Unfortunately, at higher doses, SAMe becomes too expensive for many people. However, since SAMe combines well with all other antidepressants, it is possible to take a smaller dose of SAMe in conjunction with a reduced dose of a prescription antidepressant. This is a particularly useful strategy for reducing the side effects of prescription antidepressants to a tolerable level while adding a more affordable dose of SAMe.

SAMe to Augment Antidepressants

SAMe can increase the effectiveness of prescription antidepressants and speed the onset of action. In an open trial, researchers at Massachusetts General Hospital gave SAMe (800–1,600 mg/day) to 30 depressed patients who had failed to respond to either SSRIs or venlafaxine (Effexor) (Alpert, Papakostas, Mischoulon, Worthington, Petersen et al., 2004). The addition of SAMe resulted in a response rate of 50% and a remission rate of 43%. Gastrointestinal symptoms and headaches were reported as side effects in these subjects taking two antidepressants together. An earlier double-blind placebo-controlled study had shown that SAMe accelerated the response to imipramine (Berlanga, Ortega-Soto, Ontiveros, & Senties, 1992).

In a six-month study of 350 patients, SAMe improved antidepressant response to imipramine. SAMe augmentation was also studied in 500 patients on benzodiazepines, 60 on monoamine oxidase inhibitors (MAOIs), 445 on anticonvulsants, and 18 alcoholics on antidepressants or anticonvulsants. The addition of SAMe caused no adverse reactions. SAMe reversed or prevented liver toxicity, as indicated by elevation of gamma-glutamyl-transpeptidase, in all patients taking MAOIs, anticonvulsants, or antidepressants (Torta, Zanalda, Rocca, 1988).

Case 2—SAMe With an Antidepressant

Barbara, a 48-year-old special education teacher, had been taking venlafaxine (Effexor-XR) 300 mg/day for recurring episodes of major depression. Over the years she had been on numerous antidepressants including fluoxetine (Prozac), sertraline (Zoloft), paroxetine (Paxil), nefazodone (Serzone), bupropion (Wellbutrin), citalopram (Celexa), and escitalopram (Lexapro). Each medication had worked for some period of time, and then the effects just petered out. She had been doing well on Effexor for two years until the start of the school year when her student assignments almost doubled. Her trusted classroom assistant was out on maternity leave and had been replaced by a woman who was inexperienced and disorganized. Barbara, who prided herself on her organization and professionalism, felt overwhelmed, stressed out, and on the verge of tears. After breaking down and crying in the teachers' lounge, she became afraid of losing control. When her physician tried to increase the dose of Effexor, her blood pressure rose by 10 points and she became anorgasmic. She was interested in trying SAMe but worried about the cost of taking it at higher doses as a monotherapy. She opted to continue Effexor while adding SAMe 400 mg twice a day. On this combination, there were no side effects. Her mood improved and she felt able to handle the challenges at work.

Depression, Arthritis, and Fibromyalgia
Patients with arthritis often suffer from depression exacerbated by the multiple stressors of chronic progressive pain, disrupted sleep, aging, increased debilitation, and side effects from anti-inflammatory and pain medications. Twelve studies have shown that SAMe has analgesic and anti-inflammatory effects in osteoarthritis. Six studies reported that SAMe improved both depression and pain in patients with fibromyalgia at doses equivalent to 800 mg/day with no side effects (Ernst, 2003; Grassetto & Varatto, 1994; Ianiello, Ostuni, Sfriso, et al., 1994; Tavoni, Vitali, Bombardieri, & Pasero, 1987). For a more detailed discussion, see Chapter 8.

Depression and Liver Disease
Patients with liver diseases often have comorbid depression that may be primary, secondary to the hepatic dysfunction, or due to medications being used to treat the medical condition (e.g., interferon for viral hepatitis or HIV/AIDS). Moreover, psychotropic medications, particularly SSRIs, can cause elevations of liver function tests (LFTs) or exacerbate preexisting liver dysfunction. Alcohol abuse depletes the liver of SAMe and causes the oxidative stress that contributes to tissue damage.

Numerous studies have shown that SAMe improves liver function and reverses biochemical markers (abnormal LFTs) in patients with cirrhosis or hepatitis due to alcohol, drugs, toxins, infections, or gallstones (including during pregnancy; Frezza, Centini, Cammareri, Le Grazie, & Di Padova, 1990; Friedel, Goa, & Benfield, 1989; Lieber, 1999; Mato et al., 1999; Milkiewicz, Hubscher, Skiba, Hathaway, & Elias, 1999). In a two-year double-blind randomized placebo-controlled (DBRPC) study of alcohol-induced liver cirrhosis, Childs Class A and B cases, SAMe 1,200 mg/day increased survival and delayed the need for liver transplants (Mato, Camara, Fernandez de Paz, Caballeria, Coll et al., 1999). SAMe also prevented increases in liver enzymes and restored liver functions to normal in patients treated with antiseizure medications and MAOIs (Torta et al., 1988). Prescription antidepressant medications, particularly SSRIs, can cause elevated liver functions, especially in patients who have less than normal liver reserves due to previous injury, such as alcohol abuse or hepatitis.

Many cases of undiagnosed hepatitis are discovered when LFTs become elevated in patients placed on SSRIs for depression. Discontinuation of the prescription antidepressant and initiation of SAMe usually restores LFTs to normal range. For mildly elevated LFTs, use SAMe 800 mg in the morning (except in bipolar patients). In bipolar patients, Ease-2 or Ease-Plus, Chinese herbal preparations containing bupleurum, may be used. Hepatoprotective effects of *Bupleurum kaoi* include anti-inflammatory, antifibrotic, enhanced glutathione production, and liver cell regeneration (Yen, Weng, Liu, Chai, & Lin, 2005). For sharp increases or LFTs greater than three times normal, use SAMe 1,200–1,600 mg/day enhanced with polyenolphosphatidylcholine. SAMe is depleted during the conversion of phosphatidyl-ethanolamine to phosphatidylcholine (see Figure 2.1). Taking polyenolphosphatidylcholine replenishes phosphatidylcholine supplies, reducing the consumption of SAMe. As the SAMe reserves increase, more glutathione is produced to counteract oxidative damage to the liver (Aleynik & Lieber, 2003; Lieber, 2001, 2005). In patients with serious underlying liver disease with documented fibrosis, adding B vitamins and alpha-lipoic acid can enhance response. If LFT elevations persist, betaine (trimethylglycine) can augment the

---

CLINICAL PEARL

In depressed patients with abnormal liver function, SAMe can alleviate depression, protect the liver, and help restore hepatic function.

response to SAMe by elevating glutathione (antioxidant), protecting the liver from chemical damage, and improving the liver's capacity to break down its own fats (Barak, Beckenhauer, & Tuma; Efrati, Barak, Modan-Moses, Augarten, Vilozni et al., 2003; Kharbanda, Rogers, Mailliard, Siford, Barak et al., 2005).

Depression and Parkinson's

Levodopa (Sinemet) is a common treatment for Parkinson's disease, a progressive degenerative condition that is characterized by difficulty initiating movements, dyskinesias, stiffness, tremor, rigidity, masklike facies (loss of facial expression), and unsteady gait. It often leads to withdrawal and the loss of all spontaneous activity and communication. The patient may just sit in a chair unless prompted by others to move.

It is not well known that levodopa (L-dopa) depletes brain stores of SAMe. In addition to the depressive reaction to having a debilitating illness, the depletion of SAMe is probably one of the causes of depression in patients with Parkinson's. When depression occurs with Parkinson's, it is highly resistant to treatment with standard antidepressants. In a double-blind crossover study of 21 patients with Parkinson's disease, depression improved significantly in 8 of the patients given SAMe 1,200 mg/day (Carrieri, Indaco, & Gentile, 1990). Depression also improved in 11 out of 13 subjects in an open series of Parkinson's patients given SAMe 1,600–4,000 mg/day (Di Rocco, Rogers, Brown, Werner, & Bottiglieri, 2000). At these doses, some cases also showed improvement in neurological symptoms such as dyskinesias.

Case # 3—Depression and Parkinson's

Leonard, a 68-year-old retired lawyer, had been treated with levodopa for the past three years for Parkinson's disease. When his wife, Amelia, reported that he wasn't eating or sleeping well, that he seemed tired, and that he had no interest in visiting their friends, his neurologist arranged a psychiatric evaluation. Amelia guided Leonard to a chair where he sat staring at the floor, expressionless and disinterested, giving perfunctory responses when questioned. His history included hypertension, coronary artery disease, right bundle

---

CLINICAL PEARL

Levodopa depletes brain stores of SAMe. Depletion of SAMe is probably one of the causes of depression in patients with Parkinson's, and high doses of SAMe may alleviate their depression.

---

branch block, and hyperlipidemia. He was on three antihypertensive medications plus statins.

The following considerations were weighed in deciding to treat Leonard:

1. Parkinson's patients do not respond well to standard antidepressants.
2. Levodopa tends to deplete central nervous system SAMe.
3. Presence of coronary artery disease, hypertension, and a conduction defect.
4. Use of medication such as statins that burden liver metabolism.

Leonard was treated with gradually increasing doses of SAMe, which were well tolerated. At 2,000 mg SAMe per day, his appetite and sleep improved. Over the next six weeks, he appeared more energetic and alert. His family and friends were relieved to see him reengage in social activities. He was even able to enjoy being the guest of honor at a dinner party given by his former colleagues.

Depression and HIV/AIDS

About 30–50% of HIV-positive patients experience depressive disorders associated with low immune response, disease progression, decreased survival, and lower quality of life. SAMe deficiency has been found in HIV-infected patients. An open eight-week study of 20 patients with HIV and major depression given SAMe 400 mg twice a day with folic acid (800 mcg/day) and B_{12} (1,000 mcg/day) found significant improvement in depression by week 4 (Shippy,

Mendez, Jones, Cergnul, & Karpiak, 2004). For further details, see Chapter 8.

Depression in Children

Parents who are familiar with SAMe sometimes ask about using it for depression in their children. Unfortunately, there are no published controlled studies on the safety and efficacy of SAMe in children. However, SAMe has been used successfully to treat depression in children and adolescents in clinical practice. Three cases were reported including two sisters, ages 8 and 11, and one boy, age 16. (Schaller, Thomas, & Bazzan, 2004). The parents of the girls both had strong family histories of depression and credited SAMe with providing full relief of their own depressions. They did not want to expose their children to side effects from prescription medications. The girls had developed serious major depression including crying, withdrawal, sadness, and preoccupation with themes of death. The 11-year-old was started on 200 mg/day SAMe and when her dose was increased to 600 mg/day her depression rapidly and completely remitted with no side effects. Her 8-year-old sister's depression also remitted on 200 mg SAMe twice a day The third child was a 16-year-old male with an 18-month history of major depression and oppositional defiant disorder who refused to take prescription medication because he viewed drugs as foreign to the body. He was irritable, bored, uninterested in all activites except computer games, sad, fatigued, hopeless, slept excessively, and had difficulty concentrating. His grades had dropped from Bs to Ds. The physician convinced him to try SAMe. The boy was willing because SAMe was presented as a natural substance that was already made in the body. When the dose was raised to 800 mg in the morning and 400 mg after school, his mood, energy, and school performance returned to his baseline before the depression.

Quality and Potency of SAMe Brands

SAMe rapidly interacts with other molecules in hundreds of essential metabolic pathways. It is the most avid methyl donor in the body. SAMe also rapidly oxidizes when exposed to air. In order to stabilize this highly interactive substance, SAMe is combined with a salt molecule and the tablets are given an enteric coating. The quality of the

SAMe and of the tablet is critical for maintaining potency over time. If the manufacturing is flawed, tablets lose most of their potency while sitting on shelves. Unfortunately, many companies are producing low-grade SAMe and selling it at bargain prices. Not only do these products lack efficacy, they can also cause more side effects. When you recommend SAMe to your patients, advise them to purchase products of proven quality and those in which each tablet is protected within its own foil blister pack (to preserve full potency longer).

In Appendix A, the reader will find a list of reliable SAMe products. SAMe should not be stored in the refrigerator because the tablets can be damaged by the condensation of water inside the blister packs. Also, the tablets should not be split because the enteric coating protects them from degradation by digestive enzymes.

HERBS FOR MOOD DISORDERS

Herbs contain numerous bioactive substances in their leaves, flowers, and roots. The concentration of medicinal compounds in herbal preparations may be affected by growing conditions, time of harvest, method of drying, and extraction procedures. For many herbs the medicinal activity of individual compounds is not yet known. For others, a single measurable component has been found to correlate with clinical effects, for example, hyperforin for St. John's Wort.

St. John's Wort (*Hypericum perforatum*)

St. John's Wort, an extract of the flowers and leaves of *Hypericum perforatum*, has had a controversial role in the treatment of depression. In 1996, a meta-analysis of 23 studies of St. John's Wort found that in 13 studies, it outperformed placebo with no increase in side effects (Linde, Ramirez, Mulrow, Pauls, Weidenhammer et al., 1996). It was later recognized that the concentration of one component, hyperforin, was a critical marker for effectiveness.

Subsequent rigorous research used better quality standardized St. John's Wort extracts. A six-week double-blind, randomized study of 209 hospitalized patients with severe major depression found that although imipramine (150 mg/day) worked faster (3–6 weeks) than St. John's Wort (Kira LI 160 at 600 mg t.i.d.; 6–12 weeks), St. John's

Wort was as effective as imipramine and caused fewer side effects (Vorbach, Arnoldt, & Hubner, 1997). A randomized six-week study of 240 patients with mild to moderate depression found that St. John's Wort (Remotiv or ZE 117, 500 mg/day) was as effective as fluoxetine (Prozac) 20 mg/day (Schrader, 2000). Furthermore, there were far fewer side effects with St. John's Wort (mild gastrointestinal upset) than with Prozac (vomiting, dizziness, anxiety, and erectile dysfunction). This study was funded by the medical insurance system of Germany.

As noted above, Vorbach had demonstrated that in order to treat severe depression with St. John's Wort, higher doses (1,800 mg/day) would have to be given for a longer period of time (6–12 weeks). Nevertheless, a well-publicized double-blind, randomized, placebo-controlled multicenter U.S. study of 200 hospitalized patients with extremely severe depression who were given St. John's Wort (Kira 900 mg/day) for four weeks and then 1,200 mg/day for four weeks (Shelton, Keller, Gelenberg, Dunner, Hirschfeld et al., 2001) concluded that St. John's Wort was no better than placebo. This study was overinterpreted considering that St. John's Wort had been given in subtherapeutic doses to extremely depressed subjects. Kira LI-160 (same as Jarsin 300 mg in Germany) is an extract of St. John's Wort manufactured by Lichtwer Pharma, Berlin, Germany and sold by Abkit, Lichtwer Healthcare (www.iherb.com). Each 300 mg tablet contains 900 mcg hyperforin. As with other herbs in Germany, high quality manufacturing standards are maintained by the German Komission E.

The cards were also stacked against St. John's Wort in another study in which severely depressed patients were given subtherapeutic doses (900–1,500 mg/day) and compared to patients given subtherapeutic doses of sertraline (Zoloft 50–100 mg/day; Hypericum Depression Trial Study Group, 2002). In this study, neither sertraline nor St. John's Wort did any better than placebo. Several reviews of this study reported that St. John's Wort was no better than placebo while failing to mention that sertraline had also performed no better than placebo.

Numerous studies support the efficacy of St. John's Wort in treating patients with mild to moderate depression (Gastpar, Singer, & Zeller, 2005) and moderate to severe depression (Kasper, Anghelescu, Szegedi, Dienel, & Kieser, 2006; Philipp, Kohnen, & Hiller, 1999). For example, a double-blind randomized placebo-controlled study found that 71% of patients with moderate to severe depression in psychiatric primary care practices responded to hypericum extract Ws5570 (900–1,800 mg/day) in comparison to 60% given paroxetine (Paxil 20–40 mg/day; Szegedi, Kohnen, Dienel, & Kieser, 2005).

Side Effects of St. John's Wort

St. John's Wort has potential side effects that should be discussed with clients before starting treatment. The rate of side effects increases with higher doses. St. John's Wort can cause phototoxic rash in less than 1% of people taking 900 mg/day or more. At higher doses, St. John's Wort has side effects that are milder but similar to those of SSRIs, including nausea, heartburn, loose stools, sexual dysfunction, bruxism (teeth clenching), and restless legs. Combining St. John's Wort with other serotonergic antidepressants may increase the risk of serotonin syndrome. St. John's Wort can induce mania in bipolar patients. A review of data from 35 double-blind randomized trials found that dropout and adverse effects rates in patients receiving hypericum extracts were similar to placebo, lower than with older antidepressants, and slightly lower than with SSRIs. In 17 observational studies, including 35,562 patients, dropout rates due to side effects varied from 0% to 5.7%. No studies reported serious adverse effects.

Because St. John's Wort induces cytochrome P450 3A4 and 1A2 enzymes and induces intestinal wall P-glycoprotein, it can interfere with the metabolism and absorption of numerous medications. It has been found to reduce levels of digoxin, warfarin, phenprocoumon, HIV protease inhibitors, reverse transcriptase inhibitors, indinavir, irinotecan, theophylline, amitriptyline, cyclosporine (Knuppel & Linde, 2004), alprazolam, dextromethorphan, simvastatin, and oral contraceptives. St. John's Wort should be discontinued two or three weeks prior to surgery because it can affect heart rate and blood pressure during anesthesia.

How to Use St. John's Wort in the Treatment of Depression

For mild to moderate depression, St. John's Wort can be helpful. However, many people require higher doses (1,500 mg/day or more) for remission or in cases of severe depression. At these doses, it is less advantageous because of the increased incidence of side effects similar to those associated with SSRIs. Nevertheless, in some settings St. John's Wort is particularly beneficial, for example, in mild depression with wintertime seasonal affective disorder (Cott & Fugh-Berman, 1998; Hansgen, Vesper, & Ploch, 1994; Wheatley, 1999).

While we do not usually recommend St. John's Wort as a first-line or solo treatment for depression, one exception is the patient with a history of good response to low-dose SSRI (e.g., 5 mg/day Prozac or 20 mg/day Paxil) but intolerable side effects such as weight gain or sexual dysfunction. Such a patient may do well on St. John's Wort. In addition, this herb can be useful for mild depression, combined with other treatments, when there is need for an incremental boost in antidepressant effect, if there is seasonal affective disorder, or when somatic symptoms are prevalent.

Deciding whether to use St. John's Wort involves weighing the risks of SSRI-like side effects, photosensitivity, and drug interactions against the potential benefits.

Case 4—Depressed Patient With Side Effects on Prescription Antidepressants

Maggie, a 26-year-old graduate student, had been depressed for as long as she could remember. She was first put on fluoxetine (Prozac) at age 15. It relieved her depression but caused loss of libido and anorgasmia. At 16 she was switched to sertraline (Zoloft) but it had the same side effects. Lexapro led to sexual dysfunction and tachycardia (rapid heartbeat). A trial of bupropion (Wellbutrin) caused panic attacks, stuttering, and tachycardia. Venlafaxine (Effexor) made her extremely angry. There was a family history of bipolar disorder (often associated with hostile reactions in patients given antidepressants). On buspirone (Buspar) she felt "spacey" and "out to lunch." She tried lamotrigine (Lamictal) for nine months, but had persistent headaches and nausea. On her own, she tried SAMe, but developed constant gastrointestinal upset. Eventually she responded to *Rhodiola rosea* (Rosavin) 450 mg/day with St. John's Wort (Perika) 600 mg

---

CLINICAL PEARL

While St. John's Wort may ameliorate depression in both men and women, in clinical practice, the authors find that the patients most likely to benefit are women whose depression responded to SSRIs, but who are sensitive to side effects from prescription antidepressants.

---

b.i.d. On this combination, her depression resolved with no complaints of weight gain, tachycardia, or sexual dysfunction.

St. John's Wort Augmentation of Antidepressants

St. John's Wort can be useful in augmenting response to antidepressants such as tricyclics, buproprion (Wellbutrin), venlafaxine (Effexor), and SAMe. However, St. John's Wort should not be combined with MAOIs. There is a possibility of serotonin syndrome if high doses of St. John's Wort are added to other serotonergic psychotropics. At this time, there are no published studies on combining St. John's Wort with other antidepressants.

Somatoform Disorders

St. John's Wort is useful in somatoform disorders. In a double-blind randomized placebo-controlled study, 151 patients with somatoform disorder were given either St. John's Wort 600 mg/day or placebo for six weeks. Very significant improvements occurred in those taking St. John's Wort whether or not there were depressive symptoms (Volz, Murck, Kasper, & Moller, 2002). Another six-week double-blind placebo-controlled parallel study of 184 outpatients with somatoform disorders found that 45% of those given St. John's Wort 600 mg/day responded as compared to 21% on placebo. Those with autonomic instability obtained greater benefit. St. John's Wort caused no more side effects than placebo (Muller, Mannel, Murck, & Rahlfs, 2004).

Seasonal Affective Disorder

St. John's Wort may be beneficial for seasonal affective disorder (SAD). A preliminary placebo-controlled study of 20 patients with SAD found that hypericum plus weak light (placebo) was as effective as hypericum with bright light therapy in reducing symptoms of SAD (Kasper, 1997). In an eight-week 11-item postal survey of members of the SAD Association in the UK (Wheatley, 1999), those who used Kira 900 mg/day (n = 168) had significant improvements in SAD symptoms that were comparable to improvements in those using Kira 900 mg/day plus light therapy (n = 133). Limitations of this study include lack of randomization or blinding, and lack of information about the quantity and intensity of light therapy used by the subjects. Although controlled clinical trials are needed to establish the efficacy of hypericum for SAD, preliminary data are supportive.

Quality and Potency of Brands

Exercise care in choosing a quality brand of St. John's Wort. Standardized extracts usually contain 0.3–0.5% hyperforin. Check the label for details. Because there is such variability in the quality of St. John's Wort products, we recommend brands that are standardized and that have proven efficacy based on their use in clinical trials (see Appendix A for quality brands).

Rhodiola rosea: Arctic Root, Golden Root

Although the primary clinical uses of *Rhodiola rosea* (see Chapter 4) are for physical and mental energy, cognitive disorders, memory, and performance under stress, it can be useful in the treatment of depression.

R. rosea has been shown to increase transport of tryptophan and serotonin into the brain. The first study of R. rosea for depression was done in the former Soviet Union in 1987. In this study, 128 patients with mixed types of depression were given 150 mg t.i.d. of R. rosea or placebo. Two thirds of those on R. rosea improved significantly (Brichenko & Skorokhova, 1987). Although the report of this study does not fulfill today's methodological standards, it suggests that further study would be worthwhile.

In a more recent study, a standardized extract (SHR-5 from Swedish Herbal Institute) of R. rosea rhizomes was used in a double-

---

CLINICAL PEARL

As a complementary treatment in depression, *Rhodiola rosea* can enhance energy, well-being, the impetus to get out of bed, and the motivation to become engaged in activities.

---

blind randomized placebo-controlled six-week study with parallel groups (Darbinyan, Aslayan, Embroyan, Gabrielian, Malmstrom et al., 2007). Adults between 18 and 70 years of age who met *Diagnostic and Statistical Manual of Mental Disorders* (*DSM-IV*) criteria for mild to moderate depression and whose initial Hamilton Depression Scale scores were between 12 and 31 were randomly assigned to one of three groups. Group A received moderate doses, SHR-5 (340 mg/day). Group B received SHR-5, 680 mg/day. Group C was given placebo tablets. At the end of six weeks, mean Hamilton scores dropped significantly in Groups A (from 24.52 to 15.97) and B (from 23.79 to 16.72), but not in Group C (from 24.7 to 23.4). No serious side effects were reported in any group. SHR-5 showed modest but significant effectiveness in treating patients with mild to moderate depression when administered over six weeks in doses of 340 or 680 mg/day.

We routinely use *R. rosea* as a complementary treatment in depression because it increases mental and physical energy, which are often low. It also improves mood and stress tolerance. Prescription antidepressants tend to alleviate negative mood states, but often fall short of producing a positive mood. Many patients report that with the addition of *R. rosea*, they experience a sense of well-being with increased impetus to get up and do things. In our clinical experience, patients with neurasthenia, mental as well as physical fatigue, respond well to *R. rosea*.

Depression and Menopause

Menopausal women with depression, fatigue, and memory decline find *Rhodiola rosea* to be particularly beneficial. Some patients find that it restores a sense of joyfulness and excitement about life (for further discussion, see Chapter 6).

Side Effects of Rhodiola rosea

Rhodiola rosea has an energizing or mildly stimulating effect. Unlike prescription stimulants (e.g., amphetamines), *R. rosea* does not cause addiction, habituation, or withdrawal symptoms. Individuals who are sensitive to stimulants such as caffeine may initially feel more anxious, agitated, jittery, or wired on *R. rosea*. Patients should reduce their intake of caffeine when using this herb because the stimulating effects can be additive. For those who are sensitive, it is possible to give a fraction of the usual dose and then increase gradually as tolerated. For mild to moderate depression, we recommend starting with 100–150 mg the first two days and then increasing by one capsule every three to seven days to a maximum of 500 mg/day. As an adjunctive treatment for depression, *R. rosea* is usually effective in doses of 200–400 mg/day. As a solo treatment, higher doses up to 750 mg/day may be needed.

R. *rosea* should be taken in the early part of the day to avoid interference with sleep. Some people report vivid dreams during the first two weeks. Occasionally, the herb may cause mild nausea. This can usually be managed by taking two ginger capsules 20 minutes before the *R. rosea* dose or by drinking ginger tea. In menopausal women who have been amenorrheic for less than one year, *R. rosea* may cause resumption of normal menses. In perimenopausal women with irregular menses, the herb may regularize the menstrual cycle or postpone menopausal changes. It is possible that it may increase fertility in women of childbearing age. Theoretically, women who rely upon birth control pills may be at greater risk for pregnancy. Although no cases of unwanted pregnancy have been reported, it is advisable to use an additional barrier method of birth control.

Although *R. rosea* has been shown to bind to estrogen receptors, it has not been shown to activate those receptors (see Chapter 5). *R. rosea* has not been associated with increased cancer risks, but women with a personal or family history of breast cancer should be informed that the possibility of increased risk for estrogen-sensitive breast cancer has not yet been adequately investigated. Chapter 8 reviews the evidence for anticarcinogenic effects of *R. rosea*.

Clinical Applications

In clinical practice, we have found R. *rosea* to be beneficial in a wide range of disorders of mood, memory, cognition, and fatigue (see

Chapter 4). *R. rosea* can improve energy in patients complaining of fatigue due to stress, depression, aging, medications, or medical illnesses.

Quality and Potency of Rhodiola rosea *Brands*

The roots of the *R. rosea* plant contain hundreds of medicinal compounds. No one has been able to identify what combination of these is responsible for its many effects. The methods of drying the root and extraction affect which compounds are preserved and which may be volatilized. Therefore it is important to use only those brands that have been proven to be clinically effective.

Unfortunately, some herbal manufacturers use species other than *R. rosea* as fillers to reduce costs. In looking for a good-quality brand of *R. rosea*, be sure that the product is labeled with standardization of at least 3% rosavins and at least 1% salidrosides. However, even the presence of these marker compounds may not guarantee efficacy because, depending on the source of the raw material and the method of extraction, other essential compounds may be missing. Therefore, it is particularly important for clinicians and researchers to use products containing only those *R. rosea* extracts that have proven to be effective in animal and/or human studies. You will find quality brands listed in Appendix A.

VITAMINS FOR MOOD DISORDERS

The most important vitamins and nutrients for mental health are those that are essential for the functioning of nerve cells and those that are likely to be depleted due to poor nutrition, malabsorption, rapid utilization, or deterioration due to age, illness, or environmental stress. The B vitamins (including folate) and omega-3 fatty acids fulfill these criteria.

Dietary folate and folic acid (supplemental form) must be converted into L-methyltetrahydrofolate for use in metabolic pathways. The final step in this conversion depends upon the enzyme methyltetrahydrofolate reductase (MTHFR), which is also required for the production of methionine from homocysteine (see Figure 2.1). Polymorphisms (commonly occurring gene mutations) of the MTHFR gene can lead to a reduced conversion of methylene-tetrahydrofolate

SIDEBAR 2.1 **MTHFR POLYMORPHISM, FOLATE, HOMOCYSTEINE, SAMe, AND DEPRESSION**

On the MTHFR gene, a mutation at the 677-base position due to a substitution of a cytosine base (C) by a thymine (T) results in a less active form of the enzyme, a C→T polymorphism. The normal genotype C/C has 100% enzyme MTHFR activity. However, MTHRF activity declines to 71% with C/T and 34% with T/T genotypes. The consequences of a C/T or T/T polymorphism are an increased level of homocysteine (approximately 20%) and lower folate concentrations. About 40–50% of the population has the C/T mutation, while 10–12% has the T/T mutation. The increase in homocysteine is associated with greater risks for cardiovascular disease. In addition, SAMe production may decline. The reduction in SAMe and folate along with the increase in homocysteine may contribute to depression and poor response to antidepressant medication.

to L-methylfolate (see Sidebar 2.1) resulting in increased levels of homocysteine (an independent risk factor for cardiovascular disease). For an in-depth discussion of the relationship between folate, other B vitamins, and homocysteine in depression, see the scholarly work of Teodoro Bottiglieri (2005).

One particular polymorphism with a 677C to T transition in the MTHFR gene results in an alanine to valine substitution in the polypeptide chain, which is associated with a thermolabile enzyme. The MTHFR 677TT genotype is common, occurring in 12% of the Caucasian and as high as 22% of the Latino or Mediterranean population. It has been suggested that supplementation with L-methyltetrahydrofolate would be more effective than folic acid because this would bypass the need for the final MTHFR conversion step. L-methyltetrahydrofolate is the form that is absorbed at the intestinal level and transported across the blood-brain barrier by specific receptors located in the choroid plexus. It is required for the synthesis of methionine and S-adenosylmethionine and it contributes to the synthesis of neurotransmitters. In a double-blind randomized placebo-controlled study of 123 patients with acute psychiatric disorders (major depression or schizophrenia), 33% had borderline folate deficiency (red cell folate < 200 mcg). Patients were maintained on standard psychotropic medication while given augmentation with 15 mg/day methylfolate or placebo. Those who took methylfolate showed significantly greater clinical and social recovery compared to those given placebo (Procter, 1991). Oral supplements containing L-methylfolate are now available (see Table 2.1 at the end of this chapter and Appendix A for a list of some quality products).

In depressed patients and in the elderly, low levels of B_{12} (cyanocobalamin) and folate have been associated with disorders of mood, memory, and cognition (Bottiglieri, 1996; Crellin, Bottiglieri, & Reynolds, 1993). Studies of B vitamins and folate as solo treatments for depression have shown mixed results. However, a group of 14 geriatric patients being treated with tricyclic antidepressants showed improved response when B complex (B_1, B_2, and B_6) and folate were added (Bell, Edman, Morrow, Marby, Perrone et al., 1992). The discovery that nonresponse to antidepressant medication was associated with low levels of folate led to a double-blind randomized placebo-controlled study of 127 patients on fluoxetine (Prozac) supplemented with either 400 mcg/day of folate or placebo (Coppen & Bailey, 2000). Of the women given fluoxetine plus folate, 94% had a good response versus 61% of those given fluoxetine plus placebo.

In addition to polymorphism, other factors that may reduce folate levels include chronic disease, diabetes, cancer, smoking, alcohol use, poor diet, and medications such as mood stabilizers, L-dopa, statin drugs, oral antidiabetic drugs, and chemotherapy drugs. Methylfolate and B vitamins are generally quite safe and low in side

---

CLINICAL PEARL

Recent evidence indicates that folate with B vitamins can accelerate occlusion of cardiac stents in men with baseline homocysteine levels less than 15 μmol/liter.

effects. Allergic reactions may occur. Safety in pregnancy and breast feeding has not been established. Elevated levels of homocysteine are associated with increased risk of cardiovascular disease. Folate combined with B vitamins has been shown to reduce homocysteine levels. A six-month double-blind, randomized placebo-controlled study of the effects of folate combined with B_6 and B_{12} in 636 patients, who had undergone successful coronary artery stenting, found an 8% increase in the incidence of restenosis in the group given the vitamins. However, there was no increase in restenosis in women, patients with diabetes, and patients with high baseline homocysteine levels (< 15 µmol/liter) (Lange, Suryapranata, De Luca, Borner, Dille et al., 2004). By stimulating endothelial proliferation, B vitamins and folate may contribute to occlusion of cardiac stents in some patients.

Vitamin D may be of benefit in seasonal affective disorder (SAD). Reduction of light exposure during winter months results in a decrease in production of vitamin D by skin. The relationship between sun exposure, vitamin D levels, and SAD has been explored by several small randomized studies with mixed results (Dumville, Miles, Porthouse, Cockayne, Saxon et al., 2006; Gloth, Alam, & Hollis, 1999). Since vitamin D tends to be low in winter and considering its many health benefits, it could be used as an adjunct in the treatment of SAD.

NUTRIENTS FOR MOOD DISORDERS

Omega-3 fatty acids and certain amino acids are vital to the functioning of neural tracts involved in mood regulation.

Omega-3 Fatty Acids

Our cell membranes are not as fluid as they were a century ago when omega-3 polyunsaturated fatty acids (omega-3FAs) were higher in our diets. Marine-based omega-3FAs provided eicosapentanoic acid (EPA) and docosahexanoic acid (DHA), which maintain cell membrane fluidity. In addition, EPA and DHA reduce production of inflammatory eicosanoids and the release of proinflammatory cytokines. As we consume more and more saturated fats from domesticated animals and more omega-6 polyunsaturated fatty acids (omega-6FAs) from cultivated vegetables (corn, safflower, and soybean), cell membranes acquire increasing proportions of omega-6FAs. Fish used to be a prime source of omega-3FAs until farmers started feeding them vegetable oils with omega-6FAs. Once a rich source of omega-3FAs, now most farm-bred fish contain higher levels of omega-6FAs and relatively lower levels of omega-3FAs. Although fish, particularly fatty fish such as salmon, are still an important source of omega-3FAs, they should no longer be the only source because one would have to consume fish so often that one might accumulate excess amounts of PCBs (polychlorinated biphenyls) or mercury that contaminate our food supply. Therefore, we recommend supplementation with fish oil in liquid or capsule form. Quality brands with reduced PCBs and no fishy aftertaste are available.

Flax seeds contain alpha-linoleic acid (ALA), but they must be ground to enable the ALA to be absorbed. ALA can be converted to the omega-3FAs, EPA and DHA, but the conversion is inefficient and varies among individuals. Additional sources of small amounts of ALA include nuts, seeds, and canola or flaxseed oil.

Omega-3 Fatty Acids and Depression

Data suggest that the substitution of omega-6FAs for omega-3FAs in cell membranes is associated with unipolar and bipolar depression. This may be due to loss of membrane fluidity and flexibility affecting membrane proteins (enzymes, receptors, ion channels) with changes in neurotransmission as well as increased eicosanoids and proinflammatory cytokines. A study of 12 bipolar women found that those treated with omega-3FA showed significant improvement in membrane flexibility (Hirashima, Parrow, Stoll, Demopulos, Damico et al., 2004).

Parker and colleagues (2006) wrote an excellent review of studies on omega-3FA for depression. The mixed results found in these studies may reflect differences in the dose and proportions of EPA and DHA, patient selection, and other factors. Omega-3FA deficiency has been associated with increased risk of suicide (Sublette, Hibbeln, Galfalvy, Oquendo, & Mann, 2006). A postmortem study compared the omega-3FA content of orbitofrontal cortex (Brodmann area 10) from 15 patients with major depressive disorder with 27

CLINICAL PEARL

A dose of 2–3 g total omega-3FA per day, including a 2:1 ratio of EPA to DHA, may augment the antidepressant effect of medication in many cases.

age-matched normal controls. DHA, the only fatty acid found to be significantly different from the controls, was 32% lower in the orbitofrontal cortex of female patients with major depression and 16% lower in males with major depression (McNamara, Hahn, Jandacek, Rider, Tso et al., 2007). Overall, there is sufficient evidence of efficacy to support the use of omega-3FAs as adjunctive treatments in unipolar depression and bipolar disorders (Freeman, Hibbeln, Wisner, Davis, Mischoulon et al., 2006). Furthermore, omega-3FAs are uniquely suited to treat these disorders during pregnancy and postpartum because they are safe and beneficial for maternal health as well as for infant development. The association between low fish consumption and depression is even stronger in women than in men (Timonen, Horrobin, Jokelainen, Laitinen, Herva et al., 2004).

Augmentation of standard antidepressants significantly lowered scores on depression ratings in a double-blind, placebo-controlled study of omega-3FA (4.4 g EPA plus 2.2 g DHA) for major depression (Su, Huang, Chiu, & Shen, 2003) and in a parallel-group, double-blind placebo-controlled study of 2 g/day ethyl-EPA in recurrent unipolar depression (Nemets, Stahl, & Belmaker, 2002). Ethyl-EPA is a form of EPA used in the United Kingdom that is awaiting approval in the United States. A double-blind randomized placebo-controlled study of DHA as a monotherapy for major depressive episodes found no difference between DHA alone and placebo.

Omega-3 Fatty Acids and Bipolar Disorder

Greater seafood consumption has been linked to lower lifetime prevalence of bipolar disorder, particularly bipolar II (Noaghiul & Hibbeln, 2003). In a double-blind randomized placebo-controlled study omega-3FAs (6.2 g EPA plus 3.4 mg DHA) reduced symptoms

---

CLINICAL PEARL

Given the high safety profile and positive preliminary evidence for omega-3FAs as an adjunctive treatment for bipolar disorder, and considering the serious risks associated with residual bipolar symptoms, it is worth recommending this suppliement to patients with bipolar disorder.

---

and relapse rates in bipolar patients, most of whom were taking mood stabilizers (Stoll, Severus, Freeman, Rueter, Zboyan et al., 1999).

Depressive symptoms were the target of a one-month open pilot study of bipolar I patients. Eight out of 10 subjects given 1.5–2.0 g EPA showed 50% or greater decrease in depression scores (Osher, Bersudsky, & Belmaker, 2005).

Ethyl-EPA (1–2 g/day) was used as an adjunctive treatment for depression in a double-blind randomized placebo-controlled study of 75 bipolar patients, most of whom were being treated with mood stabilizers, antipsychotics, antidepressants, and anxiolytics. Addition of ethyl-EPA significantly reduced scores for depression on the Hamilton Rating Scale for Depression and Clinical Global Impression scale. No significant differences were noted between the 1 g and the 2 g/day doses (Frangou, Lewis, & McCrone, 2006). Although there have been some reports of omega-3FAs triggering manic symptoms, this did not occur in the studies by Stoll, Osher, or Frangou, and it may be related to the ratio of EPA to DHA used.

A four-month randomized adjunctive study in patients with bipolar disorder and rapid cyclers who were receiving mood stabilizers found no significant differences in depressive symptomatology or on the Young Mania Rating Scale between those given EPA 6 mg/day and those given placebo (Keck, Mintz, McElroy, Freeman, Suppes et al., 2006). The lack of efficacy may have been due to the use of EPA without DHA.

While doses of 1–2 mg/day omega-3FAs ameliorated symptoms of depression in studies of bipolar disorder, we recommend higher doses for patients with mixed symptoms of mania and depression and for rapid cyclers. Stoll used a total of 9.6 g (EPA plus DHA) augmentation to stabilize bipolar patients in his preliminary study (Stoll et al., 1999). In practice, many patients have difficulty tolerating more than 6 g total EPA plus DHA because of gastrointestinal symptoms and the number of pills that must be taken. However, we suggest 8–10 g/day total EPA plus DHA for those who can tolerate it.

In general, omega-3FAs are mildly helpful in reducing manic symptoms and mildly to modestly helpful for depression in bipolar disorder. However, we have seen some cases of marked improvement in both manic and depressive symptoms, enabling a reduction in the maintenance dose of prescription medications. See Chapter 6 for a discussion of omega-3FAs for treatment of depression and bipolar disorder in pregnancy and postpartum.

Bipolar Disorder in Children and Adolescents

In an open-label trial, 20 children, 6 to 16 years of age, with bipolar disorder and Young Mania Rating Scale scores (28.9 ± 10.1) were given EPA 1,290 mg plus DHA 4,300 mg daily for eight weeks. A modest, but statistically significant drop in scores occurred by endpoint with Young scale scores of 19.1 ± 2.6. A few mild adverse effects occurred, mainly gastrointestinal. Overall, 35% of subjects had more than 50% decrease in Young scale scores (Wozniak, Biederman, Mick, Waxmansky, Hantsoo et al., 2007). Such modest improvements in manic symptoms among child bipolars can be quite helpful. Omega-3FAs can be considered a low-risk adjunctive treatment in pediatric patients with bipolar disorder. Further trials are warranted.

Omega-3 Fatty Acids for Borderline Personality Disorder and Self-Injury

An eight-week placebo-controlled study of 30 women with borderline personality disorder who did not meet criteria for major depression showed that those taking 1 g ethyl-EPA per day had greater reduction in depressive symptoms and aggression (Zanarini & Frankenburg, 2003). Although more studies are needed to confirm this finding, clinicians may consider a trial of omega-3FAs in borderline patients.

In a 12-week clinical trial, 49 patients with a history of self-harm were randomized to receive either 1.2 g EPA plus 0.9 g DHA per day or placebo in addition to standard psychiatric treatment. Those given omega-3FAs had significantly greater improvements in depression (Beck Depression Inventory 21 and Hamilton Rating Scale for Depression), suicidality, and stress. However, there was no impact on scores for aggression, impulsivity, or hostility (Hallahan, Hibbeln, Davis, & Garland, 2007).

Side Effects and Risks

The most common side effects of omega-3FAs are gastrointestinal: nausea, heartburn, stomach pain, belching, bloating, or diarrhea. These are more likely to occur at high doses and can be minimized by using high-quality refined fish oil preparations.

The possibility of triggering manic episodes is probably low but should be kept in mind.

Since omega-3FAs reduce platelet aggregation, there is some concern about the possibility of bleeding. Patients on anticoagulant medications should be monitored more closely when taking omega-3FAs.

Environmental toxins such as mercury and PCBs have contaminated much of the fish supply, even in farmed fish. Consumption of fish more often than once a week can lead to accumulation of these pollutants. Concern about PCBs in fish oil has led to increased awareness of the need to purchase products documented to be low in PCBs and mercury.

A review of studies of fish oil supplements in the *Medical Letter* found evidence that eating fatty fish (e.g., salmon) twice a week or taking over-the-counter fish oil capsules (1,000–1,500 mg/day) reduced mortality in patients with acute coronary disease but not in those with chronic coronary disease ("Fish Oil Supplements," 2006). In some of these studies, eating fish was more protective than taking fish oil capsules. This may reflect differences in quality and in EPA and DHA content. It is best to refrigerate fish oil products to prevent the oils from becoming rancid.

Brands of Omega-3 Fatty Acids

The FDA has approved a prescription form of fish oil, omacor (Reliant), for treatment of hypertriglyceridemia ("Fish Oil Supplements," 2006). Each 900 mg capsule contains 465 mg EPA and 375 mg DHA. The cost per month of one capsule a day is about $35. The cost of an equivalent supply of nonprescription fish oil would range from $12 to $30 per month, depending on the brand. The US Pharmacopeia (www.usp.org) tested a few over-the-counter brands and identified several brands that contained no measurable mercury, heavy metals, or contaminants. ConsumerLab found that most of the 42 brands of fish oil they tested did not contain contaminants and were accurately labeled (www.ConsumerLab.com). Vital Nutrients makes high-quality refined fish oil in concentrated liquid form. It has a light, nonfishy taste and is less likely to cause gastrointestinal side effects but is more expensive than many other products.

Choline for Bipolar Disorder

Choline bitartrate was found to reduce mania in several case reports. A study of six treatment-refractory bipolar patients on lithium found that the addition of 2,000 to 7,200 mg/day of free choline resulted in clinical improvement, though the effect on depression was variable (Stoll, Sachs, Cohen, Lafer, Christensen et al., 2006).

Inositol

Inositol, a glucose isomer precursor of phosphatidyl inositol, part of the second messenger system coupled to neurotransmitters, has been found to be more beneficial than placebo in several studies of depression, panic, and obsessive-compulsive disorder at doses ranging from 12,000 to 20,000 mg/day (Benjamin, Agam, Levine, Bersudsky, Kofman et al., 1995; Fux, Levine, Aviv, & Belmaker, 1996). Unfortunately, at therapeutic doses it can cause gastrointestinal side effects and one case of mania has been reported. Compliance can be a problem because of frequent flatulence. Therefore, inositol should be considered to be a third-line augmentation.

Inositol may be useful in bipolar disorder. One double-blind randomized placebo-controlled study of 24 bipolar adults failed to show a significant effect. However, a trend toward greater improvement was evident on the Montgomery-Asberg Depression Scale, suggesting that larger studies would be worthwhile (Chengappa, Levine, Gershon, Mallinger, Harden et al., 2000).

A randomized trial comparing augmentation of mood stabilizers with lamotrigine (Lamictal), inositol, or risperidone (Risperdal) in 66 bipolar I and II patients with treatment-resistant depression found that the rate of recovery was 23.8% with lamotrigine, 17.4% with inositol, and 4.6% with risperidone (Nierenberg, Ostacher, Calabrese, Ketter, Marangell et al., 2006). The fact that inositol ran a close second to lamotrigine suggests that it could be considered as an augmentation in bipolar patients whose depression has not responded to standard treatment with mood stabilizers and antidepressants.

5-Hydroxy-L-Tryptophan

The rationale for using the amino acid 5-hydroxy-L-tryptophan (5-HTP) for depression is based on its role as the immediate precursor for the synthesis of serotonin, 5-hydroxytryptamine. As a dietary supplement, 5-HTP is being widely used by consumers for depression, insomnia, and fibromyalgia. 5-HTP replaced L-tryptophan, which was taken off the market in 1989 after a contaminated product from a single manufacturer was linked to eosinophilia malignant syndrome. Extensive studies of 5-HTP have found no evidence of toxicity (Das, Bagchi, Bagchi, & Preuss, 2004).

The efficacy of 5-HTP in depression has been reviewed (Das et al., 2004; Turner, Loftis, & Blackwell, 2006). Out of 27 studies reviewed, 11 were double-blind placebo-controlled. Of these 11 studies, 7 reported that 5-HTP performed better than placebo, with only 5 of these showing statistical significance. Several studies have shown that the addition of 5-HTP to prescription antidepressants such as nialamide, clomipramine, and nomifensin significantly improved antidepressant response. The average dosage of 5-HTP in adults is 200–300 mg/day given in divided doses BID or TID. Overall, studies suggest that 5-HTP may have limited benefit for depression with some support for its use as an augmentation.

Side Effects, Risks, and Interactions of 5-HTP

Common side effects with 5-HTP include nausea, vomiting, and diarrhea. Less frequent side effects include headache and insomnia. Rodent studies have shown that doses below 50 mg/kg/day produce no toxicity, but above 100 mg/kg/day induce serotonin syndrome. No cases of serotonin syndrome have been reported in humans using 5-

HTP alone or in combination with SSRIs. Studies combining 5-HTP with MAOIs report no adverse effects. The use of a peripheral decarboxylase inhibitor such as levodopa may increase the level of 5-HTP in serum 14-fold (Gijsman, Van Gerven, de Kam, Schoemaker, Pieters et al., 2002).

N-Acetylcysteine for Bipolar Disorder

N-acetylcysteine (NAC) is a precursor for the synthesis of glutathione, the most important antioxidant in the brain. In animal studies, oral administration of NAC over time increased peripheral glutathione levels, protected against depletion of glutathione, and reduced markers of oxidative stress. Increased oxidative stress and disturbed glutathione metabolism have been associated with bipolar disorder and depression. Mood stabilizers, such as valproate (Depakote) and lithium improve oxidative status in bipolar patients. In a six-month double-blind randomized controlled study of 75 patients with bipolar disorder, the addition of NAC 2 g/day to the usual treatment regimen resulted in significant improvements on measures of depression, mania, quality of life, and social and occupational functioning compared to placebo. Positive effects appeared after eight weeks of daily NAC and faded after discontinuation with a one-month washout of NAC. As in previous trials, NAC was well tolerated with no significant side effects (Berk, 2007; Tucker, 2007). Although this study will require further follow-up, it shows that NAC is promising and safe as an augmentation for bipolar patients who are already on medication.

In animal studies, NAC protected rat striatum from oxidative stress and lipid peroxidation due to an antipsychotic medication, haloperidol (Haldol; see Sidebar 2.2). Psychotropic medications, particularly antipsychotics, can damage fibers in the striatum, leading to the development of tremors, stiffness, or abnormal movements. This raises the possibility that NAC could protect patients from some of the adverse effects of treatment with antipsychotic medications such as haloperidol.

NAC has also been used to treat acetaminophen (Tylenol) overdose and to reduce the risk of respiratory infections and flu. Because NAC is safe, well tolerated, and has additional possible health benefits, clinicians may find it a useful complementary treatment for

SIDEBAR 2.2 **THE STRIATUM AND BASAL GANGLIA**

The striatum, consisting of the caudate nucleus and the putamen, is part of the basal ganglia, anatomical structures within the cerebral cortex and midbrain with feedback loops to the substantia nigra, thalamus, and cerebral cortex. This feedback system maintains and coordinates the tone of muscles that oppose one another to stabilize joint position, coordinate movements, or inhibit the tone of certain muscles during the initiation of movement. Damage to any part of this system results in loss of control with oscillatory movements appearing as tremors. For example, degeneration of dopaminergic fibers from the substantia nigra to the striatum leads to the tremors, stiffness, and other motor symptoms of parkinsonism.

patients with bipolar disorder. The patient will need to be informed that it usually takes at least eight weeks of daily doses (2 g/day) for a positive response.

AYURVEDIC MEDICINE

Ayurvedic medicine is an ancient system of healing based upon balancing the constitutional elements of each individual through the use of yoga, herbs, massage, cleansings, lifestyle changes, specific diets, and other treatments (see Chapter 8; Prathikanti, 2007). Although Ayurvedic medicines have been used widely to treat depression, particularly among Indian populations, there are few controlled clinical studies. The Ayurvedic system does not lend itself easily to controlled studies because most treatments involve multiple herbs in conjunction with changes in diet and other interventions, making it difficult to identify the curative factors. Also, treatments are individualized and target the entire person rather than an isolated symptom. The effects of Ayurvedic herbs tend to be mild and slow in onset, often taking many months. Patients who have difficulty tolerating prescription medications sometimes fare better with the gentler action of medicinal herbs.

In routine cases, Western practitioners are more comfortable using treatments that are supported by evidence based on the system of medicine that they understand. The safe and effective use of complex herbal systems, particularly for patients with serious psychiatric disorders, requires collaboration with a well-trained Ayurvedic specialist. We have found that in several cases of treatment-resistant bipolar disorder, particularly in women with subtle hormonal abnormalities such as endometriosis or irregular menses, who continue to do poorly after decades of multiple well-documented adequate trials of all appropriate combinations of prescription medications (mood stabilizers, antipsychotics, and antidepressants) and psychotherapy, referral to an Ayurvedic specialist ultimately led to significant clinical improvement. The treatments took about a year and included changes in diet and lifestyle, the daily practice of yoga postures and breathing, meditation, panchakarma detoxification, and other techniques. The results were substantial improvements in mood and capacity to function. Maintenance doses of psychotropic medications were sharply reduced. This approach required patience and persistence, but the results were deeply appreciated by the patients and their families.

HOMEOPATHY

A systematic review of homeopathy in the treatment of depression found limited evidence due to a paucity of high-quality clinical studies. Of the two randomized controlled trials, one had only six subjects completing the study; the other had numerous design problems and was rated 45 out of 100 for methodological rigor. The reviewers noted many uncontrolled trials and case studies reporting positive results, particularly in studies of cancer patients with various degrees of anxiety and depression. Interestingly, the patients reported high levels of satisfaction with their homeopathic treatments (65–75%). Side effects were generally mild, transient exacerbations of previous symptoms. Interpretation of the findings was further complicated by the use of different kinds of homeopathy: individualized prescribing, limited list prescribing, and standardized complexes (Pilkington, Kirkwood, Rampes, Fisher, & Richardson, 2005).

Fourteen faculty of homeopathy doctors participated in a six-month uncontrolled feasibility study by reporting on a total of 960 patients treated for a wide range of conditions. The two conditions most frequently treated were depression (n = 55) and anxiety (n = 41). Positive outcome scores were reported most frequently in the treatment of irritable bowel syndrome (73.9%; n = 23), depression (63.6%), and anxiety (61.0%). There was no intent-to-treat analysis and it was not possible to identify which components of the treatment and patient encounters were most responsible for the outcomes (Mathie & Robinson, 2006).

Homeopathic remedies are probably safe in high dilutions when administered by trained professionals. The evidence base is insufficient to develop guidelines for the use of homeopathy in the treatment of depression. If patients come to treatment and are already taking homeopathic remedies that they feel are helpful, the clinician may wish to review the list of ingredients to identify potential interactions and, if there are none, support the patient's decision to continue with homeopathy. However, if the clinician is in the process of developing the treatment regimen, it may be simpler to ask the patient to postpone trying new homeopathic treatments in order to allow for the separate assessment of the effects of each intervention.

HORMONES FOR MOOD DISORDERS: DEHYDROEPIANDROSTERONE AND 7-KETO DHEA

Dehydroepiandrosterone (DHEA), an androgen produced in the adrenal glands, tends to decline during midlife in men and women. Lower levels of DHEA have been found in depressed patients, and mood elevation has been noted in men and women given DHEA supplementation. An increase in its metabolite, DHEA-sulfate, has been associated with improvement in depression and dysthymia (Bloch, Schmidt, Danaceau, Adams, & Rubinow, 1999; Wolkowitz, Reus, Keebler, Nelson, Freedland et al., 1999). DHEA should be used with caution and only in low doses in bipolar patients because it can exacerbate mania, irritability, and aggression.

Side Effects: 7-Keto DHEA has fewer side effects than DHEA

DHEA is generally well tolerated. However, it can sometimes cause significant elevations in testosterone levels with symptoms of acne, oily skin, hair loss, hirsutism (excess body hair), effects on the prostate, elevation of estrogen with increased risk of uterine or breast cancer, vaginal bleeding, endometrial hyperplasia, or venous thrombosis. In contrast, 7-keto DHEA does not convert to testosterone, estrogen, or progesterone and it is not associated with these side effects. 7-Keto DHEA appears to exert its effects through a different pathway because it does not elevate levels of DHEA or DHEA-sulfate.

DHEA for Depression

In a double-blind randomized placebo-controlled crossover study at the National Institute of Mental Health Midlife Outpatient Clinic, 23 men and 23 women with midlife onset of major or minor depression were treated for six weeks with DHEA, 90 mg/day for three weeks, 450 mg/day for three weeks, and six weeks of placebo. After six weeks of DHEA, 23 subjects showed a 50% or greater reduction in Hamilton Depression Rating Scale (HAM-D) as compared with 13 subjects after placebo. Taking DHEA was also associated with improved scores on a scale for sexual functioning (Schmidt, Daly, Bloch, Smith, Danaceau et al., 2005).

Case 5—7-Keto DHEA for Dysthymia and MajorDepression

Elena had suffered from dysthymia and major depression most of her adult life. She had a course of electroconvulsive therapy in her 40s that improved her mood but left her with a persistent marked memory loss. At age 51, she was treated for breast cancer with radiation, chemotherapy, surgery, and extensive breast reconstruction. As often occurs, chemotherapy precipitated menopause and worsened her memory impairment and depression. Over the next 10 years, she failed many trials of antidepressants and augmentation. Norpramine (Desipramine), phenelzine (Nardil), and bupropion (Wellbutrin) made her agitated. Fluoxetine (Prozac) made her nauseous. She had no response to robust doses of sertraline (Zoloft), paroxetine (Paxil), lithium, valproate (Depakote), carbemazepine (Tegretol), thyroid hormone, venlafaxine (Effexor), SAMe or *Rhodiola rosea*. She had slight improvement on aripiprazole (Abilify) and tianeptine (Stablon), a French serotonin reuptake accelerator antidepressant that does not cause sexual dysfunction or weight gain). Based on the history of worsening depression after menopause, her DHEA-sulfate level was checked and found to be extremely low. Elena's oncologist agreed to a trial of 7-keto DHEA (which does not elevate estrogen). After one week of 7-keto DHEA 50 mg, she felt that her mood, energy, and cognitive functions were much better. When her dose was increased to 75 mg/day she slept better and had 100% remission of her depression. She was maintained on tianeptine (Stablon) 25 mg/day. When she was tapered off Effexor, she began to have hot flashes again. Maintaining Effexor 37.5 mg/day was sufficient to control the hot flashes. She did well for several years until the stress of caring for two close family members who had become ill led to recurrence of moderate but not disabling depression. Increasing the 7-keto DHEA to 200 mg/day and the Stablon to 25 mg b.i.d. significantly improved her mood.

DHEA for Depression in HIV/AIDS Patients

Subsyndromal major depression and dysthymia (depression lasting more than two years) are far more common than major depression in the general population and in those with HIV/AIDS. Nevertheless, relatively few studies have been done that support the effectiveness of prescription antidepressants in such cases. Patients with less severe depression who suffer from HIV/AIDS are often reluctant to take standard antidepressants due to concerns about side effects and interactions with antiretroviral medication.

A double-blind randomized placebo-controlled trial in 145 HIV-positive adults with subsyndromal depression or dysthymia showed a response rate (defined as a decrease in HAM-D > 50%) of 64% for those given DHEA (100–400 mg/day) as compared to 38% for those on placebo among the patients who completed the eight-week trial (Rabkin, McElhiney, Rabkin, McGrath, & Ferrando, 2006). The mood response appeared to be maintained at eight-month follow-up. There was no relationship between baseline DHEA-sulfate serum levels and response rates. However, among the patients given DHEA, those whose DHEA-sulfate levels rose by 100% or more had a significantly higher rate of response (70%). There was a high degree of acceptance of DHEA supplementation and a low dropout rate. DHEA side effects were comparable to placebo. Because there is wide variation in the content and quality of over-the-counter DHEA supplements, the investigators used micronized DHEA prepared by a pharmacy with documented content.

7-Keto DHEA for PTSD and Bipolar Disorder

Sageman and Brown (2006a) reported five cases of women with severe chronic post-traumatic stress disorder (PTSD) due to childhood abuse who remained highly symptomatic and unresponsive to many years of cognitive behavioral therapy and psychotropic medications. Prior to treatment, three of the women were tested and found to have low DHEA-sulfate levels. All three showed marked improvement in mood and symptoms of PTSD as well as rapid progress in interpersonal and vocational functioning when treated with 25-50 mg/day 7-keto DHEA. The other two cases with moderate pretreatment DHEA levels also experienced better mood and less severe PTSD symptoms. One patient with comorbid bipolar II disorder and dissociative identity disorder had a baseline DHEA-sulfate of 70. When she was treated with DHEA, her dissociative symptoms decreased. The administration of 7-keto DHEA does not result in elevation of serum DHEA, testosterone, estrogen, or progesterone levels.

MIND–BODY APPROACHES FOR MOOD DISORDERS

A considerable amount of scientific research has been conducted on the role that yoga and other mind–body practices can play in alleviating depression. Unfortunately, many of the studies were uncontrolled, used small samples, or had flawed methodology. Because a myriad of yoga practices are being studied, it is difficult to amass a substantial body of information about any single practice. Nevertheless, it is possible to draw some parallels because many mind–body practices use a common set of basic practices with a variety of technical modifications.

Yoga for Depression

A review of research evidence for depression found that five randomized controlled trials of yoga for depression reported positive findings. However, some methodological details were missing in these reports. An optimistic but cautious interpretation of these studies was suggested (Pilkington, Kirkwood, Rampes, & Richardson, 2005).

Yoga can bring positive changes in mood not only to people suffering from clinical depression but also to healthy normals. For example, a study of 71 normal adults compared visualization and relaxation techniques with 30 minutes of yoga postures and breathing techniques. Participants in the yoga group experienced significantly greater improvements in mental and physical energy, alertness, enthusiasm, and positive mood (Wood, 1993).

In a pilot study, 113 psychiatric inpatients participated in a Hatha Yoga–based 45-minute program once a week. Classes focused on slow, gentle stretching and strengthening exercises with attention focused on deep breathing, awareness of body sensations, and relaxation. The group included 43 patients with mood disorders (bipolar, major depression, dysthymia), 36 with psychotic disorders (schizophrenia, schizoaffective, schizophreniform, delusional disorder, brief reactive psychosis), 9 with borderline personality, 5 with adjustment disorder, and 20 with other diagnoses. Scores on the Profile of Mood States declined significantly following participation in the first yoga class. Significant improvements occurred on five of the negative emotion factors: tension-anxiety, depression-dejection, anger-hostility, fatigue-inertia, and confusion-bewilderment (Lavey, Sherman, Mueser, Osborne, Currier et al., 2005). This study suggests that yoga may benefit patients during hospitalization for depression and other diagnoses.

Most people who take yoga classes report improvements in mood and well-being. Many factors affect mood including genetic predisposition, environmental circumstances, attitudes, stress, tension, fatigue, cognitive style, habitual patterns of thinking and judging, psychological defenses (for example, turning anger against the self in the form of harsh self-judgment), excess expectations of oneself, inability to accept limitations and disappointments, and tendencies to dwell on negative thoughts. Yoga postures and stretches are most effective in ameliorating the factors that contribute to depression when they are combined with yoga breathing, positive affirmations, psycho-philosophical-spiritual development, and cognitive restructuring. These elements can be found in the major schools of yoga. For a clinical exploration of yoga practices that addresses many facets of depression, we refer the reader to Amy Weintraub's *Yoga for Depression: A Compassionate Guide to Relieve Suffering Through Yoga* (Weintraub, 2004).

Iyengar Yoga

B. K. S. Iyengar popularized a structured yoga practice focused on yoga postures (asanas) assisted by props (ropes, chairs, cushions) to support the positions for novices and to progressively train them in the correct techniques (Iyengar, 1966, 1988). Classes emphasize awareness of muscular activity and joints. Coordination with breath practices, attention, and concentration are key elements. Iyengar recommended certain postures for relief of depression, including chest opening (backward bending), inversions (head down), and rigorous leg stand positions.

A randomized wait-list control study of 28 mildly depressed adults (who were not formally diagnosed), less than 30 years old, showed that those who engaged in two 1-hour Iyengar yoga classes per week for five weeks had significant reductions in Beck Depression Inventory and Spielberger State Trait Anxiety Inventory scores compared with the control group (Woolery, Myers, Sternlieb, & Zeltzer, 2004).

David Shapiro and colleagues (2007) studied the effects of Iyengar Yoga on depressed patients who were taking antidepressant medication but who were only in partial remission. They also analyzed the traits and physiological factors that distinguished those who achieved full remission with the addition of yoga from those who did not. Out of 27 subjects, 17 completed 20 Iyengar Yoga classes over a period of 8 weeks in this single-group outcome study. While yoga postures were the predominant method, they included breath coordination and there were brief periods of rest and breath practices. Significant reductions were found in depression; average HAM-D17 dropped from 12.5 at baseline to 6.2 after yoga intervention ($p < 0.001$). Scores also improved significantly on SCL ($p < 0.4$), Spielberger AngerOut Scale (ANGOUT) ($p < 0.05$), Spielberger Trait Anxiety Inventory ($p < 0.005$), and Pittsburgh Sleep Scale ($P < 0.2$). In

CLINICAL PEARL

Severely depressed patients may require more intensive, frequent, and prolonged yoga practices. The role of the health care provider in encouraging and supporting the patient's motivation to persist with yoga training is critical for a successful outcome.

addition to psychological assessments, physiological measures showed changes in autonomic function associated with depression and emotion regulation. Heart rate variability (HRV) was measured in low frequency (LF-HRV, 0.075–0.125) and high frequency (HF-HRV, 0.125–0.50 Hz) bands. LF-HRV reflects the influence of the sympathetic nervous system and the parasympathetic nervous system (PNS) on heart rate. HF-HRV primarily indicates the effects of PNS on the heart. Among the 17 completers, the average LF-HRV was significantly reduced ($p < 0.05$). However, HF-HRV did not increase, suggesting a relative lack of parasympathetic modulation. Out of 17 completers, 11 achieved remission (defined as HAM-D17 <7). Remitters tended to engage in more regular exercise, had higher levels of HRV at baseline, and had greater capacity for emotional regulation compared with nonremitters. No adverse effects occurred. The authors suggested the possibility that in those with lower resting vagal tone (nonremitters) the yoga intervention may not have raised the level of vagal activity enough to achieve remission of depression. They wondered if a longer period of treatment would have been more effective. These possibilities are consistent with our clinical observations that more severely depressed individuals often require two or three times as many sessions of Sudarshan Kriya Yoga (see below) per week for relief compared with those who are less depressed.

Shavasana
Khumar and colleagues studied Shavasana (relaxation and rhythmic breathing) in a group of university students who were mildly depressed (Khumar & Kaur, 1993). Students were randomized to practice Shavasana for 30 minutes daily or to no intervention for 30

days. Significant reductions in scores on the Amritsar Depression Inventory and the Zang Depression Self-Rating Scale were found in those who did Shavasana compared with the control group. Methodological details were not adequately reported. No adverse events were noted.

Hatha Yoga

Hatha Yoga focuses on yoga postures coordinated with breath practices. In a naturalistic study, 87 college students volunteered to take a class in swimming, Hatha Yoga (which included postures and breathing), or lectures on health. Those who engaged in yoga showed greater acute decreases in scores for anger, tension, and fatigue than those in the swim class or the leading control group (Berger & Owen, 1992). Caution should be used in extrapolating findings in normal populations to patients diagnosed with depression.

Qigong

Qigong is an ancient Chinese and Korean practice, which includes meditation, breath exercises, and body movements. *Qi* translates as "vital energy" and "breath." The word *gong* means "work."

In a 16-week rater-blinded study of Qigong for elderly patients (over age 65) with depression, 82 subjects were randomly assigned to either three Qigong (Baduanjin) sessions per week (30–45 minutes) plus 15 minutes/day unsupervised home practice or a newspaper reading group. Patients who participated in the Qigong program showed significant improvements on the Geriatric Depression Scale ($p=0.041$), Chinese General Self-efficacy Scale ($p < 0.001$), Personal Well Being Index ($p < 0.001$), and General Health Questionnaire ($p < .042$). The use of a newspaper discussion group nullified the effects of attention from the instructor or group socialization on outcomes. The authors concluded that 8 to 12 weeks of Qigong can relieve depression in elderly subjects (Tsang, Fung, Chan, Lee, & Chan, 2006). Daily practices and regular sessions with an instructor are necessary to maintain the benefits.

Yoga Breathing: Sudarshan Kriya Yoga

Several studies suggest antidepressant effects with a yoga breath practice called Sudarshan Kriya Yoga (SKY). In Chapter 3, SKY is described in greater detail. Briefly, SKY includes five breath practices (victorious breath or Ujjayi, bellows breath or Bhastrika, AUM, Sudarshan Kriya or cyclical breathing, and alternate nostril breathing). Courses also teach yoga postures, meditation, relaxation, some yoga philosophy, and psychoeducation in stress reduction.

A small pilot study used SKY breathing (Ujjayi, Bhastrika, and Sudarshan Kriya) to treat 30 patients—15 with dysthymia (a disorder that is somewhat less severe but more chronic than major depression) and 15 with major depression. The researchers found that SKY significantly improved symptoms of depression in all 30 participants (Naga Venkatesha Murthy, Janakiramaiah, Gangadhar, & Subbakrishna, 1998).

In a larger three-month follow-up study, 46 outpatients with dysthymia were taught SKY breathing and then instructed to practice every day at home. Of those patients who kept up with regular practice (at least three days a week) for the first month, 68% recovered from their depression. Those who did not practice as regularly improved less. Interestingly, the attitude of the participants toward yoga breathing—whether they were skeptical or enthusiastic—had no impact on the results (Janakiramaiah, Gangadhar, Murthy, Harish, Shetty et al., 1998).

In a study of severely depressed patients on a psychiatric ward, 45 adults were assigned to three groups. The first group was given only SKY breath training and no medication. The group processes and the yoga knowledge that are part of SKY courses were eliminated from this program in order to distinguish the effects of the breathing from these other factors. The second group was given 150 mg/day of an antidepressant, imipramine. The third group was treated three times a week with unipolar electroshock therapy. At the end of four weeks, the patients were retested, using the Hamilton Depression Scale and the Beck Depression Inventory. The group given SKY breath training showed as much improvement in their depression scores as the group given imipramine. SKY and imipramine groups did almost as well as the electroshock group (Janakiramaiah, Gangadhar, Murthy, Harish, Subbakrishna et al., 2000). One limitation was that the method of group assignment was not reported.

The practice of SKY was found to increase serum levels of brain-derived neurotrophic factor, an indicator of neuroplasticity (Pan,

Liao, Jiang, Wang, & Huang, 2006). In a randomized controlled trial of depressed patients, A-Min Huang and colleagues found that SKY practice increased BDNF and that the increase correlated with improvement in depression (Pan, Brown, Gerbarg, Liao, Jiang et al., in process).

Depressed people tend to feel isolated, to have low self-esteem, and to dwell on regrets and guilt about the past. SKY helps to alleviate these aspects of depression by promoting feelings of connectedness, by teaching people to focus on the present moment rather than ruminate about the past, by reducing self-blame and criticism, and by helping people experience and come to terms with their feelings.

As an adjunctive treatment, SKY can reduce the need for medication, facilitate the therapeutic process, and enhance feelings of joy and connectedness with others. While we do not find enough evidence yet to consider SKY to be a substitute for medication or psychotherapy, we have found in clinical practice that many people are able to overcome depression using SKY without prescription medications.

SKY can lead to greater progress in psychotherapy. It is well known that during psychotherapy, people can become stuck at a certain point in the process, the therapeutic impasse. Some people are unable to reach deeper levels of insight and may be held back by their need to block out intense emotions. SKY can help overcome an impasse by catalyzing fresh insights, deeper emotions, and effective action (Gerbarg, 2007; see Chapter 3).

Case 6—SKY for Geriatric Depression and Anxiety

An 80-year-old physician was basically in good physical health, except for high blood pressure and chronic arthritic pain, which were controlled through medication. Living alone, she was experiencing a great deal of stress, anxiety, and depression. On the advice of a colleague, she took the SKY breathing course to deal with these problems—both the depression and the chronic pain—and she was very pleased with the results. The three-stage Ujjayi breathing and Sudarshan Kriya greatly relieved her depression, reduced her chronic pain, and increased her mobility. Two years later, she continued to practice yoga breathing every morning, and found that it prevented her from feeling stressed, depressed, or anxious. She is still working, feels calmer, and has a greater sense of control. She now recommends SKY to her patients.

Exercise for Depression

Early research on the effects of exercise on depression was fraught with methodological problems. However, a meta-analysis of 11 more recent randomized controlled trials, found exercise to be a promising treatment for moderate depression in subjects who engaged in two to four exercise sessions per week for 12 weeks (Blumenthal, Babyak, Moore, Craighead, Herman et al., 1999). Another meta-analysis found that most studies supported the benefits of exercise for depression regardless of the age or gender of subjects, the severity of depression, or the type of exercise (Craft & Landers, 1998). While no specific mechanism of action has been proven to account for the efficacy of exercise, neurochemical changes (increases in serotonin, norepinephrine, endorphins, and other neuromodulators), improved well-being, stress resilience, and self-efficacy probably contribute to the observed benefits (Otto, Church, Craft, Greer, Smits et al., 2007).

COMPLEX CASES: MULTILAYERED APPROACHES FOR INTEGRATIVE TREATMENTS

Many patients present with more than one problem and require a combination of psychotherapy, prescription medications, and CAM treatments for recovery. Here we present a complex case to illustrate the construction of a multilayered integrative treatment approach in a highly motivated patient who was not willing to settle for less.

Case 7—Depression, premenstrual syndrome, anxiety, obsessive personality, and inability to attract men: Timing, layering, and integration of CAM with psychoanalysis

Ms. W. failed to pass her law boards because of depression, procrastination, and obsessive thinking. During college she had suffered three episodes of major depression with premenstrual mood exacerbations. Although partially improved on SSRIs (Prozac, Zoloft, and Paxil), she hated the side effects, which included a 50-pound weight gain and sexual dysfunction.

Although she was quite attractive, Ms. W. had never had a close boyfriend. She worked on relationship issues during three years of psychoanalysis. Fluoxetine (Prozac) helped the depression and enabled her to function better in school, but it caused anorgasmia. Buproprion (Wellbutrin) made her irritable. Sertraline (Zoloft) improved the depression but caused sexual dysfunction and eventually lost its effectiveness. The history revealed symptoms of possible attention-deficit disorder (type 2 inattentive) or bipolar II. Relatives on both sides of the family had depression and the mother had obsessive-compulsive disorder.

The first layer of integrative treatment included citalopram (Celexa) and light therapy (which improved sleep). Citalopram had just been released in 1999 and was being marketed as the new SSRI less likely to cause weight gain or sexual side effects. Contrary to this claim, the patient's weight went up to 185 pounds. Citalopram also caused sexual dysfunction. In order to stop the weight gain, she was tapered off citalopram while adding 7.5 mg/day of buspirone (Buspar) for anxiety and then SAMe starting with 800 mg/day. Her depression started to improve with increasing response as the dose increased to 2,000 mg/day SAMe. Eventually the antidepressant effect was maintained on 1,200–1,600 mg/day SAMe depending on her degree of depression. Weight loss was accelerated by using 10 mg/day Meridia, which acts on serotonin and dopamine to reduce appetite. Over the next two years, Ms. W. gradually lost 60 pounds. However, her premenstrual syndrome and obsessive symptoms persisted.

It took six months to assess the effects of SAMe (about 60% improvement in depression). The discontinuation of citalopram only partially relieved the sexual dysfunction. The second layer of treatment, the addition of *Rhodiola rosea* 600 mg/day, restored the patient's sexual function to normal. She began actively looking for men using the Internet and speed dating, in which singles briefly meet numerous potential partners. Coincidentally, the *R. rosea* markedly relieved her anxiety.

For the third treatment layer, St. John's Wort 600 mg was added to address the obsessive symptoms. Ms. W. had an unusually robust response, stopped procrastinating, and was able to keep up with her workload for the first time in her adult life. When she tried to discontinue St. John's Wort, obsessional symptoms recurred. However, the 600 mg/day of St. John's Wort reduced the intensity of her orgasms. She settled on a compromise, using 300 mg/day St. John's Wort and increasing to 600 mg/day when under pressure to write legal documents.

With her weight down to 125 pounds and her anxiety under better control, Ms. W. discontinued Meridia and buspirone. She continued taking SAMe, *R. rosea*, and St. John's Wort. Ms. W. began meeting many men through speed dating. After the first encounter, despite her physical attractiveness, the men never asked for a date. In trying to understand this problem, she solicited feedback from people she knew. Her friends said that it was difficult to be around her, but they could not pinpoint the reason. It seemed that her high level of tension was a turnoff for men.

The fourth level of treatment, designed to help overcome this handicap, was a trial of pheromones (bioactive compounds that may activate receptors in the olfactory epithelium and enhance innate attraction; www.athenainstitute.com; Cutler & Genovese, 2002). The validity of two studies showing increased sociosexual behaviors with synthetic pheromones was questioned due to statistical and sampling errors (Winman, 2004). Though we could not entirely rule out a placebo effect, the results were spectacular. Ms. W.'s dating increased from zero up to six or seven days a week, and sometimes several dates in one evening. Men were very attracted to her sexually, but the dates never led to a relationship. Ms. W.'s tendencies to be tense, anxious, and overreactive were still interfering with her ability to develop a close relationship.

On the assumption that the patient's residual tension,

anxiety, and overreactivity were due to autonomic imbalance (overactivity of the sympathetic nervous system and underactivity of the parasympathetic nervous system) the fifth level of treatment was recommended, a mind–body intervention, the Art of Living Basic Course in yoga breathing. After taking this course and practicing the yoga breathing, Ms. W. became much less anxious with fewer episodes of overreactive tachycardia. She felt much better when she performed her daily yoga breath practices consistently. The effect was evident in that she would deteriorate rapidly when she skipped her yoga practice for more than four consecutive days. More important, yoga breathing relaxed her. She became emotionally softer and more appealing. As a result, men wanted to develop relationships with her.

Her only remaining complaint was PMS with depression and irritability. With the sixth layer of treatment, light therapy (10,000 lux) for 30 minutes every morning, the residual PMS symptoms completely remitted.

Concurrently, in psychotherapy Ms. W. worked on residual resistances to having a relationship. Her therapist thought she was being too picky. She wanted to have a child and was concerned that at age 37 her biological clock was ticking. She overcame her last resistances and developed a serious relationship with one man. Eventually they lived together in her first long-term relationship.

Although this case is complex, it has features often seen in clinical practice. Over time, an integrative treatment including SAMe, *Rhodiola rosea*, St. John's Wort, pheromones, psychotherapy, and yoga breathing, with temporary use of buspirone and Meridia, brought the patient a greater degree of recovery, 95% improvement in depression, and greater satisfaction in her personal and professional life.

Integrative Approach to Treat Depression

1. Evaluation and diagnosis including nutritional status, comorbid mental and physical disorders, medication side effects, and sub-

stance abuse. Ascertain the patient's past and current use of CAM and preferences.

2. Inform patient of options for standard and CAM treatments including risks and benefits. Document this discussion in the patient chart.

3. Laboratory studies (if they have not been done within the previous year): complete blood count, thyroid functions, chemistry panel, DHEA and DHEA-sulfate (over age 40), and coenzyme Q10 level (if the patient is taking statins). For individuals living in northern climates who may have inadequate sun exposure, check serum vitamin D level.

4. Correct nutritional deficiencies through dietary education and supplements: multivitamin, B_{12} 1,000 mcg/day, folic acid 800–1000 mg/day, omega-3 fatty acids 1,000 mg b.i.d. (preferably from fish oil). In men with cardiac stents, and baseline homocysteine less than 15 μmol/liter, avoid B vitamins and folate supplements as they can increase the risk of obstruction.

5. If the patient is having incomplete response to an antidepressant but no side effects, consider increasing the dose of the antidepressant, switching antidepressants, or augmentation with CAM. Document the reasons for your choices of CAM and standard treatments as you proceed.

6. For patients who have failed numerous adequate trials of antidepressants and talk therapies due to nonresponse or intolerable side effects, begin CAM trials with SAMe starting with 400 mg/day and increasing to 1,600 mg/day as tolerated.

7. When the patient is able to comply with mind–body practices, refer for program of yoga breathing and yoga postures or Qigong.

8. If symptoms of depression persist, add *R. rosea* starting with 150 mg and increasing up to 400 mg a.m. plus 350 mg midday as tolerated. On doses above 500 mg/day, watch for bruising or bleeding.

9. If symptoms of depression persist, continue CAM trials as described in this chapter.

Integrative Approach to Treat Bipolar Disorder

1. Follow steps 1–4 above.

5. If the patient is having incomplete response to prescription mood

stabilizers but no side effects, check for adequate medication serum levels. Next consider increasing the doses and switching or adding other mood stabilizers or antidepressant cautiously.

6. For patients who have failed numerous adequate medication trials and talk therapies due to nonresponse or intolerable side effects, begin CAM trials.

7. Omega-3 fatty acids (preferably fish oil) start with 1,000 mg b.i.d. and increase to 8,000 to 10,000 mg/day in divided doses with meals as tolerated. Watch for gastrointestinal side effects.

8. A trial of N-acetylcysteine 2 g/day may be given. Response usually does not occur for at least eight weeks.

9. For bipolar patients who are primarily depressed and who are not prone to becoming manic, trials of R. rosea and 7-keto-DHEA may be beneficial. Begin with low doses and increase gradually while monitoring for signs of overstimulation, agitation, or hostility. The authors have found that if the patient has a relatively low DHEA or DHEA-sulfate (lower half of the normal range according to laboratory standards) they are more likely to respond to 7-keto DHEA, although this is not always the case, and it has not yet been documented in clinical trials.

TABLE 2.1 Mood Disorders Treatment Guidelines

CAM	Clinical Uses	Daily Dose	Side Effects, Drug Interactions,* Contraindications
B vitamins	depression, energy	B$_{12}$ 1,000 mcg folate 800 mcg	Rare: activation Caution: cardiac stents**
Choline	mania	2,000–7,200 mg	Excess doses: depression
DHEA	depression	25–200 mg	hirsutism, acne Caution: bipolars Contraindications: estrogen-sensitive cancer, prostate cancer
7-keto DHEA	depression	25–200 mg	Caution: bipolars Contraindications: estrogen-sensitive cancer, prostate cancer
Inositol	depression	12–20 g	Gas, loose bowels, mania
Omega-3 fatty acids	bipolar, unipolar: augmentation borderline: augmentation	6–10 g	GI distress, belching, loose stools May affect glucose metabolism in diabetics
Rhodiola rosea	depression	150–900 mg	Agitation, insomnia, anxiety, headache. Rare: palpitations, chest pain
S-adenosyl-methionine (SAMe)	depression, fibromyalgia, arthritis, liver disease, Parkinson's	400–1,600 mg 600–1,200 mg 800–1,600 mg 1,200–1,600 mg 800–4,400 mg	Nausea, loose bowels, activation, anxiety, mania in bipolar, headache, occasional palpitations

TABLE 2.1 *Continued*

CAM	Clinical Uses	Daily Dose	Side Effects, Drug Interactions,* Contraindications
St. John's Wort (*Hypericum perforatum*)	mild–moderate depression, somatoform disorders, seasonal affective disorder	300–600 mg t.i.d.	Nausea, heartburn, loose bowels, jitteriness, insomnia, fatigue, bruxism, phototoxic rash, mania in bipolar. Affects CYP 3A4, 1A2 P-glycoprotein: decreases digoxin, warfarin, indivir, cyclosporine, theophylline, oral contraceptives D/C: during pregnancy and 10 days prior to surgery
Bio-Strath B Vitamins + antioxidants	mood, energy	1 Tbsp b.i.d. 3 tabs b.i.d.	Caution: cardiac stent**
L-methylfolate Deplin	mood, energy		Caution: cardiac stent**
Natural Balance 100 mg *R. rosea* + 350 mg St. John's Wort	mild–moderate depression	3–6 pills	Side effects of both *R. rosea* and St. John's Wort as above
Metanx 2.8 mg L-methylfolate 25 mg pyridoxal 5'-phosphate 2 mg methylcobalamin	cardiovascular risks, elevated homocysteine		Minimal Caution: cardiac stent**

D/C = discontinue; GI = gastrointestinal

* Common side effects are listed. There are additional rare side effects. Individuals with high blood pressure, diabetes, pregnancy (or during breast-feeding), or any chronic or serious medical condition should check with their physician before taking supplements. Patients taking anticoagulants should consult their physician before using supplements.

** May increase risk of restenosis of cardiac stents in men only with baseline homocysteine less than 15µmol/liter.

CHAPTER 3 OUTLINE

1. **Stress Response Systems and Complementary Treatments**

2. **Mind–Body Practices**: Research and Clinical Evidence

3. **Simple, Effective Breath Practices for Anxiety**

4. **Post-Traumatic Stress Disorder (PTSD)**
   a. veterans and military personnel
   b. survivors of mass disasters
   c. victims of emotional, physical and sexual abuse

5. **Phobias, Obsessive Compulsive Disorder, Sleep Disorders**

6. **Yoga Facilitates Psychotherapy**

7. **Precautions, Contraindications, Risk Reduction**

8. **Hormones**
   a. melatonin, REM behavior disorder, and jet lag
   b. 7-Keto DHEA for PTSD and bipolar disorder

9. **Herbs and Nutrients**: kava, *Rhodiola rosea*, valerian, lemon balm, passionflower, theanine, GABA, ginkgo, chamomile, St. John's Wort, omega-3 fatty acids, picamilon S-adenosylmethionine, homeopathy

Anxiety Disorders

This chapter focuses on neurophysiological aspects of anxiety and emotion regulation that can be influenced by complementary and alternative treatments, including the stress response system, fear and anxiety regulatory circuits, fear extinction, interoception (internal somatosensory perceptions of trauma experiences and memories), trauma schemas, and neuroplasticity. While there are some herbs that are helpful in anxiety disorders, in clinical practice, the authors find that specific mind–body practices are far more effective because they can ameliorate the underlying pathogenic mechanisms and provide rapid relief with minimal side effects. Therefore, this chapter begins with a discussion of mind–body practices followed by herbs and nutrients.

STRESS RESPONSE SYSTEMS

Anxiety, in its myriad physical and mental expressions, can be triggered by any internal or external stressor. When the mind perceives or contemplates threats of the past, present, or future, the stress response systems are activated, releasing neurotransmitters and neurohormones that prepare for fight, flight, or freeze behaviors. The

SIDEBAR 3.1 AUTONOMIC PATHWAYS—EMOTION, COGNITION, ATTENTION, AND CONSCIOUSNESS

The autonomic nervous system consists of the sympathetic nervous system (SNS) and the parasympathetic nervous system (PNS). The nerve tracts of the SNS run through the spinal cord and synapse with peripheral nerves in ganglia, clusters of nerves along both sides of the vertebral column. A few tracts of the PNS also run through the spinal cord, but the main pathways are through the right and left vagus nerves (10th cranial nerves). The effects of the right and left vagus nerves on the body have been known and studied for decades, but only recently have their extensive effects on the brain and mind–body communication been recognized.

The vagus nerves exit from the brainstem and meander through the chest and abdomen, sending branches to innervate the pharynx, heart, lungs, gastrointestinal tract, liver, pancreas, kidneys, adrenal glands, urinary tract, genitals, and blood vessels. (The word *vagus*, derives from *vagare* meaning "to wander.") The vagus nerves are bidirectional (see Figure 3.2). Only 20% of vagal fibers (efferents) carry messages from the brain to the body, whereas 80% of vagal fibers (afferents) carry information from the body up to the brainstem nuclei. From there, pathways ascend to the limbic system (emotion-processing structures), thalamus, and broad areas of the cerebral cortex (including the prefrontal cortex), influencing how we experience our bodies, our emotions, and our state of consciousness.

human stress response systems evolved for survival in the time of hunters and gatherers when the day was spent in routine quiet physical activity punctuated by sudden episodic dangers, and the long dark nights were spent in sleep. Today many people experience long periods of personal and professional stress in an environment that often feels unsafe. Periods of rest and relaxation are not sufficient for rebalancing of the stress response system. The result is chronic overactivation of the sympathetic nervous system (SNS). While the SNS releases excitatory neurotransmitters, the hypothalamic-pituitary-

SIDEBAR 3.2 **THE STRESS RESPONSE SYSTEM**

Parts of the stress response system located within the central nervous system are in the hypothalamus, medulla, and brainstem. The hypothalamus contains specialized cells that release corticotrophin hormone (CRH) and arginine-vasopressin. CRH nerves are also in the medulla. Cells that releas norepinephrine are found in the locus ceruleus and elsewhere in the brainstem.

The peripheral branches of the stress response system are the hyothalamic-pituitary-adrenal axis (HPA), the efferent sympathoadrenal system (SAS), and the parasympathetic nervous system (PNS). While the HPA is responsible for long-term adaptation to stress, the SAS switches on the acute stress response and general adaptation. Since the main actions of the PNS are to counteract the SAS, during acute stress the PNS may withdraw some of its effects, thereby allowing the SNS to dominate even more (the SNS is usually dominant).

Neurochemical mediators of the stress response system act at the system, organ, and cellular levels. CRH from the hypothalamus triggers the pituitary gland to release adrenocorticotrophic hormone (ACTH) and beta-endorphin. ACTH regulares adrenal release of cortisol and glucocorticoids. Maintaining the balance between the switch-on (SNS) and switch-off (PNS) parts of the stress response system is critical in order to protect the organism from overreacting, for example, preventing damage from excess levels of cortisol and excitatory neurotransmitters, such as glutamate.

adrenal axis releases adrenaline and cortisol. The task of the parasympathetic nervous system (PNS) is to counterbalance these effects by slowing the heart and respiration, calming the mind and emotions, and replenishing the energy consumed by the SNS activity (see Sidebars 3.1 and 3.2).

Unfortunately, in people who suffer from anxiety disorders the PNS is underactive while the SNS is overactive (Beauchaine, 2001; Berntson, Sarter, & Cacioppo, 2003; Carney & Ellis, 1988; Mezzacappa, Tremblay, Kindlon, Saul, Arseneault et al., 1996, 1997; Porges,

2001; Thayer & Brosschot, 2005). The net result is that the PNS is unable to counteract the effects of the stress response system. This is a fundamental neurophysiological problem in anxiety disorders. While psychotropic medications used to treat anxiety dampen the SNS, they have not been shown to increase the activity of the PNS. Many psychotropic medications dull cognition, blunt emotions, and interfere with mental functioning. In contrast, adaptogens (see Chapter 4, sections on *Rhodiola rosea* and adaptogens) enhance the activity of both the SNS and the PNS, improving the ability to respond to stress appropriately and then terminate the response when the danger is over. Furthermore, adaptogens have been shown to improve cognitive functions (Panossian & Wagner, 2005).

Measuring the Activity of the Parasympathetic Nervous System

Until recently, the role of the PNS was vastly underestimated and there were no noninvasive procedures to measure its activity. However, since the advent of technology for analyzing heart rate variability (HRV) as a Fourier transformation derived from electroencephalogram recordings of beat-to-beat intervals, it has become possible to indirectly measure the effects of various interventions on the PNS. HRV is the rate at which the heartbeat rate changes (see Sidebar 3.3 and Figure 3.1). Changes in heart rate are linked with the respiratory cycle. When you inhale, heart rate increases and when you exhale, heart rate decreases. Respiratory sinus arrhythmia (RSA) refers to the normal heart rate increase during inspiration and decrease during expiration. RSA and HRV are used to measure SNS and PNS activity. Young healthy individuals tend to have higher HRV, whereas low HRV is associated with increased risk of cardiovascular disease, sudden death, and mortality from all causes. One can increase HRV by breathing more slowly or by increasing the activity of the PNS through vagus nerve stimulation and mind–body practices as described below.

Activating the Parasympathetic Nervous System

One way to activate the PNS is to stimulate the vagus nerves (10th cranial nerves), which exit the brainstem and carry most of the pathways of the PNS to the major organs and tissues of the body. Elec-

SIDEBAR 3.3 **HEART RATE VARIABILITY**

The amplitude of the HRV reflects the tone and responsiveness of the autonomic nervous system (the relative activity of the sympathetic and parasympathetic systems) and the cardiopulmonary system. HRV amplitude is the peak heartbeat rate minus the lowest heartbeat rate. When stress and sympathetic activity are high, the amplitude of the HRV tends to be low. HRV is the rate at which the heartbeat rate changes. Coherence is a measure of the regularity of the overall heart rate variability cycle (see Figure 3.1).

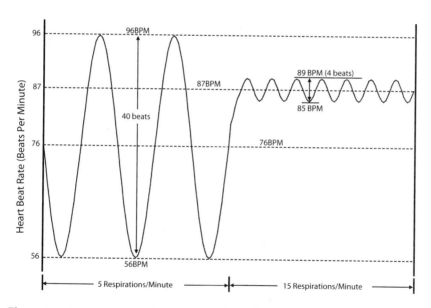

Figure 3.1 Heart rate variability. HRV amplitude is 40 beats at a respiratory rate of five breaths per minute. HRV amplitude is only four beats at a respiratory rate of 15 breaths per minute. Reproduced with permission of Stephen Elliot (Elliott & Edmonson, 2005).

tronic vagal nerve stimulation (VNS) is an invasive procedure requiring surgical placement of a wire to deliver electrical impulses to the left vagus nerve only. VNS is expensive and can cause side effects, including diaphragm spasms, hiccups, voice changes, and gastrointestinal disturbance. VNS cannot be used on the right vagus nerve because that could cause fatal arrhythmia. There are, however, simpler and safer methods to stimulate the vagus nerve using electrical stimulation of the left outer auditory ear canal (Kraus, Hosl, Kiess, Schanze, Kornhuber et al., 2007) or through mind–body techniques, particularly yoga breathing. For example, slow breathing and prolonged expiration enhance vagal nerve activity and slow the heart rate via a cardiorespiratory reflex. One can further stimulate the vagus nerves by modifying other aspects of respiration such as breathing against airway resistance and using short breath holds. Enhanced PNS function is one of the essential mechanisms underlying the physical and mental calming induced by yoga and meditative practices. Yoga practices not only enhance the capacity to modulate appropriate stress responses and to terminate those responses when they are no longer needed, but also to recover and restore energy and homeostasis.

The respiratory apparatus, including the lungs, airways, diaphragm, chest wall, and blood vessels contain thousands of sensory receptors, pressure receptors, and chemoreceptors ($pO2$ and $pCO2$). Mechanoreceptors, which are stretch sensors, respond to alveolar inflation and deflation, with electrical discharges that encode information sent to vagal afferents (Yu, 2005). This input goes to the homeostatic system as an important form of peripheral feedback (from the body to the brain), influencing emotional and cognitive processing, as described by Craig (2003) and Damasio (1999) (see Sidebar 3.3). Alterations in respiratory patterns, registered by sensory receptors, change the visceral somatosensory input carried by vagal afferents to the brain. This may explain how different yoga breath techniques can lead to rapid changes in emotional states, cognitive processing, representations of bodily feeling states, and the reactions and behaviors linked to those feeling states.

Over time, yoga breathing tends to normalize SNS activity and increase PNS tone (see Figure 3.1). The central autonomic network includes higher centers such as the medial prefrontal cortex (mPFC) that inhibit lower centers such as the amygdala (Thayer & Brosschot, 2005). When the mPFC is hypoactive and the amygdala is hyperactive, as occurs in depression and post-traumatic stress disorder (PTSD), the inhibitory mechanisms may fail to modulate emotions such as fear and anger, leading to dysregulation of emotional responses and behaviors. Dysfunction in the circuits between the prefrontal cortex, amygdala, and thalamus may contribute to fear-related symptoms in PTSD (Das, Kemp, Littell, Olivieri, Peduto et al., 2005; LeDoux, 2000). Poor affective information processing, deficits in working memory, and impaired executive function have been associated with underactivity of the PNS (low HRV) and prefrontal cortex.

Peripheral Models of Emotion: Interoception

James Lange's theory of emotion emphasized the role of peripheral feedback, afferent information from muscles and viscera, in the sensory and motivational components involved in the generation of feelings. Peripheral models of emotion have been extended to include motivational behavior, decision making, emotional and social behavior, and self-awareness (Damasio, 1994, 1999). Interoception is the perception of "feelings" (pain, temperature, sensual touch, muscular and visceral sensations, vasomotor activity, and air hunger) that reflect the state of the body and that have their primary representation in the dorsal posterior insula, located inside the prefrontal cortex. The metarepresentation of interoceptive information, primarily in the right anterior insula, has been postulated as a substrate for emotional awareness (Craig, 2003). Damasio hypothesized that areas of the brain involved in the mapping and regulation of internal states (homeostasis) contribute to representational images of the body state and constitute a basis for awareness of feeling states (Critchley, 2005; Gerbarg, 2007).

Interoceptive information about moment-to-moment changes in the state of the airways, lungs, and respiratory apparatus travels up the vagus nerves and is delivered to the insula along with other messages from chemoreceptors and baroreceptors. This information constitutes the peripheral feedback that can influence emotional processing. Yoga breathing is based on the volitional change of breathing patterns. As such, it provides a unique opportunity to deliberately alter interoceptive feedback to the brain. Through intro-spection and by external measurements, it is possible to observe spe-cific shifts in cognitive and emotional processing induced by yoga breath practices and potentially to identify specific therapeutic breath techniques.

Most forms of yoga and meditation begin with breath awareness and gradual slowing of the respiratory rate. This initiates activation of the PNS, quiets the mind (through ascending afferent vagal path-ways to the central autonomic network), and relaxes the body through efferent pathways as well as neuroendocrine release (see Figure 3.2). A neurophysiological theory of yoga breathing and its use in treating anxiety, aggression, PTSD, and depression have been presented (Brown & Gerberg, 2005a, 2005b).

MIND–BODY PRACTICES

Mind–body practices can significantly affect the autonomic nervous system. Particular yoga and meditation practices quiet or excite the SNS and the PNS. For the purpose of treating anxiety disorders, it is important to not only strengthen the PNS but also to increase the flexibility of the entire stress response system. One problem in anxi-ety disorders is that the individual becomes conditioned to set off inappropriate excess reactions to stimuli or inappropriate underreac-tions (e.g., emotional numbing). Hyperarousal, hypervigilance, over-reactivity, and numbing reflect dysfunction within the autonomic nerve system (see the review of meditation techniques in the treat-ment of medical illness in Arias, Steinberg, Banga, & Trestman, 2006).

For patients with anxiety disorders, it is crucial to calm the patient and control anxiety reactions as quickly as possible to prevent the repeated experiences of anxiety or panic from reinforcing overre-activity and generating more anxiety, leading to exhaustion, depres-sion, and avoidance. Mind–body techniques that focus on yoga breath practices can provide rapid reduction in anxiety. In contrast, anxious patients have difficulty meditating. Response tends to take longer and to be weaker. However, once the patient has learned to induce a relaxed calm state through yoga breathing, meditation becomes easier and can be beneficial. It is important to understand

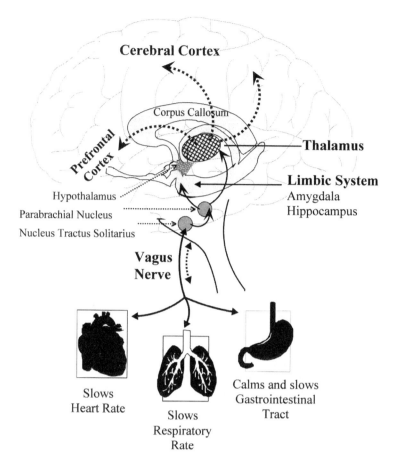

Figure 3.2 Vagus nerve effects. The vagus nerves are bidirectional. Afferent fibers bring interoceptive information from the body to relay stations in the brainstem: the parabrachial nucleus and the nucleus tractus solitarius. From the brainstem, pathways diverge to the limbic system, hypothalamus, and the thalamus. Within the limbic system and forebrain, emotion processing is affected. From the thalamus, vagal input is transmitted to cortical areas including the prefrontal, frontal, parietal, and occipital. The vagus nerves influence alertness, attention, cognitive processes, emotion regulation, and stress response.

the different kinds of yoga breathing and to know which forms are utilized by different mind–body programs. For example, mindfulness meditation includes some very simple slow breath practices. Breath work is included in Buddhist meditation and in programs that focus on yoga postures, such as Iyengar, Hatha, and Tai Chi. However, the programs that incorporate more powerful breath practices as central elements are Qigong, Sudarshan Kriya, Kundalini, and Santhi Kriya. These programs are widely available and are more likely to be efficacious in anxiety disorders and PTSD.

Anxious patients are often desperate for the immediate relief they expect to find in a pill. It is helpful for the health care provider to reassure the patient and to show them that yoga breathing can alleviate anxiety within minutes. The sections below on coherent or resonant breathing and Ujjayi breathing describe simple practices that can be learned quickly. When patients experience rapid physical relaxation and mental calming, they become more motivated to work with their breath rather than become more dependent on medication.

By voluntarily altering the pattern of breath, it is possible to influence emotional states (Philippot, Gaetane, & Blairy, 2002). Neural pathways for breathing and emotion are intricately intertwined. Low respiratory sinus arrhythmia (reflecting low vagal activity) is associated with negative states of mind, fear and depression in infants, aggression and antisocial behavior in adolescent boys, depression, anxiety disorder, and panic disorder (Beauchaine, 2001; Carney et al., 1995; Mezzacappa et al., 1997).

Research on Mind–Body Practices for Anxiety Disorders

Research on mind–body techniques has been limited by the use of older methodologies, small numbers of subjects, nonrandomization, and lack of placebo controls. A review of meditation for anxiety disorders found that only 2 out of 50 studies met inclusion criteria (Krisanaprakornkit, Krisanaprakornkit, Piyavhatkul, & Laopaiboon, 2006; Raskin, Bali, & Peeke, 1980; Shannahoff-Khalsa, Ray, Levine, Gallen, Schwartz et al., 1999; Shannahoff-Khalsa, 2003). As with any treatment, the relationship with the patient, the discussion and timing of the intervention, the capacity to adapt the intervention to the individual's needs, and the integration with concurrent treatments are critical for positive results.

Coherent Breathing or Resonant Breathing

A modern adaptation of the ancient practice of breathing at approximately five breaths per minute has been called coherent breathing by Stephen Elliot (Elliott & Edmonson, 2005). Breathing at approximately five to six breaths per minute, also called resonant breathing by Paul Lehrer, promotes sympathovagal balance and cardiorespiratory resonance (Song & Lehrer, 2003; Vaschillo, Vaschillo, & Lehrer, 2006). Inspiration and expiration are each approximately six seconds in duration. Qigong masters use this rate to train beginners and Zen Buddhist monks use it during deep meditation. Coherent breathing usually induces healthy alpha rhythms in the brain and optimal ventilation-perfusion ratios during rest or light activity (Elliott & Edmonson, 2005; Lehrer, Sasaki, & Saito, 1999).

In the authors' experience, coherent breathing is a safe and easily accessible method to reduce anxiety, insomnia, depression, fatigue, anger, aggression, impulsivity, inattention, and symptoms of PTSD. Patients can obtain a CD called *Respire 1* that paces respirations to five per minute using sound cues (www.coherence.com). Those who are able to learn Ujjayi breathing can be instructed to use the *Respire 1* CD with Ujjayi for even greater effects. Coherent breathing with or without Ujjayi has no adverse effects and can be used in children, geriatric patients, patients with medical illnesses, and during pregnancy and breast-feeding.

Case 1—Explosive Rage, PTSD, Insomnia

A 27-year-old construction worker, Mike had recurring problem with his wife and at work due to explosive rages, a pattern in three generations of men in his family. He was among the first rescue workers during the 9/11 World Trade Center attacks and spent many months at Ground Zero. After 9/11, he developed PTSD with increased dysphoria, distress, insomnia, and worsening rage attacks. The problems at home escalated. Trials of psychotherapy, debriefing, cognitive behavior therapy, selective serotonin reuptake inhibitors, and mood stabilizers were completely ineffective.

Mike was unwilling to participate in a yoga breath course. However, he agreed to try Ujjayi (see Sudarshan Kriya yoga below) and coherent breathing. He was instructed to start with 10 minutes b.i.d. of Ujjayi with the coherent breathing (Respire 1) CD and to gradually increase it to 20 minutes b.i.d. over the next month. He had an excellent response. At 10-month follow-up he was using Ujjayi with the CD 40 minutes twice daily. Mike reported that for the first time in his life he was able to control his temper and that he no longer had problems with anger despite the ongoing stresses at home and on the job. Although his external life circumstances were more stressful than before, he was happier than ever. By shifting into the coherent breathing with Ujjayi,

---

CLINICAL PEARL

1. Coherent breathing or resonant breathing is a safe, easy, accessible, inexpensive method for relief of anxiety, avoidance, insomnia, PTSD, anger, impulsivity, depression, and ADD.

2. It is appropriate for all patients, including children, adults, geriatric and medically ill patients, and women who are pregnant or breast-feeding.

3. Ujjayi breathing further enhances the benefits of coherent breathing.

4. In poststroke and demented geriatric patients, coherent breathing helps to reduce agitation, daytime fatigue, and insomnia.

5. In patients with Parkinson's disease, coherent breathing may reduce the frequency of "off" periods.

6. Over time, patients can learn to do coherent breathing throughout the day.

7. Coherent breathing prepares the patient to respond more rapidly and to obtain better results from biofeedback and more advanced yoga breathing.

whenever he felt stressed during the day, Mike was able to remain calm.

Case 2—Child Attention-Deficit Disorder, Anxiety, Avoidance, Insomnia

A woman with anxiety and depression and her husband, who had ADD and bipolar II disorder, sought advice regarding their 10-year-old son, Ethan. Their son was difficult to manage because of severe anxiety, insomnia, avoidance, ADD, and school problems. He had failed multiple therapies (including cognitive behavioral therapy) and reacted adversely to prescription stimulants. They could not afford biofeedback or neurotherapy treatments. The mother was instructed to do coherent breathing with her son every day. Ethan liked it so much that he began to do it on his own. After three months, the parents reported that he was doing coherent breathing for one hour at bedtime and that it enabled him to fall asleep. He learned to pace his breathing without the CD during the day whenever he felt stressed or uncomfortable. Consequently, his anxiety, avoidance, adjustment to school, and overall behavior improved. His ability to focus his attention at school and during homework increased.

Qigong

Qigong is an ancient Taoist and Chinese system of yoga used for health and longevity. Internal Qigong uses primarily concentrated attention with inhalation, exhalation, and breath holds to stimulate the circulation of blood and the vital life energy, *qi*. Basic Qigong exercises are generally done while breathing at a rate of approximately five breaths per minute, as in resonant breathing (see above). External Qigong focuses on physical movements, breathwork, and internal quiescence. It is best to learn from a qualified teacher who can ensure that the techniques are being done correctly. However, patients with social phobia or agoraphobia may not be able to attend classes. In such cases, videotapes and DVDs are available for those who are motivated to practice at home. The beginning practices are mild, nonstrenuous, and unlikely to cause harm even if not done perfectly.

Most studies of Qigong are of limited value because of methodological limitations and small sample sizes. However, the effects of Qigong on HRV were assessed in 20 healthy sedentary adults compared with 20 healthy Qigong trainees. During controlled respiration, Qigong training increased high-frequency power and decreased the low-frequency/high-frequency power ratio of HRV, indicating increased cardiac parasympathetic tone and lower SNS tone. Moreover, experienced Qigong trainees had higher HRV than age-matched sedentary controls (Lee, Huh, Kim, Ryu, Lee et al., 2002).

Sudarshan Kriya Yoga

Sri Sri Ravi Shankar created Sudarshan Kriya Yoga (SKY), a comprehensive course offered at beginner and advanced levels that includes an advanced form of Ujjayi breathing, Bhastrika, AUM chant, Sudarshan Kriya (cyclical breathing at varying rates), alternate nostril breathing, yoga postures, meditation, relaxation, psychoeducation in stress reduction, yoga philosophy, and group processes. For more detailed discussion of the neurophysiological basis and clinical applications of SKY, see articles by Brown and Gerberg (2005a, 2005b). A nonrandomized, six-week study in Sweden compared the effects of a six-day Sudarshan Kriya Yoga Course, called SK&P, in 55 adults to the effects of simple relaxation in an armchair (with the mind gently focused on breathing) in 48 yoga-naïve university students. In comparison to the control group, the SK&P group showed greater improvements on measures of anxiety, depression, and stress, as well as increased optimism. Limitations of this study were the nonrandomization and the short length of follow-up. The amount of prior yoga experience of the SK&P group was not explained, whereas the control group was described as "yoga-naïve." While these methodigical issues make interpretation of this study difficult, the test results did show significant within subject improvements in the SK&P group (Kjellgren, Bood, Axelsson, Norlander & Saatcioglu, 2007).

Ujjayi breathing creates a sound using contraction of laryngeal muscles with partial closure of the glottis, permitting fine regulation of the respiratory rate while increasing airway resistance, intrathoracic pressure, baroreceptor stimulation, HRV, RSA (Calabrese, Perrault, Dinh, Eberhard, & Benchetrit, 2000), and stimulation of somatosensory afferents in the pharynx, lungs, chest wall, and diaphragm. When done at a slow rate (2–6 breaths per minute) with expiration longer than inspiration, Ujjayi is physically and emotionally calming. Slow yoga breathing (including Ujjayi) increases RSA, HRV, PNS activity (Cappo & Holmes, 1984; Song & Lehrer, 2003), arterial baroreflex sensitivity, and oxygenation. Advanced forms of Ujjayi using breath holds further increase PNS activity (Telles & Desiraju, 1992).

Bhastrika uses rapid (30 breaths per minute) forceful breaths for short bursts (less than one minute) leading to SNS activation and CNS excitation followed by emotional calming with mental alertness. It is similar to Kapalabhati. Omkar, chanting "Om" or "AUM," may increase vagal tone and decrease SNS activation.

Sudarshan Kriya consists of sets of cyclical breathing (no pause between inhalation and exhalation) at three rates (slow, medium, and fast). The practice of SKY was found to elevate serum levels of brain-derived neurotrophic factor (BDNF), an indicator of increased neuroplasticity (Pin et al., 2006). Neuroplasticity refers to the processes by which short- and long-term changes in the brain occur, for example the configuration of synapses. In a randomized controlled trial of depressed patients, A-Min Huang and colleagues found that SKY practice increased BDNF and that the increase correlated with improvement in depression (Pan et al., in process). Complex neurophysiological effects, including increasing HRV and possibly increased electroencephalogram (EEG) coherence and synchrony, have been studied in SKY practitioners.

Sudarshan Kriya Yoga Affects EEG Coherence and Synchrony

In a pilot study of 10 SKY practitioners with different levels of experience, Stephen Larsen and colleagues (Larsen, Ye, Gerbarg, Brown, Gunkelman et al., 2006), continuously recorded electrocardiogram, HRV, EEG (19 cortical sites), and respirometry during five-minute baseline, 70 minutes of SKY, and 20 minutes of post-SKY rest.

In general, EEGs of beginners, who had completed their first SKY course one week prior to the study, showed small pockets of synchrony, but little "whole-brain synchrony" (Fehmi & McKnight, 2001). Synchrony involves the degree of similarity in the amplitude, frequency, and phase of wave forms when comparing EEG recordings over one region of the brain with recordings over another region (Robbins, 2000). Coherence analysis of the degree of synchrony is used to assess communication between distant brain regions. During rapid breath cycles, EEG disorganization increased and synchrony decreased. During rests after each set of breath cycles, synchrony increased. In practitioners who had done SKY for at least 18 months, baseline synchrony was higher and less subject to disruption during breath practice. In the most advanced subjects (four years or more), alpha bands remained stable over central and peripheral areas with very high degrees of continuous whole-brain synchrony across all 19 channels during breath practices and rest periods (see Figure 3.3). These findings are consistent with pilot studies showing increased EEG coherence with SKY (Bhatia, Kumar, Kumar, Pandey, & Kochupillai, 2003; Shnayder, Agarkova, Liouliakina, Naumova, & Shnayer, 2006).

The daily practice of SKY appears to increase coherence and high-amplitude synchrony (Larsen et al., 2006). Increases in high-amplitude gamma synchrony were observed in long-term meditating Tibetan Buddhist monks (Lutz, Greischar, Rawlings, Ricard, & Davidson, 2004), and have been associated with improved cognitive functioning (Mizuhara, Wang, Kobayashi, & Yamaguchi, 2005), memory, long-term coding of information (Guderian & Duzel, 2005), and neuroplasticity. Lazar and colleagues (2005) documented increased cortical thickening in brain regions associated with attention, interoception, and sensory processing (including the prefrontal cortex and right anterior insula) in long-term meditators compared with age-matched controls.

Dissociation, Splitting, and Long-Range Synchrony

Dissociation (as occurs in patients with PTSD) could reflect dysfunction in the processes necessary for integration of the components of emotion schemas (accumulated impressions and fragments of trauma-related experiences and relationships) with encoded information from other experiences preceding the traumas, concurrent with the traumas, and occurring after the traumas. One could view splitting (as in borderline personality disorders) as an inability to integrate positive and negative emotion schemas (internal represen-

Beginning Practitioner   Advanced Practitioner (5 years)

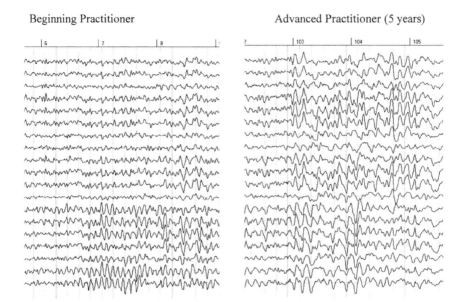

Figure 3.3 Sudarshan Kriya: Increased synchrony on EEG. After Sudarshan Kriya, high amplitude synchrony on EEG increases with length of practice. In the advanced practitioner all 19 leads show high amplitude synchronous waves. Reprinted with permission of Stephen Larsen (Larsen et al., 2006).

tations). Disturbances of long-range synchrony may also contribute to disconnection syndromes (Hummel & Gerloff, 2005). If emotional disconnection and dissociation involve analogous problems in long-range synchrony and integration, then interventions (such as yoga breathing and meditation) that enhance coherence and synchrony may be efficacious (see Case 5).

Hypothesis: Sudarshan Kriya Yoga Unlocking Trauma Configurations

We postulate that the physiological challenge of SKY temporarily disrupts established brain wave patterns and synapses in areas containing trauma-related schemas. This may occur through disentrainment of electrical activity, fluctuations in autonomic input, changes in activity within structures involved in emotional regulation, coding, and memory (limbic, thalamic, and prefrontal), shifts in pO_2 and pCO2, and neurohormonal release (oxytocin, prolactin). *Entrainment* is the process by which certain patterns of electrical activity, through repetition, become locked-in and consequently resistant to change. *Disentrainment* refers to the use of slightly higher or slightly lower frequency (compared to the entrained frequency of electrical activity) rhythmic feedback to the brain during neurotherapy to reduce the amplitude of these pathological locked-in patterns with a subsequent shift toward normalcy (Larsen, 2006; Ochs, 2006; Schoenberger, Shif, Esty, Ochs, & Matheis, 2001). SKY may unlock entrained pathological patterns and provide opportunities for new linkages and configurations to form. Under conditions of safety and relaxation, new input (experiences, concepts, emotions) with positive affective valence may gain access to previously closed areas (containing trauma schemas), promoting permanent structural change and recovery (McCormick, 2002).

Santhi Kriya Yoga

Santi Kriya Yoga includes yoga movements, a variety of yoga breath forms (pranayam), and rounds of cyclical breathing in two rhythms, one faster and one slower. While resting supine, practitioners also perform a body scan and meditate on the chakras (centers of psychic energy, part of the yogic concept of consciousness) and sensory organs. In a small study of eight subjects, 30 days of practicing Santi Kriya led to increased alpha synchrony in prefrontal and occipital areas of the cerebral cortex (Satyanarayana, Rajeswari, Rani, Krishna, & Rao, 1992). Total cortical alpha is associated with a state of relaxation, calmness, and enhanced awareness. Santhi Kriya has not been studied in patients with anxiety disorder, but it may also help shift their EEG patterns toward a state of greater relaxation.

Kundalini Versus Cognitive Behavior Therapy

Kundalini Yoga consists of different combinations of physical postures, eye postures, breath patterns, and mantras. Mental activity aims for thoughtless awareness and transcendent states to attain higher levels of spiritual energy. Most of the clinical literature on Kundalini contains anecdotal observations, with limited objective study. Nevertheless, Kundalini is a powerful, complex, multilayered system with a long history of use for healing and personal growth.

Patients who find the practices too complicated and time consuming may have difficulty with compliance. One of the practices, unilateral forced nostril breathing (UFNB), involves closing one side of the nasal passage while breathing slowly through the opposite side throughout inhalation and exhalation. It has been postulated that UFNB stimulates sympathetic dominance on the ipsilateral (same side) of the brain and body, while activating the parasympathetic system on the contralateral side (Schiff & Rump, 1995; Shannahoff-Khalsa, 2007; Werntz, Bickford, & Shannahoff-Khalsa, 1987). For a thorough discussion of Kundalini Yoga and clinical cases, see *Kundalini Yoga Meditation* by David Shannahoff-Khalsa (2006b).

A four-month randomized trial compared a stress management program for Swedish employees based on cognitive behavior therapy versus a Kundalini Yoga program (yoga postures with yoga breathing; Granath, Ingvarsson, von Thiele, & Lundberg, 2006). Both groups showed significant improvement on self-rated measures of stress, anger, exhaustion, and quality of life with medium-to-high effect sizes. No significant differences were found between the groups.

Iyengar Hatha Yoga

B. K. S. Iyengar developed a program of physical postures using props such as ropes to support various positions. Hatha Yoga includes different levels of physical postures, breathing exercises, and relaxation. While the yoga literature recommends numerous postures for relief of psychological symptoms, research evidence is very limited.

A 90-minute biweekly three-month Iyengar Hatha Yoga class was given to a group of women who perceived themselves as emotionally distressed in a nonrandomized wait-list control study (Michalsen, Grossman, Acil, Langhorst, Ludtke et al., 2005). Those who participated in the yoga intervention showed significant improvements in self-rated measures of perceived stress, anxiety, mood, and physical well-being compared to controls. Significant decreases in salivary cortisol levels (reflecting reduction in the stress response of the hypothalamic-pituitary-adrenal axis) were found in the yoga group.

Tai Chi Chuan

Tai Chi is a Chinese system of meditation and breath practice during smooth movements. It may be considered a branch of Qigong. Tai

Chi Chuan was found to reduce psychological and physical indicators of stress and anxiety in a nonrandomized comparison study of 33 experienced and 33 beginning practitioners before, during, and after the practice (Jin, 1989). Compared to baseline Profile of Mood States, ratings of tension, depression, anger, fatigue, and confusion were significantly lower during and after Tai Chi. However, state anxiety was significantly lower before than during Tai Chi [$f(1.60)$, $0 < 0.001$]. Larger trials are needed to confirm these observations.

Sahaja Yoga

Sahaja Yoga includes thoughtless awareness, self-affirmations, and breathwork. It is being studied in epileptic patients, but has not yet been studied in anxiety disorders (Panjwani, Selvamurthy, Singh, Gupta, Thakur et al., 1996; Ramaratnam & Sridharan, 2000).

Ha Breath of Hawaii

The knowledge of Ha Breath has been passed down through generations of kahunas, island priests, in Hawaii. Breath techniques with postures and arm movements include a form similar to Ujjayi called *Ou ka Leo O ka Pu,* meaning the voice of the shell sounds, the sound of a seashell held up to an ear. Ha breathing is a health practice for well-being, meditative contemplation, enlightenment, and the storing of energy (Kahn, 2004).

Mantra Repetition and Meditation

A mantra is a word or phrase with special meaning that can be repeated mentally or out loud to help focus the mind during meditative practice. An open study of a five-week program of silent mantra repetition for stress management in 30 veterans and 36 hospital employees using a telephone interview (critical incident interviewing technique) to elicit qualitative data identified 147 incidents in which participants used their mantra to manage emotions, stress, insomnia, and unwanted thoughts three to six months after course completion (Bormann, Gifford, Shirely, Smith, Redwine et al., 2006). While this study suggested that mantra repetition may provide some benefit, randomized controlled trials with objective measures are needed to clarify specific benefits.

A brief program of meditation training was studied in healthy adults interested in learning meditation stress reduction. Subjects were evaluated for effects on perceived stress and negative emotion. A single-group, open-label, pretest, posttest design was used. Out of 200 subjects, 133 (76% females) completed at least one follow-up visit and were included in data analyses. Participants were taught a simple mantra-based meditation technique in four, 1-hour small-group meetings, with instructions to practice for 15 to 20 minutes twice daily. Subjects were evaluated at baseline and monthly follow-up measures using Profile of Mood States, Perceived Stress Scale, State-Trait Anxiety Inventory (STAI), and Brief Symptom Inventory (BSI). After instruction, significant improvement was noted on all four outcome measures with reductions from baseline that ranged from 14% (STAI) to 36% (BSI). Higher baseline neuroticism scores were associated with greater improvement. Those most prone to experience negative emotions appeared to benefit the most from the intervention. Preliminary evidence suggested that brief instruction in a simple meditation technique can improve negative mood and perceived stress in healthy adults interested in learning meditation (Lane, Seskevich, & Pieper, 2007).

Buddhist Meditation

In Thai Buddhism, the emphasis is on the mindfulness of breathing as taught in the Anapanasati Sutta, part of the Tipitaka or Pali canon (250 B.C.), the compiled teachings of Buddha. According to the Tipitaka, the pursuit and development of mindfulness of in-and-out breathing leads to the culmination of the four frames of reference: focus on the body, the feelings, the mind, and mental qualities. The four frames of reference bring the seven factors for awakening (Brown & Gerbarg, 2008).

Although Tibetan Buddhism includes breath practices and movements called *trul-khor*, they have not been studied by Western researchers and are taught by only a few masters in the United States. *Trul-khor* movements and breath practices are used to stabilize the mind and clarify meditation. Exhalation with sounds of *Ha* and *Phat* are used to break through mental obstacles. Yantra, a branch of trul-khor, employs healing movements with corresponding breath practices that put the whole body into mudras (postures) to circulate and rejuvenate energy. Mudras are symbolic gestures, usually of the hands, that impart a particular quality to the practitioner. The practice of trul-khor is believed to purify karma, eliminate negativity, and engender peace.

Yoga Postures, Breathing and Meditation

A three-month study of medical students compared a program of yoga postures and breathing, prayer, visualization, and meditation with a control reading group. The yoga group had significant mean reduction on the State-Trait Anxiety Inventory the day of examinations (-34%) versus control (+3.4%; p < 0.001; Malathi & Damodaran, 1999).

A randomized controlled trial of 25 adolescents with irritable bowel syndrome assigned to either one hour of yoga instruction (yoga postures with deep breathing) followed by four weeks of daily home practice or a wait-list control found that those in the yoga group showed significantly lower scores on gastrointestinal symptoms and emotion-focused avoidance (Kuttner et al., 2006).

Musicians were offered a yoga and meditation program in a nonrandomized, self-selected study. Those who did not choose yoga served as controls. Musicians in the yoga program (n = 10) reported improvement in performance anxiety compared with control (n = 8); Khalsa & Cope, 2006).

Mindfulness Meditation and Mindfulness-Based Stress Reduction

In an open pilot study of mindfulness meditation for generalized anxiety disorder, and panic disorder 24 participants were screened using the Structured Clinical Interview for DSM-III-R, Beck Anxiety Inventory (BAI), Beck Depression Inventory, Hamilton Rating Scale for Anxiety (HAM-A), Hamilton Rating Scale for Depression (HAM-D), and ratings of panic attacks (Kabat-Zinn, Massion, Kristellar, Peterson, Fletcher et al., 1992). The intervention included an eight-week course in meditation, followed by a weekly two-hour class, daily meditation up to 45 minutes, and a 7.5-hour silent retreat two weeks before the program ended. Meditation included body scan, sitting meditation, and mindful Hatha Yoga (postures with breath control). Significant declines were found in scores on HAM-D, HAM-A, BAI, and frequency of panic attacks over the course of the intervention and at three-month follow-up. A follow-up study of 18 of the original subjects three years later showed that most subjects continued mindfulness practices and maintained improvements on HAM-A and BAI (Miller, Fletcher, & Kabat-Zinn, 1995). This study supports the short- and long-term benefits of the intervention, but requires validation by larger randomized controlled trials.

A review of controlled research (15 studies) on the effects of mindfulness-based stress reduction found the evidence for benefits in anxiety and depression to be equivocal. In studies using an active control group, mindfulness-based stress reduction showed no effect. Most studies did not report on adherence to a daily practice routine. Analysis of those studies that assessed program adherence found that the relationship between practicing mindfulness and symptom improvement was equivocal (Toneatto & Nguyen, 2007).

Transcendental Meditation

In an 18-week randomized controlled trial of 31 subjects with anxiety neurosis (*DSM-II*), Transcendental Meditation was compared to muscle biofeedback and relaxation. The three interventions were equally effective in reducing anxiety but did not alleviate insomnia. The dropout rate was 44% (Raskin, Bali & Peeke, 1980).

Open Focus Meditation

The most common habitual attentional mode in our society is narrowly focused attention. Narrowness and exclusiveness of attention require effort, tension, and orientation to task completion. Narrow focus may be directed either toward or away from an internal or an external event. You may notice as you are reading that when your attention is narrowly focused on the text, you understand and absorb the content. You can also open your focus to include passing thoughts, emotions, body sensations, sounds, sights, smells, and other perceptions. Open focus is a technique developed by Lester Fehmi, PhD, for learning how to increase the flexibility of attention, that is, the ability to shift between narrow and open focus. Open focus meditation increases awareness of the element of space within and around the body. The increased awareness of space and of perceptions leads to open focus and is associated with large-amplitude healthy alpha waves on EEG. Meditations on internal and external space are also part of advanced practices in yoga and Buddhism. Freud used the term "evenly hovering attention" to describe the ideal state of mind for a psychoanalyst to become aware and able to observe many levels of information simultaneously, including conscious, unconscious, transference, and somatic elements coming from the patient as well as those from the analyst. The authors find similarities between open focus and evenly hovering attention (Fehmi & McKnight, 2001).

Open Focus CDs and workshops for stress and pain reduction are available at www.openfocus.com. Over time, the practice of open focus for 20 to 30 minutes twice a day may increase flexibility of attention. This requires the patient to be persistent and compliant with daily practice. It may also be beneficial for pain relief.

MIND–BODY TECHNIQUES IN CLINICAL PRACTICE

For patients with anxiety disorders, it is best to begin with a discussion of the basic concepts regarding how imbalances in the stress response systems underlie anxiety symptoms and the ways that mind–body practices may correct these imbalances. Once patients understand the connection between, for example, breath patterns and anxiety regulation, they are more likely to comply with a recommendation for daily breath practices.

Simple, Safe, Effective Breath Practices

One of the simplest effective introductory practices is coherent breathing (see above). It is easy for patients to purchase the Respire 1 CD (www.coherence.com), follow the paced breathing at five breaths per minute, and experience gentle relaxation with no adverse effects. Prescribe 10 or 20 minutes twice a day plus additional practice if needed.

For stronger effects, the patient will need to learn Ujjayi breathing or alternate nostril breathing. In most cases, this will induce a calm, relaxed state of mind and body in 5 to 10 minutes. The authors find that combining Ujjayi with the Respire 1 CD to pace respirations increases the benefits. Health care practitioners should learn coherent breathing before prescribing it. One very effective method is to observe areas of tension in the face, neck, shoulders, and chest while instructing the patient to gently relax and breathe without straining.

Ujjayi Breathing for Anxiety

In clinical practice, the authors find that basic Ujjayi breathing is the single most rapidly effective breath intervention for anxiety symptoms in patients diagnosed with anxiety disorders. It is preferable for the therapist to teach Ujjayi or alternate nostril breathing during the session. Patients will immediately experience a calmer, clearer state of mind, enhancing their motivation to continue. It usually takes about 20 minutes to teach this technique and requires one or two follow-up visits to correct and refine the practice. Certain patients, particularly some who are elderly, those who have difficulty following instructions, and those with significant nasal obstruction may not be successful. This technique can be learned in yoga courses taught by the Art of Living Foundation and other organizations. However, if a patient is unable to comply or not suitable for such courses, it can be taught individually by a yoga instructor or health practitioner who has been well trained in this technique. The patient who is taught Ujjayi breathing will usually experience a profound sense of physical and mental calmness within five to 10 minutes of doing this technique. The following cases illustrate the use of Ujjayi breathing as an adjunctive treatment for anxiety disorders. After the patient has established a daily practice for several weeks and continued to see benefits, referral for the complete Sudarshan Kriya Yoga course may be indicated if the patient is able to tolerate the group setting. Patients with significant dissociative symptoms, borderline personality, bipolar disorder, psychotic disorders, seizures, or pregnancy may not be suitable for group classes.

Case 3—College Student Stress

Ed was a popular football player and a good student in high school. During his first semester at college, he felt overwhelmed by the workload and missed the support of the close friends he had known for years in his hometown. His anxiety interfered with his concentration, making it harder for him to study. When he used alcohol to calm himself down, he became more depressed. One night he became so intoxicated that his friends had to take him to an emergency room. He was sent home without completing the semester. Once home, Ed suffered from anxiety, insecurity, shame, and feelings of failure. In weekly psychotherapy he began to understand why he was feeling so pressured and worked on self-acceptance. Although he made progress in recovering his self-esteem, Ed was still having significant anxiety. His psychologist referred him for a medication consultation. Ed was reluctant to start medication, which he saw as a last resort. He was offered the alternative of trying to use Ujjayi breathing first. Ed learned Ujjayi quickly and felt relief within a few minutes. He liked the way it relaxed his body and quieted his worried thoughts. Doing Ujjayi gave him a sense that he could actively control his anxiety, a more positive image than seeing himself as dependent on medication. He was highly motivated and used the Ujjayi breathing 10 minutes twice a day plus more as needed for anxiety. Ed's anxiety improved without medication. He returned to school and completed the next semester.

Case 4—Generalized Anxiety Disorder and Insomnia

April was always a worrier, overly conscientious, trying to make everything perfect. After three years of psychotherapy, her anxiety was under reasonable control. However, when her teenage daughter developed diabetes, she became severely anxious about her daughter's condition. Every time the phone rang, she jumped with fear that her daughter was in crisis. She worried constantly, could not sleep, and finally returned to treatment. April was given Buspar 10 mg t.i.d., which helped reduce the anxiety, but she was still symptomatic. Because she had not tolerated SSRIs in the past, she was taught Ujjayi breathing. On the first follow-up visit, it became evident that she was doing the yoga breathing too forcefully, tensing up her body instead of relaxing. This was corrected with instructions to breathe slowly without straining and to relax her shoulders. The following week she reported significant relief from anxiety and worry. It became easier for her to make progress in her psychotherapy without the interference of the extreme anxiety. She was able to use Ujjayi to stop the obsessive nighttime worrying that had been keeping her awake. With better sleep, she felt more energetic and resilient.

Alternate Nostril Breathing

Alternate nostril breathing is used in many yoga traditions. It is easy to learn and generally has a calming effect within 10 minutes. With the eyes closed, the second and third fingers rest on the bridge of the nose for support. The remaining fingers are used to gently press the side of the nose, alternately closing one nostril or the other. The practitioner exhales slowly and then inhales slowly through the open nostril, switching sides after each complete breath cycle. The authors usually recommend 10 to 20 minutes of alternate nostril breathing twice a day plus as needed for anxiety. Five to 10 minutes of the technique prior to meditation enhances meditative or prayer practices. Using a certain number of counts for each breath phase produces different effects. For example, most beginners find that slowly counting to six during expiration and four during inspiration is comfortable and beneficial.

POST-TRAUMATIC STRESS DISORDER

Mind–body practices can be highly effective in reducing symptoms of PTSD in military personnel, survivors of war and other mass disasters, and victims of abuse. These practices can be used to develop greater stress resilience.

Veterans, Military Personnel, and Civilian Survivors of War

Military deployment and exposure to combat entail increased risks for mental health problems, including depression, PTSD, substance abuse, impaired social functioning, and difficulty reintegrating after returning home. Studies suggest that as many as one fourth of the service members returning from Afghanistan, Operation Enduring Freedom, and Operation Iraqi Freedom are experiencing some level of psychological injury, which may or may not yet be visible (Mood,

2007). Lessons from previous wars, such as World Wars I and II, the Korean War, the Vietnam War, Bosnia, and Desert Storm, indicate that when left untreated, these injuries can stretch into long-term disability. Many veterans who have received standard treatments, including medication, individual and group therapy, cognitive behavior therapy, and others, are left with symptoms of chronic PTSD.

War zone stresses include feeling helpless to prevent potentially lethal events; witnessing friends killed or injured; killing enemy combatants and innocent bystanders, including women and children; unpredictable life-threatening attacks, including improvised explosive devices, ambushes, and suicide bombers; handling the remains of U.S. personnel, civilians, or soldiers; exposure to dying men and women; and observing communities devastated by combat. Such combat experiences can lead to severe symptoms of PTSD with secondary substance abuse, family discord, loss of belief in values, and an altered sense of identity. Many individuals, including medical staff returning from combat zones, do not seek care because of shame or fear that disclosure would adversely affect their military careers (Hoge, Auchterlonie, & Milliken, 2006). In order to destigmatize these conditions and to include nonmilitary personnel involved in combat operations, the term *combat-operational stress injury* has been proposed (Figley & Nash, 2007).

Complementary and alternative treatments can be of benefit to veterans and military personnel. Such approaches may be more acceptable to veterans because they do not involve formal psychiatric diagnoses and are not associated with psychiatric treatments. Mind–body practices can relieve symptoms of depression, anxiety, and PTSD. Multimodal programs that include yoga postures, breath practices, relaxation techniques, group processes, and psychoeducation on stress reduction are particularly beneficial.

In severe anxiety disorders and PTSD, slow, deep, or abdominal breathing is usually insufficient, as the following study illustrates. A randomized controlled trial comparing relaxation (simple instructions to relax in a reclining chair), relaxation with deep breathing (gradual filling of the lungs and slow complete exhalation), and relaxation with deep breathing and thermal biofeedback in 90 Vietnam veterans with PTSD found all interventions to be mildly therapeutic. Addition of deep breathing and thermal biofeedback did not produce further improvements on PTSD scales (Watson, Tuorila, Vickers, Gearhart, & Mendez, 1997). More intensive yoga breathing using advanced techniques is necessary to ameliorate anxiety and PTSD.

In an open trial, 139 war-traumatized high school students in Kosovo were given an eight-week mind–body skills program including meditation, biofeedback, movement, guided imagery, breathing techniques, autogenic training, drawing, family genograms, psychoeducation about stress, and group discussions of their experiences (Gordon, Staples, Blyta, & Bytyqi, 2004). Scores on an Albanian version of the PTSD Reaction Index (16 dichotomous questions derived from *DSM-III*) (Pynoos, Frederick, Nader, Arroyo, Steinberg et al., 1987). were significantly reduced after the mind–body skill program and remained reduced at 9- and 15-month follow-up. This study lacked a control and had other methodological limitations. It is difficult to evaluate which of the many components were essential for the therapeutic effect. Nevertheless, it suggests that a multimodal program of mind–body practices may reduce symptoms of PTSD.

The Australian government provides extensive services and psychological support for veterans, many of whom served as advance scouts and survived heavy combat. Thirty-five years later, many Australian Vietnam veterans remain permanently disabled due to chronic PTSD complicated by substance abuse or medical problems.

A six-week Iyengar Yoga program was given to disabled Australian veterans of the Vietnam War with PTSD in four small open studies. Although the Iyengar Yoga postures improved symptoms of depression, the addition of yoga breathing (particularly Ujjayi) and Ham Su meditation significantly reduced symptoms of PTSD, including anxiety, insomnia, flashbacks, and anger outbursts (Carter & Byrne, 2004).

In a rater-blind, randomized, wait-list controlled study of 25 disabled Australian Vietnam veterans with PTSD, those given a five-day course in Sudarshan Kriya Yoga showed significantly greater reductions on the Clinician Administered PTSD Scale (CAPS) than those in the wait-list group (Carter, Byrne, Brown, Gerbarg, & Ware, in process). There was statistically significant improvement in scores on the CAPS ($p = 0.007$) in both the test group and in the wait-list control group following the SKY intervention. Statistically significant improvements in alcohol consumption and subscales of depression

(MINI-Plus) occurred in both groups following the yoga course. At six-month follow-up, average CAPS scores were about 30 points lower than at baseline. The veterans also learned how to use the yoga breathing to calm down when they awoke at night or when they felt road rage.

Survivors of Mass Disasters

In conditions of mass disaster, the physical needs of survivors for food, water, shelter, and medical care must be met first. However, the psychological needs must also be addressed to relieve immediate suffering and to prevent long-term sequelae such as chronic PTSD with severe psychological distress and impairment in interpersonal relationships and employment. Further research is needed to explore the potential benefits of mind–body practices, which can provide a relatively low-cost, low-risk means to relieve PTSD in large populations affected by mass disasters in situations where health care systems may be overwhelmed and ineffective.

McCormick (2002) described benefits of a yoga program for relief of symptoms of PTSD in children and adults following the September 11 attacks on the New York World Trade Center. The program included self-observation, group sharing and discussions of PTSD experiences, breathwork, guided meditation, body scan with relaxation, yoga stretches, and awareness of emotions. Although formal testing was not done, participants reported feeling in better control with more resilience after the yoga program. Children became more spontaneous in creative expression and physical movement activities.

Breath Water Sound (BWS) is an eight-hour course that includes Ujjayi breathing, Bhastrika, AUM chant, psychoeducation in stress reduction, and positive philosophy with group processes. Sometimes 10 minutes of Sudarshan Kriya (cyclical breathing) or alternate nostril breathing are added to the program. It is usually given free of charge by the International Association for Human Values for the psychological relief of large populations in the aftermath of mass disasters such as floods, hurricanes, earthquakes, war, and terrorist attacks (Gerbarg & Brown, 2005b).

In a wait-list comparison controlled study of 180 survivors of the 2004 Southeast Asian tsunami who were living in refugee camps in Nagapattinam district on the southern coast of India eight months after the disaster, participants were screened for PTSD using the Post-traumatic Stress Disorder Check-List (PCL-17; Descilo, Vedamurthachar, Gerbarg, Nagaraja, Gangadhar et al., 2006, 2007). Out of 240 refugees who were screened, 183 (70%) scored above 50 and were included in the study. Five camps were assigned to three groups. The first group was given a 10-hour course in BWS with 10 minutes of Sudarshan Kriya over a period of four days. The second group received the same intervention followed one week later by a one-on-one client-centered exposure treatment called Traumatic Incident Reduction (TIR). The third group served as a six-week wait-list control. All participants were given the PCL-17, the Beck Depression Inventory (BDI-22), and the Quality of Life (GHQ-12) at baseline, immediately after each intervention, at six weeks, three months, and six months. Mean scores on all measures improved significantly immediately after the four-day BWS intervention, and the improvements were maintained with additional modest gains at six-week, three-month, and six-month follow-ups. The control group showed no improvement at six weeks. At six-week follow-up, mean PCL-17 scores dropped 42.52, 39.22, and 4.61 points in the BWS, BWS + TIR and control groups, respectively. The addition of TIR did not lead to any measurable improvements in test scores, possibly due to a floor effect, the BWS having decreased the PCL-17 scores (PTSD symptomatology) below the threshold usually used to determine eligibility for TIR. However, transcripts of the TIR sessions yield qualitative evidence of benefits such as feeling freer, lighter, better about oneself, less preoccupied with memories and images of the disaster, greater acceptance, and diminished reactivity to memories and reminders. This study found BWS and BWS + TIR to be very effective in reducing symptoms of PTSD as reflected in a large effect size of 10.8 (baseline to 24 weeks) on the PCL-17.

Victims of Emotional, Physical, and Sexual Abuse

Patients with PTSD due to sexual abuse benefited when SKY breathing was combined with traditional psychiatric and psychological therapies (Sageman, 2002, 2004; Sageman & Brown, 2006a, 2006b). Yoga breathing reduces arousal, anxiety, and overreactivity, enabling the patient to recall and discuss traumatic material without feeling overwhelmed. Other beneficial components of the SKY

CLINICAL PEARL

In cases of adult-onset PTSD secondary to recent trauma in previously healthy individuals, Ujjayi breathing and brief psychotherapy may be all that is needed. However, in cases involving more severe prolonged trauma or a history of significant childhood abuse, more intense yoga breathing may be necessary in conjunction with more intensive psychotherapy and medication.

course include psychoeducation in human values of acceptance, social responsibility, and community service.

In a four-day randomized controlled trial, 40 women who had been abused by an intimate partner were randomly assigned to tell about the abuse (two 45-minute sessions of testimony with a trained listener over two consecutive days), participate in yoga breathing (two 45-minute sessions of yoga breathing including slow deep breathing with some breath holds, sound, and yoga postures), a combined testimony and yoga breathing intervention (45-minute testimony immediately followed by 45 minutes of yoga breathing), or serve as wait-list controls (Franzblau, Smith, Echevarria, & Van Cantford, 2006). Those who received both testimony and yoga breathing showed the greatest improvement on scores for self-efficacy on the Franzblau Self Efficacy Scale (FSES) 20, particularly in feelings of control, security, and confidence. This study is limited by small sample size, brief duration, and the use of only one measure, the FSES 20. Nevertheless, it highlights the potential for developing integrative treatments for psychological trauma.

Case 5—PTSD and Temporomandibular Joint Pain Due to Childhood Sexual Abuse: Somatic and Interoceptive Components

Disturbing somatic sensations, particularly interoceptive, are characteristic of PTSD. The PNS carries sensory information about the internal state of the body (visceral sensations, heat and cold, vibration, and pain) to the insula, an anatomic structure in the frontal lobe postulated to contain representations of the body and metarepresentations of the self (Craig, 2003; Critchley, 2005). The insula receives moment-to-moment information about the state of the throat, pharynx, jaw, lungs, and respiratory apparatus. Processing of somatic experiences associated with abuse would occur in the insula. Voluntary manipulation of breath using yoga techniques changes the input to the insula and may profoundly affect interoception-based perceptions of the body and their associations to emotion schemas.

Tammy was hospitalized at the age of 16 following a suicide attempt. After discharge she was treated with a mood stabilizer, an antidepressant, and a low-dose atypical antipsychotic for transient delusions. Her history included multigenerational sexual abuse, which was verified by her older aunts. She recalled that from age six to ten she was forced her to perform oral sex for her uncle. During five years of weekly psychotherapy, she became increasingly stable, maintained full-time employment, gained self-confidence, and married a man who had three young children she loved. However, she continued to complain of stress, tension, and severe temporomandibular joint pain (TMJ), which was unresponsive to all treatments short of surgery. The pain was so severe that simply walking would set it off.

The possible relationship between childhood sexual abuse and the TMJ pain was never overtly discussed in the treatment because the therapist felt that until the patient was closer to making this connection herself, such an interpretation would not be effective. One risk of a premature interpretation was that it might go no deeper than an intellectual acknowledgment. At worst, it could leave the patient feeling alienated, invalidated, or criticized, as though the therapist was telling her that the pain was not real, that it was "all in her mind."

Tammy was offered the Sudarshan Kriya Yoga (SKY) course as an adjunctive treatment to help reduce stress and tension. During the long Sudarshan Kriya she experienced relief from TMJ pain, but had no conscious reexperience of past trauma. As soon as she got home, she gathered the children and took them outside to run and play. For the first time in years she was able to run without pain. She reported that on the days when she did her home SKY practice, she had no TMJ pain, whereas on the days when she skipped the practice, some mild TMJ pain would recur.

In this case, the pain and tension in the patient's jaw was a psychosomatic link to sexual abuse. Yoga breathing broke the link between the somatic symptom and the trauma without retraumatization, through processes that bypassed conscious recall of the past experiences.

Additional components in the relief of TMJ pain may have been related to the general effects on muscle relaxation or via the vagal afferent modulation of nocioceptive (noxious or painful stimuli) transmission. Sensory nerves that discriminate noxious stimuli are termed nociceptors. Viscerosensory and somatosensory signals from pharynx, larynx, face, mouth, jaw, and TMJ overlap in the paratrigeminal nucleus, which has connections with autonomic centers in the brainstem (Saxon & Hopkins, 2006). Autonomic input may have a pain-modulating effect in the processing of craniofacial pain (Bereiter, Bereiter, & Ramos, 2002).

The authors have treated numerous cases in which yoga breathing permanently and therapeutically altered the way patients experienced the part of their body that was most bound up with their traumatic experiences (Gerbarg, 2007).

PHOBIAS AND MIND–BODY PRACTICES

Although there are no controlled studies of mind–body practices for specific phobias, case reports and clinical experience indicate potential benefits.

Case 6—Germ Phobia and Agoraphobia

Stuart had been a sickly baby, whose mother was so afraid of losing him that she drilled into him the importance of cleanliness and the fear of germs. Stuart's older brother enjoyed scaring him by pretending there were deadly germs everywhere, on a piece of cake, a baseball, the TV channel controller—on anything his brother wanted to take from him. When Stuart grew up, he realized his brother's deceptions, but the damage had already been done and he could not control his fear reactions. He had to force himself to go out among people and would return home in a state of panic. He could not drink anything but boiled, filtered water in a cellophane-wrapped paper cup, and each time he ate, his stomach knotted up with fear that he was consuming lethal bacteria. As the years passed, his symptoms worsened. After a bout of the flu, Stuart found it impossible to leave his house.

Stuart knew intellectually that his obsessive fears were ruining his life. Afraid to go out for help, he began therapy via telephone. His therapist advised medication but Stuart was afraid that the pills contained germs, so he refused to take them. Although eventually he was able to go to his therapist's office, psychotherapy did not significantly relieve his problems. Next, his therapist encouraged him to take the SKY course, but the thought of being in a room full of people and germs triggered a panic attack. Since Stuart was incapable of attending a regular yoga class, his therapist taught him Ujjayi breathing in the office. Doing the breathing every day reduced his anxiety. Finally, he was able to attend a SKY course by sitting in a remote corner away from other people's germs. The daily SKY practice reduced his anxiety enough for him to expand his range of activities. Whenever he started to feel anxious, Ujjayi breathing for 5 to 10 minutes would restore his sense of calm. Having a tool to relieve anxiety enables phobic patients to gain a sense of control needed to overcome avoidance behaviors.

Case 7—Social Phobia

Tom was a successful accountant who had suffered all his life from low self-esteem, insecurity, and social phobia (fear of talking to people in social situations). As a child, he did not know how to behave in social situations and was generally shunned or ridiculed by other kids. His adult relationships with women were marked by mutual emotional abuse. He entered therapy when violence erupted with his girlfriend. Medication, including mirtazapine (Remeron), oxcarbazepine (Trileptol), and mixed amphetamine salts (Adderall), combined with intense psychotherapy, stabilized his mood, improved his attention, and enabled him to end a destructive relationship. After four years of therapy, Tom found a new girlfriend and formed a more caring, healthy relationship. However, when he encountered people in social situations, he would become speechless and embarrassed, withdraw into a quiet corner, and just wait to go home.

When Tom attended a SKY course, the caring environment and small group discussions put him more at ease. He began opening up to other group members. During Sudarshan Kriya breathing he experienced warm feelings in his heart. He felt more deeply connected with other people. Tom repeated the course and each time he was able to talk more freely. Although he continued to dislike large crowds, he became able to carry on conversations at social events and to actively enjoy small dinner parties. Tom continued to progress in therapy, further helped by advanced courses in yoga breathing and meditation.

OBSESSIVE-COMPULSIVE DISORDER

Several scientific studies, particularly of Kundalini Yoga, have found yoga practices to be beneficial in obsessive-compulsive disorder (OCD). There are no formal studies of SKY for OCD. Our clinical experience and that of our colleagues suggests that yoga breathing is a promising adjunctive treatment for OCD.

In a 12-month study, 22 patients with OCD were randomized into two groups. The first group (n = 12) received Kundalini Yoga (eight practices including slow, 1 bpm, left-nostril breathing with breath holds, mantra meditation, and yoga postures). The comparison control group (n = 10) was given relaxation and mindfulness meditation. The Kundalini Yoga group showed significant mean reduction (-38.4%) on the Yale-Brown Obsessive-Compulsive Scale (Y-BOCS) versus the control group (-13.9%). No adverse events were reported (Shannahoff-

Khalsa, Ray, Levine, Gelloen, Schwartz et al., 1999). Subsequently, both groups merged for an additional year of the Kundalini program. After 12 months, the 11 completers had a mean improvement of 70.1% on Y-BOCS compared to baseline (Shannahoff-Khalsa, 2003).

SLEEP DISORDERS

Pharmacotherapy for insomnia in geriatric populations is associated with problematic side effects including confusion, motor incoordination, intellectual and memory impairment, syncope, increased risk of falls and fractures, daytime sleepiness, and dysphoria. Mind–body techniques may be particularly helpful in that they are safer in the elderly population. In a randomized controlled trial, 118 men and women between the ages of 60 and 92 were assigned to either Tai Chi or low-impact exercise 60 minutes, three times a week for 24 weeks (Li, Fisher, Harmer, Irbe, Tearse et al., 2004). Those in the Tai Chi group showed significant improvements in sleep quality, sleep-onset latency, sleep duration, sleep efficiency, and sleep disturbances compared to the exercise control group on self-rated measures (Pittsburgh Sleep Quality Index). In the Tai Chi participants, sleep-onset latency decreased about 18 minutes per night and sleep duration increased about 48 minutes per night. While these results support the benefits of a thrice weekly Tai Chi program for improving sleep, self-ratings of sleep are subject to recall bias.

In a randomized controlled trial, 69 residents in a home for the elderly (over the age of 60) were randomly assigned to three groups: a six-week yoga program (postures, relaxation, breath practice, and lectures on yoga philosophy); an herbal Ayurveda preparation, Rasayana Kalpa (composed of *Withania somnifera* root 2 g, *Emblica officianalis* 1 g, *Sida cordifolia* 0.25 g, and *Piper longum* 0.5 g); or a wait-list control (no intervention; Manjunath & Telles, 2005). On a self-rating sleep questionnaire, the yoga group showed significant decrease in the time to fall asleep (average decrease of 10 minutes, $p < 0.05$), increase in the number of hours slept (average increase 60 minutes, $p < 0.05$), and improved feelings of being rested ($p < 0.05$) compared to no change in the Ayurveda or wait-list control groups. Findings from subjective self-assessments suggest that yoga programs may be safe and effective for sleep disorders in the elderly.

PRECAUTIONS AND CONTRAINDICATIONS FOR MIND-BODY PRACTICES: HOW TO MINIMIZE RISKS AND MAXIMIZE BENEFITS

Most people are able to experience yoga breathing courses without difficulty. However, clinicians should be aware of the following precautions and contraindications.

Pregnancy

Pregnant women should not do rapid, forceful breath practices or breath holds, as are used in Qigong, Kundalini, Kapalabhati, Bhastrika, and Sudarshan Kriya yoga. They may do gentle Ujjayi breathing with no straining, alternate nostril breathing, coherent or resonant breathing, and meditation.

Medical Conditions

Patients with uncontrolled hypertension, migraine headaches, severe chronic obstructive pulmonary disease (COPD), acute asthma symptoms, recent injuries of the neck, shoulders, or chest, or recent myocardial infarction should not do breath holds, Bhastrika, or any rapid or forceful yoga breathing. Gentle basic Ujjayi (without breath holds), alternate nostril breathing, coherent breathing, and meditation are safe and soothing. Although patients with mild COPD or mild asthma may have some initial symptom exacerbation, they often benefit from yoga breathing in the long run with increased respiratory capacity. Yoga breathing should not be done during acute asthma attacks. Collaboration among the health care providers, the yoga teacher, and the patient may be necessary to guide the patient more gradually through practices depending on their tolerance level in order to obtain long-term benefits. The use of yoga postures and meditation to reduce anxiety can also be beneficial.

Seizure Disorders

Yoga breathing is generally contraindicated in seizure disorders. Specific yoga postures, meditation, and breath forms have been used to treat patients with seizure disorders, but there is insufficient data to recommend such practices at this time.

Bipolar Disorders

Bipolar patients may be triggered to become manic, particularly from Bhastrika, Kapalabhati, Kundalini, or rapid cycle breathing. In general, bipolar I patients should not undertake training in yoga breathing. Even slow Ujjayi or alternate nostril breathing can induce mania and therefore must be done cautiously in bipolar I patients. Bipolar II patients whose mood swings are under good control on medication may do yoga breathing under supervision if they avoid Bhastrika and rapid cycle breath forms. However, if they become agitated or anxious, the yoga breathing should be discontinued. Bipolar II patients who have developed a strong therapeutic alliance and who have consistently relinquished the excitement of mania can take responsibility for monitoring their own level of agitation during yoga breathing practices. They can learn to slow down their breath rate whenever they notice themselves becoming agitated. Working closely with such patients, clinicians who are knowledgeable about yoga breathing effects can enable their bipolar II patients to benefit from yoga breathing while minimizing the risks.

Yoga breathing can increase excretion of lithium, causing a drop in serum lithium levels. Bipolar patients being treated on lithium alone should not undertake yoga breath training. Patients on lithium in combination with other mood stabilizers who begin yoga practices should have lithium levels monitored and adjusted if necessary.

Severe Character Disorders, Such as Borderline Personality

Severely character disordered patients may not be suitable for the group setting, particularly if there is a history of self-injury, suicide attempts, or manipulative behavior. Such patients should be in a stable, ongoing psychotherapy program before undertaking yoga training. Individual instruction in calming practices such as gentle yoga postures, coherent breathing, Ujjayi, or alternate nostril breathing may be helpful.

Psychosis

Psychosis is a general contraindication for yoga breathing. Psychotic patients may overuse rapid breath techniques to induce altered states of consciousness. Some schizophrenic patients benefit from gentle basic Ujjayi, alternate nostril breathing, and gentle yoga postures (see Chapter 7).

Anxiety Disorders

Patients with anxiety disorders, particularly those who tend to hyperventilate and have panic attacks, need preparation before taking a yoga breathing course. When they begin to do rapid breathing, if they start to worry about having a panic attack, their own worry may bring one on. The clinician should explain the purpose of the course and review the activities that will be encountered. It is extremely helpful to explain to patients that they will be learning fast and slow breath techniques and that if at any time during the fast breathing they begin to feel anxious, they can simply slow the respirations down to a medium or even a slow rate. It is not necessary to do all of the rapid breathing in order to benefit from the training. If they begin to experience lightheadedness, paresthesias (tingling sensations), or cramping in their hands or feet, they should exhale less forcefully to avoid blowing off too much carbon dioxide. Breathing more gently will relieve the uncomfortable sensations. Careful preparation will enable patients to avoid triggering a panic attack and to obtain a sense of control. Over time they will become able to tolerate more. Patients should be assured that they will be taught controlled breath techniques which are different from uncontrolled hyperventilation and that the breath training will help to reduce their anxiety. Voluntary hyperventilation has been used for desensitization in patients with panic attacks (Meuret, Ritz, Wilhelm, & Roth, 2005).

Post-Traumatic Stress Disorder

Individuals with PTSD primarily due to recent trauma or trauma during adulthood (e.g., accidents, illness, war, or natural disasters) usually do well with SKY. Patients with chronic PTSD from childhood abuse can benefit from SKY if they do not have significant dissociative symptoms. The therapist should contact the teacher, prepare the patient, and help process trauma-related material that may emerge.

Patients with the more severe forms of PTSD may be fearful, mistrustful, overreactive, and prone to reexperiencing trauma memories and flashbacks. Mind–body practices that include intense or rapid yoga breathing, such as Qigong, SKY, or Kundalini, can be beneficial, but they may occasionally trigger reexperiencing, retraumatization, or regression. In order to minimize the risk of adverse reactions while gaining the maximum benefits, the following steps are recommended.

1. Carefully assess the patient's flashbacks, dissociative episodes, and capacity to maintain a sense of reality. If the patient tends to get lost in severe flashbacks that last more than 20 minutes, is unable to come out of the flashbacks, or acts out violently during flashbacks, it may not be safe for the patient to take a group course. If dissociative episodes are prolonged or involve uncontrolled switching into alters as in dissociative identity disorder, the patient should not do intense yoga breathing because it can lower the threshold to enter altered states of consciousness.

2. Carefully assess potential for self-injury or suicide attempts. If there is significant risk of harm, then the patient should be given individual instruction in calming practices such as coherent breathing, Ujjayi, or alternate nostril breathing while undergoing further psychotherapy until the patient is more stable and at less risk. Gentle breathwork is likely to reduce anxiety and overreactivity while enhancing progress in psychotherapy.

3. The patient should have an established mental health treatment relationship. The primary therapist should be involved in the decision to start the mind–body practice, to monitor the patient during and after the practice, and to be available to discuss whatever the patient may experience, including the emergence of trauma-related memories and somatic experiences. In most cases, reexperiencing during SKY is not traumatic and can lead to more rapid therapeutic resolution. However, a backup plan should be in place to handle adverse reactions that may occasionally occur. In some cases, it is helpful to establish a means of communication between the mental health provider and the yoga instructor.

4. The patient should be given extra preparation before taking mind–body courses. Since PTSD patients tend to fear the unknown and to react badly to the unexpected, they do better with a clear explanation of what will occur during the course.

5. Patients who show severe autonomic instability or intense over-reactivity, for example some veterans of war, may need to do one to three months of coherent breathing with Ujjayi 10 to 20 minutes twice daily and possibly 20 minutes of alternate nostril breathing per day to strengthen the parasympathetic nervous system and reduce the risk of overwhelming reactions before undertaking the SKY course.

HOW YOGA CAN FACILITATE PSYCHOTHERAPY AND PSYCHOANALYSIS

Sigmund Freud (1930) was interested in the effects of yoga on states of consciousness and body awareness. In *Civilization and Its Discontents* he wrote, "It is very difficult for me to work with these almost intangible qualities. Another friend of mine . . . has assured me that through the practices of yoga, by withdrawing from the world, by fixing the attention on bodily functions and by peculiar methods of breathing, one can in fact evoke new sensations. . . . He sees in them a physiological basis, as it were, of much of the wisdom of mysticism." (pp. 72–73).

Mind–body practices can facilitate psychotherapy and psychoanalysis in several ways. When patients acquire tools for reducing anxiety, they are better able to tolerate the painful memories and emotions that arise during therapy sessions as well as in their outside daily life. Yoga philosophy and techniques are compatible with most psychotherapeutic approaches in that they teach nonjudgmental awareness and dispassionate observation of thoughts, feelings, and sensations. Patients learn how to observe themselves, how to direct their attention, and how to shift between experiencing emotions and observing from a safe distance. In cases where intensive psychotherapy or psychoanalysis have achieved only partial improvements with persistent blockage from traumatic material, emotional numbing, or isolation of affect, yoga can sometimes move the treatment forward.

Most psychotherapies rely primarily on verbal communication. However, verbal approaches often fail to access trauma-related material that has not been verbally encoded and that may not be represented symbolically. According to multiple-coding theory, nonverbal, subsymbolic elements, actions, and sensory and visceral reactions form the *affective core* of emotion schemas (Bucci, Possidente, & Talbot, 2003; Bucci, 2001). In patients with a history of neglect or trauma, pathogenic schemas with defensive dissociation are blocked from linkage to verbal coding. Such formations can be highly resistant to change. The reconstruction of emotion schemas requires access and processing of subsymbolic bodily and sensory components as well as the revision of distorted elements and affective links (Bucci et al., 2003). Psychotherapy and psychoanalysis seek to activate these schemas by free association, interpretation, transference, dream analysis, and other means.

Where traditional psychotherapeutic techniques fail to penetrate defenses surrounding trauma-related emotional schemas, messages from the autonomic interoceptive system generated by mind–body practices may succeed. Yoga developed over 8,000 years, using the

---

CLINICAL PEARL

Yoga can enhance psycotherapy and psychoanalysis:

1. Increases capacity to tolerate intense affects

2. Reduces the need to avoid emotions through repression, supression, denial, numbing , and dissociation

2. Reduces anxiety, overreactivity, and sleep difficulties

3. Brings unconscious content from trauma-related emotion schemas into consciousness

4. Improves cognitive-emotional integration

5. Reduces trauma-related somatic experiences including visceral, sensory, and painful sensations

6. Enables the patient to acquire a sense of mastery and competence rather than feeling helpless or passive

7. May help overcome a therapeutic impasse

8. Strengthens the therapeutic alliance through patient empowerment and collaboration

body's natural interoceptive system of communication between peripheral and central neural networks. This visceral internet can be carefully used to access unconscious material linked to emotional and somatic components of trauma-based schemas. As an adjunct to psychotherapy, SKY and other mind–body practices can help relieve symptoms of PTSD (Gerbarg, 2007).

Introducing mind–body techniques may also strengthen the therapeutic alliance. When the therapist encourages the patient to engage in mind–body practices, the patient is being supported to learn how to master anxiety through self-soothing. This empowers the patient toward less dependence on the therapist or medication. The patient may experience this support toward mastery and independence as caring. As the patient engages in yoga practices, greater awareness, access to memories, and new insights may emerge. The therapist has an opportunity to value this material as it is delivered into the therapy sessions, validating the patient in an active and collaborative, rather than a passive or inferior role.

How and When to Introduce Yoga as a Complementary Treatment

Factors to consider in suggesting yoga during therapy include the following:

1. The potential risks and benefits as described above
2. The patient's readiness to engage in a regular mind–body practice
3. The therapist's knowledge of available yoga programs
4. The quality of local yoga instructors
5. The target symptoms identified for the intervention: mood, energy, anxiety, insomnia, overreactivity, mental focus, pain, or other symptoms
6. The mind–body programs that may facilitate the patient's growth in psychotherapy (see Clinical Pearl above)
7. The therapist should be prepared for sudden breakthroughs and new insights

The quality of instructors teaching mind–body practices varies greatly. It is incumbent upon the health care practitioner to obtain information about the yoga teacher before referring patients. While certification by an established training program may indicate technical proficiency, it does not assure that a teacher will interact appropriately with your patients. If the teacher is overly zealous, excessively authoritarian, rigid, emotionally abusive, critical, insensitive, known to engage in boundary violations, or unresponsive to the needs and limitations of clients, then the referral may have a negative impact. A teacher who is supportive, appropriate, receptive to professional input, and able to give feedback can contribute significantly to the health and well-being of patients.

Clinicians who study mind–body practices, particularly by taking classes themselves, are best equipped to make appropriate referrals, prepare patients, and help patients overcome obstacles to maintaining regular practice over time. While most patients benefit from taking a multimodal yoga course, our clinical experience has shown that they will make better progress if they repeat the course after a few months of practice and again three to six months later. Although there are immediate gains, long-term benefits may not be evident for 6 to 12 months.

Encouraging patients to talk about their yoga experiences brings important material into the treatment. The therapist who helps the patient process these experiences is helping the patient to gain the most from mind–body practices.

CAREGIVER STRESS: HOW MIND–BODY PRACTICES BENEFIT PROFESSIONAL HEALTH CARE PROVIDERS

Health care providers and trainees are often subject to severe work stress, vicarious traumatization, and burnout. Some become casualties of substance abuse as a means to relax or escape the emotional fallout from their work. Others suffer from anxiety, insomnia, or depression. Mind–body practices can provide a healthy method to relieve physical and emotional tension. For mental health care providers, yoga and meditation can enhance the ability to remain calm during challenging sessions, increase alertness and mental focus, and improve energy.

Oncology is one of the most stressful medical specialties, particularly in research centers where the pressure to obtain grants and

CLINICAL PEARL

Health care providers may benefit from mind–body practices to improve stress resilience, mood, energy, calmness, mental focus, sleep, and stress-related physical problems. Many health care providers report that yoga practices are an antidote for professional stress and burnout. They realize that sustaining energy, enthusiasm, and equanimity are vital for their work as healers.

publish is added to the stresses of dealing with very sick and often dying patients, as well as having to break bad news to patients and their families (as many as 20,000 times in the career of an oncologist). The University of Texas M.D. Anderson Cancer Center has developed a comprehensive Faculty Development and Faculty Health program. Sudarshan Kriya Yoga workshops for faculty stress were evaluated in a qualitative survey. The 22-hour Sudarshan Kriya Yoga Workshop was given over five days to three groups, a total of 48 faculty and staff (56% female, 44% male) (Apted, 2006). The courses took place in March, July, and October 2005. Course participants were asked to complete an online survey in January 2006. There were 24 responders (50% of participants). Among those who responded to the survey, two thirds continued regular breath practices on their own and one third continued attending weekly group sessions. More than 70% of respondents reported feeling better or much better regarding anxiety, tension, ability to stay calm, and stress, while more than 50% recorded better or much better ratings for mood, sleep, anger, frustration, and optimism. Many participants reported resolution of chronic stress-related physical problems.

HORMONES FOR ANXIETY DISORDERS AND INSOMNIA

Melatonin

Melatonin (N-acetyl-5-methoxytryptamine), a hormone secreted by the pineal gland, interacts with melatonin receptors and affects sleep circadian rhythms. Melatonin is generally safe, easy to use, and beneficial in mild to moderate sleep disorders. Unlike most hypnotics, it does not disturb sleep architecture and does not lead to habituation. Double-blind randomized placebo-controlled (DBRPC) trials show that melatonin improves sleep, reduces sleep onset latency (Kayumov, Brown, Jindal, Buttoo, & Shapiro, 2001), and restores sleep efficiency (Zhdanova, Wurtman, Regan, Taylor, Shi et al., 2001) in patients with insomnia. Melatonin is particularly useful in treating delayed sleep phase syndrome (DSPS), insomnia in dementia, REM behavior disorder, insomnia in autistics, and jet lag (Pandi-Perumal, Zisapel, Srinivasan, & Cardinali, 2005).

Short- and long-term studies of melatonin for insomnia in Alzheimer's patients show improvements in sleep, mood, memory, reduced sundowning, and delay in cognitive deterioration (Srinivasan, Pandi-Perumal, Cardinali, Poeggeler, & Hardeland, 2006; Srinivasan et al., 2005). In a DBRPC study, elderly melatonin-deficient insomniacs given one week of 2 mg sustained-release melatonin effectively maintained their sleep, while one week of 2 mg fast-release melatonin improved sleep initiation. One mg/day sustained-release melatonin for two months improved sleep initiation and maintenance with no adverse effects (Haimov, Lavi, Laudon, Herer, Vigder et al., 1995). A four-week open pilot study of 11 elderly nursing home residents with dementia found that melatonin three mg h.s. reduced sundowning (agitated behaviors at night) and daytime drowsiness (Cohen-Mansfield, Garfinkel, & Lipson, 2000). A DBRPC crossover trial of 40 patients with Parkinson's disease showed significant improvements in sleep with melatonin 50 mg and 5 mg versus placebo (Dowling, Mastick, Colling, Carter, Singer et al., 2005). Furthermore, melatonin has strong antioxidant protective effects in the dopamine system.

In a DBRPC trial of 24 patients being treated with fluoxetine 20 mg for major depression and insomnia, doses up to 10 mg h.s. melatonin improved sleep quality and continuity, compared to the control group. Those taking melatonin reported no more side effects than those taking placebo (Dolberg, Hirschmann, & Grunhaus, 1998). Melatonin significantly improved sleep in a DBRPC crossover trial in schizophrenics (Shamir, Laudon, Barak, Anis, Rotenberg et al., 2000) and in a pilot study of 11 patients with bipolar disorder, manic type (Bersani & Garavini, 2000).

A review of 14 randomized controlled trials revealed that melatonin reduced sleep onset latency more in people with controlled
DSPS than in those with a diagnosis of insomnia (Buscemi, Vandermeer, Hooton, Pandya, Tjosvold et al., 2005). The distinction
between DSPS and insomnia accounted for much of the heterogeneity in the studies reviewed. Ten of the 14 trials provided reviews on
safety. These indicated a low incidence of adverse events (headaches,
drowsiness, dizziness, and nausea) with no difference between melatonin and placebo in any study. Because no study ran more than
three months, conclusions about long-term safety could not be
drawn.

REM Sleep Behavior Disorder
REM sleep behavior disorder (RBD) is a chronic progressive parasomnia. The motor paralysis that normally occurs during REM sleep
is lost such that patients may act out their dreams, thrashing and
kicking, hurting themselves or their partner. RBD often occurs in
neurodegenerative disorders and in Parkinson's patients treated with
dopamine agonists and levodopa. In patients with neurodegenerative
disease, stimulants, tricyclic antidepressants, and SSRIs can trigger
RBD (Schenck, Bundlie, Ettinger, & Mahowald, 1986). Clonazepam
(0.5–2 mg h.s.) or carbamazepine (100 mg t.i.d.), the standard treatments for RBD, can exacerbate cognitive dysfunction or lead to
ataxia (increasing the risk of falling). Other side effects of carbamazepine include hepatitis, blood cell dyscrasias, and hyponatremia.
Side effects rarely occur with melatonin, even at 9–12 mg h.s., the
doses necessary to treat RBD (Kunz & Bes, 1997; Paparrigopoulos,
2005).

Case 8—Treating REM Sleep Behavior Disorder
George is a 79-year-old retired business manager. He was
brought for evaluation by his oldest daughter because she
was worried that he would hurt Martha, her 78-year-old
mother. Martha had confided in her daughter that George
had been punching and kicking her in bed at night. The family had first taken him to a psychotherapist who explained
that the nightly attacks were due to George's subconscious
anger toward Martha. He said that because George could not

verbally express his anger, he was acting it out during his sleep. Martha was terrified, George was confused, and the family was in an uproar. There was no previous history of violence or substance abuse. George was becoming more forgetful but otherwise functioned well for his age. Martha and George had always had a solid, healthy relationship. George was treated with 3 mg rapid onset melatonin and 6 mg slow-release melatonin at bedtime for REM sleep behavior disorder. The nightly thrashings ceased and the couple slept peacefully thereafter.

Pervasive Developmental Disorders or Autism

In a DBRPC trial, 15 children with pervasive developmental disorders or autism with severe insomnia had significant improvement in insomnia, irritability, alertness, and social ability when given melatonin (Jan, Espezel, & Appleton, 1994). Eight out of 10 epileptic children with severe sleep waking rhythm pathology, ages 6 months to 10 years, showed better sleep and daytime alertness with melatonin 5 to 10 mg hs. In the same study, six of the responders gained better seizure control (Fauteck, Schmidt, Lerchl, Kurlemann & Wittkowski, 1999). In a study of 20 developmentally disabled children, sleep problems improved on melatonin (Dodge & Wilson, 2001). Two DPRPC trials in 40 and 62 children with chronic sleep onset insomnia found that melatonin 5 mg outperformed placebo (Smits, Nagtegaal, van der Heijden, Coenen, & Kerkhof, 2001).

Jet Lag and High Altitudes

Melatonin is a convenient, low-risk means for reducing symptoms of jet lag, particularly when travelers cross five or more time zones (Arendt, 1997–1998). It is easier to delay than to advance the sleep cycle more than one hour at a time. An evening dose of melatonin helps the biological clock by enhancing homeostatic sleep mechanisms. For example, flying from New York City to Europe requires a sleep phase advance of six or more hours. Using 8–9 mg fast-release melatonin for sleep on an evening flight accelerates the adjustment to European time and reduces jet lag. For some individuals, an 8–9 mg dose may cause excess sedation. In such cases, smaller doses may be sufficient. Melatonin may be preferable to prescription sedative/hypnotics such as benzodiazepines, which can impair the ability to respond to an emergency or interfere with functioning the next day. Because sedating medications reduce the tendency to move and walk during long flights, they can increase the risk of deep vein thrombosis (Herxheimer & Petrie, 2001).

A four-day DBRPC study of 320 people showed that those who were given 5 mg fast-release melatonin on a long plane trip slept better, fell asleep faster, and were more awake and energetic during the subsequent four days than comparison groups given 5 mg slow-release, 0.5 mg fast-release, or placebo (Suhner, Schlagenhauf, Johnson, Tschopp, & Steffen, 1998). In a small double-blind study, airline crews were more rested using 10 mg fast-release melatonin to sleep between flights compared to placebo. The benefits of melatonin were equivalent to zopiclone (nonbenzodiazepine sedative similar in structure to Lunesta), without next-day impairment in cognition (Paul, Brown, Bougvet, Gray, Pigeau et al., 2001).

The best recipe we have found for jet lag, a combination of melatonin and *Rhodiola rosea*, helps adjust the sleep cycle and improves daytime energy and alertness. When traveling from west to east crossing three or more time zones, the following regimen is effective for most people:

1. Five days before flying from west to east, start *R. rosea* 180–200 mg/day in a.m.
2. The day of the flight, take 300 mg *R. rosea* in a.m.
3. Take 3–9 mg melatonin at the time when people at your destination go to bed. Try to sleep on the plane using eye shades and earplugs. Do not watch movies and ask the flight attendant not to wake you (skip meals if possible).
4. Upon arrival, take *R. rosea* 300 mg at the time when people are waking up there.
5. During your stay, if you are under age 55, continue to take *R. rosea* in a.m. and melatonin in p.m. for the first five days. Those above age 55, continue *R. rosea* in a.m. and melatonin in p.m. for two weeks.

When traveling from east to west, take *R. rosea* 180–200 mg in a.m. for five days prior to flight.

1. If there is more than a three-hour time change, use the same principle as above. Wait until bedtime at your destination and then take melatonin 3–9 mg. Do your best to sleep.
2. Follow the same regimen as above.

For those traveling to high-altitude destinations, taking *R. rosea* 200–400 mg/day for one week prior to and throughout the trip can prevent altitude sickness. The addition of ginkgo 120 mg b.i.d. and/or aetazolamide (Diamox) 250 mg/day may further enhance the *R. rosea* benefits at high altitudes. Respiratory reactions to high altitude involve shifts in pH levels. Acetazolamide, a carbonic anhydrase inhibitor, readjusts the pH level in cerebrospinal fluid and serum.

Benzodiazepine Withdrawal

Many patients start benzodiazepines for sleep during a period of stress, but are unable to discontinue them due to recurrence of insomnia. Melatonin can be used to help patients discontinue benzodiazepines while maintaining sleep quality. For those unable to completely discontinue benzodiazepines, it was possible to significantly reduce the dose of benzodiazepine using melatonin (Pandi-Perumal et al., 2005).

Clinical Guidelines, Safety, and Side Effects

Consumers should choose supplements from mainstream companies with pharmaceutical-grade melatonin to avoid the possibility of impurities ("Melatonin," 1995). Side effects, including cramps, fatigue, dizziness, headache, and irritability, are infrequent and usually mild. Melatonin is a safe short-term alternative to prescription hypnotics for insomnia. In therapeutic doses, 1.0–3.0 mg h.s. (with increases up to maximum 9 mg h.s. prn), it has few side effects. Elderly patients who are susceptible to cognitive and memory impairment and daytime drowsiness from benzodiazepines may respond to melatonin with fewer adverse events. Patients should be instructed to take melatonin about 30 minutes before bedtime, get into bed, turn the lights off, and wait for it to take effect. Taking melatonin during the daytime may sensitize the eyes to damage from bright light. The safety of high-dose melatonin has not been evaluated. Very high doses (above 50 mg/day) might have long-term effects on testosterone or prolactin levels. Patients on long-term daily melatonin or Ramelteon (a melatonin analogue) should be monitored for possible adverse effects (Bellon, 2006).

7-Keto DHEA for Post-Traumatic Stress Disorder

The literature on treatment of patients with comorbid PTSD and bipolar disorder is sparse. Retrospective studies of adults with bipolar disorder find that about half have a history of severe trauma and about 35% have comorbid PTSD. Such patients tend to have more frequent and severe mood swings, a higher incidence of comorbid substance abuse, more frequent hospitalizations, and poorer response to standard treatments (Garno, Goldberg, Ramirez, & Ritzler, 2005; Leverich & Post, 2006).

A small case series (five women) with severe chronic PTSD due to severe early abuse reported rapid and substantial improvement in dissociative symptoms, emotional numbing, avoidance, irritability, energy, mood, memory, concentration, cognitive function, libido, anxiety, and insomnia when treated with 3-acetyl-7-oxo-dehydroepiandrosterone (7-keto DHEA), a metabolite of dehydroepiandrosterone (DHEA; Sageman & Brown, 2006b). These patients were symptomatic despite years of psychotherapy and pharmacotherapy. Levels of DHEA-sulfate prior to treatment were below normal or in the lower quartile of normal. Doses of 7-keto DHEA ranged from 50 to 75 mg/day. None of the five patients reported any adverse side effects. A previous study of 13 women with chronic PTSD had found that those with a higher level of DHEA in response to adrenal activation by adrenocorticotropic hormone had less severe PTSD symptomatology (Rasmusson, Vasek, Lipschitz, Vojvoda, Mustone et al., 2004). Cortisol-lowering treatments have been found to reduce the kinds of symptoms associated with PTSD. DHEA has been shown to counteract effects of circulating glucocorticoids and to improve memory, mood, and cognition. Unlike DHEA, 7-keto DHEA is not aromatized to testosterone or estrogen and therefore is unlikely to increase the risks of acne, baldness, hirsutism, prostatic changes, or increased estrogenicity (risk of uterine or breast cancer). Further trials are needed to explore the benefits of 7-keto DHEA in treating PTSD. For patients with chronic PTSD who show poor or limited response to standard treatments, 7-keto

DHEA should be considered. Serum DHEA and DHEA-sulfate levels should be obtained on patients with refractory PTSD or depression. Those with levels below normal or in the lower 50% of normal may benefit from a trial of 7-keto DHEA. The range of normal on laboratory tests of DHEA and DHEA-sulfate may not reflect the values seen in healthy age- and gender-matched controls. For guidelines see values listed under Treatment and Disease Prevention Protocols at www.lef.org.

In bipolar II cases, 7-keto DHEA (or DHEA) should be started in low doses (25 mg/day) and increased gradually while monitoring for any increase in manic symptoms such as irritability or anger. Most patients respond between 50 and 100 mg/day. Extreme caution should be used in bipolar I patients, rapid cyclers, or those with a recent history of mania. Patients should be informed of the risk of possible mania.

Case 9—7-Keto DHEA for PTSD With Bipolar Disorder

Linda is a 52-year-old machinist who was diagnosed with bipolar disorder, PTSD, dissociative identity disorder, and alcohol abuse in sustained remission. Her psychotherapist referred her for evaluation of persistent severe depression with inability to get out of bed or function at work, fatigue, and loss of memory and mental sharpness. Episodes of hypomania were characterized by rapid speech and sleep disturbance. She had been treated with lithium in the past, but her primary care physician had discontinued it because of obesity, severe coronary artery disease, diabetes, hyperlipidemia, and hypercholesterolemia. The patient was taking 60 mg/day fluoxetine (Prozac) and drinking 10 cups per day of coffee plus two six-packs of caffeinated soda.

The first step in treating bipolar disorder was to initiate a mood stabilizer while removing exacerbating factors such as destabilizing antidepressants (SSRIs) and stimulants (caffeine). Although discontinuation of fluoxetine was considered, the patient explained that although it did not control her depression, without it she would become suicidal. Avoiding mood stabilizers that were likely to cause weight gain (lithium and valproate), Linda was started on lamotrigine (Lamictal) with initial improvement. However, she developed a drug rash, necessitating a switch to oxcarbazepine (Trileptal), which also triggered an allergic reaction. A trial of gabapentin (Neurontin) 300 mg twice daily (she could not tolerate higher doses) partially relieved the depression, but left persistent mood swings, fatigue, and hypersomnia. Omega-3 fatty acids, B vitamins, and 400 mg *Rhodiola rosea* were added, but she began to deteriorate with worsening depression, suicidal ideation, and racing thoughts.

Laboratory studies showed that although Linda's DHEA was normal, her DHEA-sulfate was only 60. While laboratory reports indicate a normal range of 20–200 mcg/dl for DHEA-sulfate, it is worth treating levels below 200 in the context of PTSD, bipolar disorder, or mid- to late-life depression. After one week on 25 mg/day 7-keto DHEA, the depression began to steadily improve with increased energy, alertness, motivation, and ability to function. The patient improved further as the dose increased to 25 mg b.i.d.

Two months later, Linda ran out of 7-keto DHEA and did not take it for a week. She plummeted into a severe, sluggish depression. Resumption of 7-keto DHEA rapidly lifted the depression. Two years later, she continues to function well without depression on a combination of 7-keto DHEA, gabapentin, fluoxetine, *Rhodiola rosea*, vitamins, and omega-3 fatty acids. In addition, she has found significant relief from dissociative symptoms and made greater progress in psychotherapy.

Although the evidence for 7-keto DHEA treatment is preliminary, considering the severity of these conditions and the low risk of side effects, it is worthwhile to obtain DHEA and DHEA-sulfate levels in patients with bipolar disorder, PTSD, or mid- to late-life depression. While laboratory reports indicate a normal range of 20–200 ng/dl, if the DHEA-sulfate is below 200, it is worth a trial of 7-keto DHEA 25–50 mg/day. If symptoms persist, the dose may be gradually raised up to 200 mg/day. In patients with bipolar disorder, 7-keto DHEA may trigger mania.

HERBS AND NUTRIENTS FOR ANXIETY DISORDERS AND INSOMNIA

Kava

Kava (extracted from *Piper methysticum*) is a traditional social and ceremonial drink in the Pacific Islands. It contains alpha-pyrones (kavalactones), which have sodium and calcium channel blocking activity as well as some serotonin blocking action. The intoxicant, sedative, anxiolytic, anticonvulsant, and analgesic properties of kava have been attributed to kavalactones. There has been considerable controversy regarding the safety and efficacy of kava. A review of seven DBRPC studies of kava for anxiety concluded that it was relatively safe and superior to placebo (Pittler & Ernst, 2000). However, three of the studies involved patients with mild anxiety and short treatment periods. A meta-analysis of three DBRPC trials of kava for generalized anxiety disorder found no benefit from kava (Connor, Payne, & Davidson, 2006).

In the 1800s, ship records described kava intoxication in natives and seamen left behind by Captain Cook (Singh & Blumenthal, 1996). Among the Aboriginies in northern Australia, long-term daily kava users developed facial swelling, scaly rash, increased patellar reflexes, dyspnea, low levels of albumin, increased GGTPase, abnormal blood counts with decreased white cell and platelet counts, hematuria, and tall P waves on electrocardiograms consistent with pulmonary hypertension (Mathews, Riley, Fejo, Munoz, Milns et al., 1988). A study of 62 indigenous kava users showed increased liver enzymes, which reversed after several weeks' abstinence (Clough, Bailie, & Currie, 2003). Postmarketing studies of over 3,000 patients on kava revealed a 1.5% and 2.3% incidence of side effects, primarily gastrointestinal, allergic reactions, headache, and light sensitivity. Less common side effects included restlessness, drowsiness, lack of energy, and tremor. In four cases, kava induced dystonic reactions, oral or lingual dyskinesias, and worsening parkinsonian symptoms in a woman on levodopa, effects consistent with dopamine blocking. In one case, a 45-year-old woman developed severe parkinsonism after kava treatment (Meseguer, Taboa, Sanchez, Mena, Campos et al., 2002). Long-term safety, teratogenicity, or mutagenicity beyond six months has not been studied. Taking kava with alcohol, other sedatives, or muscle relaxants can result in coma (Almeida & Grimsley, 1996).

Since 1998, liver toxicity, including liver failure requiring transplantation, has been reported with kava extracted with acetone or alcohol. The US FDA's Letter to Health Care Professionals and a consumer advisory warned of potential liver injury (Kraft et al., 2001; U.S. Food and Drug Administration, 2002). Kava extract and kavalactones inhibit P450 enzymes (CYP1A2, 2C9, 2C19, 2D6, 3A4, and 4A9/11; Mathews, Etheridge, & Black, 2002) and CYP2E1 (Gurley, Gardner, Hubbard, Williams, Gentry et al., 2005) involved in metabolism of many pharmaceuticals. Kava has modest benefits in short-term studies of mild anxiety. Considering the risks of intoxication, abuse, dependency, and rarely severe adverse effects, the authors do not recommend kava until more compelling data on safety and efficacy become available.

Rhodiola rosea

Rhodiola rosea alone and in combinations with other adaptogens has been shown to significantly improve mental and physical performance under stress (see Chapter 4). Psychoactive constituents of root extracts from *R. rosea* and *Eleutherococcus senticosus* and berry extracts from *Schizandra chinesis* contain phenolic compounds, structurally related to catecholamines involved in sympathetic nervous system activation during stress response. Extracts from the roots of *Bryonia alba* and *Withania somnifera* contain tetracyclic triterpenoids, structurally similar to corticosteroids involved in activation of the stress system and in protection from overreaction to stress. Salidroside extracted from *R. rosea* protected PC 12 cells from glutamate toxicity (an excitatory neurotransmitter whose damaging effects have been studied in PTSD; Cao, Du, & Wang, 2006).

Adaptogenic Herbs for Military Stress: Rhodiola, Eleutherococcus, and Schizandra

Military training, active duty, and postcombat adjustment to civilian life can be extremely stressful physically and emotionally. When the intensity and duration of the many stressors of combat service exceed the capacity for recovery, troops become more vulnerable during combat as well as in the aftermath. Studies of adaptogenic herbs suggest that they could play a preventive role by enhancing resistance to the effects of stress, improving performance during stress, and enhancing recovery. In a randomized placebo-controlled study of 181 healthy military cadets with routine military service tasks (including night duty), those who were given a single dose of *R. rosea* (either 370 mg or 555 mg) showed significantly less fatigue ($p < 0.001$) on measures of mental performance and improvements in pulse rates, blood pressure, and overall well-being compared with cadets given either placebo or no capsule (Shevtsov, Zholus, Shervarly, Vol'skij, Korovin et al., 2003). Studies have shown that *R. rosea* increases the capacity of muscle and nerve cells to maintain production of the high-energy molecules, adenosine triphosphate and creatine phosphate, which are necessary to sustain cellular activities and repair mechanisms (Kurkin & Zapesochnaya, 1986).

During the Cold War, the Soviet Ministry of Defense conducted extensive tests of herbal preparations to enhance strength, endurance, and physical and mental performance in its Olympic athletes, military personnel, and cosmonauts (Vastag, 2007). Their research focused on finding the ideal combination of three herbs: *Rhodiola rosea, Eleutherococcus senticosus*, and *Schizandra chinensis*. The Swedish Herbal Institute participated in preparing adaptogen formulas for Russian research, particularly with cosmonauts. Most of this research remains in classified reports filed with the Ministry of Defense. Some of these reports were translated by Dr. Zakir Ramazanov, a professor of phytochemistry who had also been involved in designing solar panels for the Russian space program. Two of these, the Baranov Reports, document many studies demonstrating improvement in strength, endurance, alertness, SNS/PNS balance, and coordination, particularly under prolonged stress with significantly reduced recovery time after exertion (Baranov, 1994). The formula that was most extensively studied in these reports was called ADAPT. It contained the following adaptogenic herbs:

• 3 mg salidrosides (6 to 9 mg rosavins) from 50 mg of *Rhodiola rosea* root extract

• 3 mg total glycosides from 100 mg extract of *Eleutherococcus senticosus*

• 4 mg total schizandrines from 150 mg fruit extract of *Schizandra chinensis*

The Swedish Herbal Institute sells a product called ADAPT-232 containing the same combination of herbs. However, the proportions of each herb are kept as a proprietary secret.

St. John's Wort

St. John's Wort (*Hypericum perforatum*) has been shown to reduce the effects of stress in studies of rodents. Case reports and some open-label studies of patients with generalized anxiety disorder suggesting response to St. John's Wort have appeared in the literature, but controlled studies have not been supportive. A DBRPC 12-week study of 40 subjects with social phobia found no difference between those on St. John's Wort with flexible doses (600–1,800 mg/day) and those taking placebo on the Liebowitz Social Anxiety Scale (Kobak, Taylor, Warner, & Futterer, 2005). Although one open-label study suggested benefits of St. John's Wort for obsessive-compulsive disorder, a subsequent 12-week DBRPC study of 60 patients with obsessive-compulsive disorder found no difference in the mean change of scores on the Yale-Brown Obsessive-Compulsive Scale between the group given St. John's Wort LI 160 (600–1,800 mg/day) and the group given placebo (Kobak, Taylor, Bystritsky, Kohlenberg, Greist et al., 2005).

In clinical practice with anxious patients, the authors prefer to use the brand Kira (Lichtwer Pharma) rather than Perika (Nature's Way) because it is less stimulating. Perika may exacerbate anxiety and agitation. However, Perika may be more helpful in activating patients who have a sluggish depression (e.g., apathy or psychomotor retardation).

Valerian

Valerian (*Valeriana officinalis*) is thought to bind to gama-amniobutyric acid-A receptors. One review of DBRPC trials of valerian for sleep found the evidence to be encouraging but not compelling (Stevinson & Ernst, 2000). Another review found subjective improvement in sleep in six out of seven DBRPC trials with no side effects other than minimal hangover in doses of 600 to 900 mg (Krystal & Ressler, 2002). One DBRPC crossover study of 16 mild insomniacs using polysomnography reported a significant decrease in slow wave sleep onset latency and an increase in the percentage of slow wave sleep time (Donath, Quispe, Diefenbach, Maurer, Fietze et al., 2000). The effect of valerian improves over time, and maximal benefit may take two weeks.

A small study of 36 patients with generalized anxiety disorder compared valerian (mean daily dose 81.3 mg valepotriates), diazepam (mean daily dose 6.5 mg), and placebo (Andreatini, Sartori, Seabra, & Leite, 2002). There were no significant differences in this four-week randomized controlled trial among the three groups on either baseline or the change from baseline scores on the Hamilton anxiety scale. All three groups had significant reduction in Hamilton depression scale scores. However, only the diazepam and valerian groups showed significant reductions on the Hamilton anxiety scale psychic factor. In a multicenter randomized placebo-controlled parallel-group study of 184 adults with mild insomnia (Morin, Koetter, Bastien, Ware, & Wooten, 2005), the groups given valerian-hops or diphenhydramine showed modest improvements in subjective sleep parameters, most of which did not reach statistical significance. The valerian-hops produced greater, but not statistically significant, reductions in sleep latency than diphenhydramine and placebo. Quality of life improved significantly in the valerian-hops group compared to placebo, suggesting that valerian-hops may be a useful adjunct for mild insomnia. No serious adverse events occurred and there were no residual symptoms.

Reports of dystonia and hepatitis from preparations containing a mixture of ingredients (including valerian) are difficult to interpret. Valerian tea and tablets have an unpleasant taste and odor. One advantage of valerian over other sedative/hypnotics is that there have been no cases of habituation or abuse and only one case of possible withdrawal symptoms. Valerian should be avoided in pregnancy. A review and meta-analysis of 16 valerian studies concluded that it might improve sleep without causing side effects and that further studies were needed (Bent, Padula, Moore, Patterson, & Mehling, 2006).

Lemon Balm (*Melissa officinalis*)
In a DBRPC crossover study of *Melissa officinalis* using a 20-minute laboratory-induced psychological stressor, the Defined Intensity Stressor Simulation (DISS) battery, in 20 healthy volunteers, subjects were given single doses of 600 mg, 1,000 mg, 1,600 mg, or placebo (Kennedy, Wake, Saveier, Tildesley, Perry et al., 2003). The

600 mg dose significantly improved self-ratings of "calmness" on the Bond-Lader scales.

Valerian and Lemon Balm

A combination of lemon balm and valerian in three doses (600 mg, 1,200 mg, 1,800 mg) was given to 24 healthy volunteers in a DBRPC crossover trial using a 20-minute laboratory-induced psychological stressor, the DISS battery (Kennedy, Little, & Scholey, 2004). Mood and anxiety were evaluated at baseline and 1, 3, and 6 hours. The 600 mg dose significantly reduced anxiety ratings, while the 1,800 mg dose somewhat increased anxiety ratings. Within a therapeutic window, the combination of *M. officinalis* and *V. officinalis* may reduce anxiety under stress.

In a large uncontrolled multicenter study, a combination valerian–lemon balm product (Euvegal forte) was tested in 918 children under the age of 12 years with restlessness and dyssomnia (Muller & Klement, 2006). Substantial improvement occurred in 80.9% of the children with dyssomnia and 70.4% of those with restlessness. Controlled trials would be useful in assessing the safety and efficacy of herbs for children. The tolerability of Euvegal forte was evaluated as "good" or "very good" by 96.7% of the patients. No herb-related adverse events occurred in this study.

Valerian and Kava

A DBRPC internet-based study of kava and valerian reported no significant differences between kava and placebo for anxiety or between valerian and placebo for sleep disturbance (Jacobs, Bent, Tice, Blackwell, & Cummings, 2005). Subject selection was based on State-Trait Anxiety Inventory subtest (Stai-State) and on self-report of "a problem going to sleep or staying asleep over the past two weeks" rather than on standard diagnostic criteria. The negative results may have been due to selection of a heterogeneous population, comorbid conditions, inadequate doses of herbs, or other limitations of internet surveys.

Passionflower

Passionflower (*Passiflora incarnata*) has been approved by the Komission E, a government agency that closely regulates the quality of herbal supplements in Germany, for treatment of nervous restless-ness. Passionflower contains a dihydroflavone, chrysin, which binds to benzodiazepine receptors. In a DBRPC comparison trial, 36 patients with *DSM-IV* generalized anxiety disorder (Hamilton anxiety scale □□14) were given *Passiflora* extract 45 drops per day plus a placebo tablet, or oxazepam (a benzodiazepine) 30 mg/day plus placebo drops for four weeks. Although the oxazepam effect was more rapid, *Passiflora* was as effective in reducing anxiety and caused less impairment in job performance (Akhondzadeh, Naghavi, Vazar-ian, Shayeganpour, Rashidi et al., 2001). Larger studies are needed to validate these findings.

Theanine

Theanine (5-*N*-ethylglutamine or gamma-glutamylethylamide), an amino acid found in green tea (*Camellia sinensis*), may reduce anxi-ety under conditions of stress. Green tea has been used for centuries for its calming and medicinal effects. Three to four cups of green tea contain 60–160 mg of theanine. In animal studies, theanine perfu-sion into the brain increased dopamine release and possibly inhibi-tion of excitatory neurotransmission (Yamada, Terashima, Okubo, Juneja, & Yokogoshi, 2005). Studies in humans have shown mixed results. One DBRPC theanine study in 16 healthy volunteers showed some evidence of mild relaxing effects during baseline under resting conditions, but not during experimentally induced anxiety (Lu, Gray, Oliver, Liley, Harrison et al., 2004). Another DBRPC study of 12 healthy subjects given a mental arithmetic task as a stres-sor found that those given L-theanine had reduced heart rate, reduced salivary immunoglobulin A, and attenuation of sympathetic nervous system activation (Kimura, Ozeki, Juneja, & Ohira, 2007). These antistress effects could be due to inhibition of cortical excita-tion. However, studies in normal subjects may not be applicable to those with anxiety disorders. L-theanine has been reported to increase alpha waves, which are associated with a relaxed, alert state of mind. In a high-density electrical mapping study, L-theanine increased attention-related anticipatory alpha over the right parieto-occipital areas during a demanding attentional task (Gomez-Ramirez, Higgins, Rycroft, Owen, Mahoney et al., 2007).

In clinical practice, the authors find that theanine can be helpful in mild to moderate anxiety, particularly in patients who are highly sensitive to side effects of other agents. It has minimal and usually no side effects when given in a starting dose of 200 mg one to three times a day up to a maximum of six times a day. In brain-damaged patients, large doses may cause paradoxical overactivation. Green tea and theanine have numerous health benefits, including antioxidant and antiproliferative activity. Patients may simply drink green tea or take capsules for more accurate dosing. Decaffeinated green tea and capsules are available, particularly for anxious or agitated patients.

GABA (Gamma-aminobutyric Acid)

GABA (gamma-aminobutyric acid) is a major inhibitory neurotransmitter and is involved in cardiovascular regulation, pituitary function, immunity, fertilization, and renal function. Compounds that enhance GABA have been found to reduce anxiety and stabilize mood. Many foods contain small amounts of GABA and some fermented food products contain high levels. Natural GABA is being produced by fermentation and widely used as a functional food supplement in Japan.

The effects on electrocardiogram of 100 mg of GABA produced by natural fermentation (Pharma-GABA) were compared to 200 mg L-theanine and placebo in a double-blind placebo-controlled crossover study of 13 healthy adults. Alpha waves are associated with relaxed, effortless alertness. Beta waves occur in highly stressful situations and during difficulty with mental concentration. GABA intake resulted in significantly greater increase in alpha and decrease in beta compared to both L-theanine and control (Abdou, Higashiguchi, Horie, Kim, Hatta et al., 2006). The high alpha-beta ratio indicates a state of arousal with relaxation or relaxed concentration.

Low levels of immunoglobulin-A (IgA) have been found in the saliva of highly anxious individuals with further pronounced reductions in stressful situations. Relaxation leads to substantial increases in IgA. Salivary IgA levels were used as a marker of stress and immune response in a double-blind randomized placebo-controlled trial of 100 mg GABA (Pharma-GABA) in eight adults with a history of acrophobia (fear of heights). Pharmacokinetic studies had shown that oral administration of this GABA preparation led to peak concentration in 30 minutes with decline starting at 60 minutes. In order to induce stress, subjects had to walk across a narrow pedestrian suspension bridge 54 m high, 300 m long, and 2 m wide. In the placebo group, IgA levels dropped substantially when measured halfway across and at the end of the bridge. In comparison, in subjects given GABA, IgA levels dropped only slightly midway and rose above baseline by the end of the bridge. In this small preliminary study, subjects who took GABA showed significantly less reduction in salivary IgA (marker of stress and anxiety compared with controls, $p < 0.05$; Abdou et al., 2006).

Pregabalin is a synthetic structural analogue of GABA that has been approved by the U.S. FDA for treatment of neuropathic pain and partial-onset seizures. It is being considered for approval as an adjunctive treatment for generalized anxiety disorder. Several randomized controlled trials confirm that pregabalin is comparable to lorazepam (Ativan), alprazolam (Xanax), and venlafaxine (Effexor) for moderate-to-severe generalized anxiety disorder. Pregabalin is generally safe and well tolerated. Side effects include dizziness, somnolence, and headache. It shows less cognitive interference than benzodiazepines and has low potential for abuse or dependence. However, the onset of anxiolytic effects requires one week of daily treatment (Bandelow, Wedekind, & Leon, 2007).

Ginkgo (*Ginkgo biloba*)

A special extract of ginkgo (EGb 761, manufactured by Willmar Schwabe Pharmaceutical Co., Karlsruhe, Germany, and distributed in the United States as Ginkgold by Nature's Way) was found to reduce anxiety in two studies. In a DBRPC study, 170 adults (aged 18–70 years) with generalized anxiety disorder or adjustment disorder with anxious mood were given either 480 mg/day EGb 761, 240 mg/day EGb 761, or placebo for four weeks. Hamilton Rating Scale for Anxiety scores decreased significantly, by -14.2 (±8.1) ($p = 0.0003$) and -12.1 (6±9.0) ($p = 0.003$) in the higher and lower doses, respectively, compared to placebo -7.8 (±9.2). EGb 761 outperformed placebo on all secondary measures: clinical global impression of change, Erlangen anxiety tension and aggression scale, list of complaints, and the patient's global rating of change (Woelk, Arnoldt, Kieser, & Hoerr, 2007).

In a 22-week randomized controlled trial of 400 patients with dementia and neuropsychiatric features, patients were given either 240 mg/day EGb 761 or placebo. Of those treated with ginkgo, 67.5% had significant improvement in cognitive function versus 6.1% on placebo. Among the caregivers of patients on ginkgo, 36% reported less distress (related to the patient's symptoms) compared with a 4% increase for those on placebo. Scores on the Neuropsychiatric Inventory dropped significantly in the ginkgo group compared to an increase in the placebo group. The largest differences in scores were improvements in apathy/indifference, anxiety, irritability/lability, depression/dysphoria, and sleep/nighttime behavior (Scripnikov, Khomenko, & Napryeyenko, 2007).

Special extract EGb 761 has shown positive effects on anxiety in well-designed controlled trials. Whether the effects would be the same with other preparations of ginkgo remains to be seen.

Chamomile (*Matricaria recutita*)

There is little scientific evidence to support the use of chamomile for sleep or anxiety. Apigenin, a component of chamomile, has high affinity for benzodiazepine receptors, but minimal sedative or muscle-relaxant effects (Brown, 1996). People who have ragweed allergy should not use chamomile.

Omega-3 Fatty Acids

Omega-3 fatty acids (omega-3FAs) were found to be approximately 30% lower in the red cell membranes of untreated patients with social anxiety disorder with a significant inverse correlation between low omega-3FAs and scores on the Liebowitz Social Anxiety Scale (Green, Hermest, Monselise, Marom, Presburger et al., 2006). While low levels of omega-3FAs may play a role in anxiety disorders, few clinical studies have been done. In a study of test anxiety, a mixture of omega-3FAs and omega-6 FAs improved appetite, mood, mental concentration, fatigue, organization, sleep, and anxiety, as well as reducing cortisol levels (Yehuda, Rabinovitz, & Mostofsky, 2005). In a three-month DBRPC study of substance abusers with presumed poor dietary habits, 13 patients were given 3 g of n-3 PUFAS (omega-3 polyunsaturated fatty acids; eicosapentanoic acid, EPA, + docosahexaenoic acid, DHA) versus 11 given placebo. Compared to the placebo group, those given n-3 PUFAS had significant progressive decline in anxiety scores for three months (p = 0.010) and at six months (p = 0.042) (Buydens-Branchey & Branchey, 2006). Preliminary studies have also shown that omega-3FAs can reduce stress-related aggression in young and old adults as well as women with borderline personality disorder (Bourre, 2005a). One DBRPC crossover trial of EPA alone in patients with obsessive-compulsive disorder on SSRIs found no effect on Hamilton anxiety or depression scales (Fux, Benjamin, & Nemets, 2004). While this study did not find EPA to be effective against obsessive-compulsive disorder, it is possible that a combination of EPA and DHA might have been better, particularly in view of the studies described above.

Clinical Considerations in Using Herbs for Anxiety and Insomnia

Herbs are most useful in patients who:
1. Have mild to moderate anxiety or insomnia
2. Are at risk for addiction or abuse
3. Habituate to anxiolytics such as benzodiazepines
4. Are sensitive to prescription medication side effects such as excess sedation or cognitive interference (e.g., children and geriatric patients)
5. Require maximal alertness the next day
6. Have shown adverse reactions to sedative/hypnotic medications (e.g., night eating syndrome with Ambien or amnesia from benzodiazepines)
7. Have not responded to or not complied with mind–body practices or who need more time to learn them

Patients with recurrent major depression and concurrent moderate to severe anxiety or insomnia usually need more sedating medications (e.g., benzodiazepines, tricyclic antidepressants, mirtazepine, or atypical neuroleptics). Psychotherapy or cognitive behavioral therapy, lifestyle changes, mind–body practices, and daily exercise over a period of months or years are usually needed to gradually discontinue such medications.

HOMEOPATHY

Homeopathy is a widely used form of CAM founded by Samuel Hahnemann over 200 years ago. It is based on the principles of "similars" (like cures like), the vital force (animal energy), minimal doses (highly diluted remedies), laws of cure (progression of symptom resolution), and an approach based on the whole person rather than just the disease (Bell & Pappas, 2007). A systematic review of the use of homeopathy for anxiety found eight randomized controlled studies including test anxiety, generalized anxiety disorder, and anxiety related to medical conditions. Most of the literature consists of single case reports, some uncontrolled and observational studies, and surveys (Pilkington, Kirkwood, Rampes, Fisher, & Richardson, 2006). The randomized controlled trials reported inconsistent results or had methodological problems. Adverse reactions, temporary worsening of symptoms, or reappearance of symptoms were considered to be "remedy reactions."

In a DBRPC 10-week study of classical homeopathy for 44 patients with *DSM-IV* generalized anxiety disorder, significant and substantial improvement in anxiety on the Hamilton Scale was found in both the group treated with homeopathy and in the group given placebo. There was no difference in the degree of improvement between the two groups (Bonne, Shemer, Gorali, Katz, & Shalev, 2003). This study highlights some of the difficulties of research on homeopathic treatments and studies of anxiety in patients recruited by advertisement in general. A 10-week trial may be insufficient in that homeopathic treatments may take several months to a year for full effect.

A six-month uncontrolled feasibility study on a total of 960 patients undergoing homeopathic treatment for a wide range of conditions found positive outcome scores in patients treated for irritable bowel syndrome (73.9%, n = 23) and anxiety (61.0%, n = 41). There was no intent-to-treat analysis (Mathie & Robinson, 2006). There is a high rate of spontaneous remission, placebo response, and response to the reassurance of medical attention in anxiety disordered patients. These factors as well as the individualization of treatments complicate the interpretation of studies of homeopathy for anxiety.

TABLE 3.1 Treatment Guidelines for Disorders of Anxiety, PTSD, and Sleep

CAM	Clinical Uses	Daily Dose	Side Effects, Drug Interactions,* Contraindications
B vitamins B$_{12}$ folate	stress	1,000 mcg 800 mcg	Rare: activation Caution: cardiac stents**
Chamomile (*Matricaria recutita*)	minimal sedative		Ragweed family— allergic reactions D/C: pregnancy
GABA	anxiety, stress, phobias	100 mg	Minimal
Ginkgo	anxiety	240–360 mg/day	Minimal: headache Contraindication: anticoagulants D/C: 2 weeks prior to surgery
Inositol	OCD	12–20 g	Gas, loose bowels, mania
Kava (*Piper methysticum*)	anxiety, insomnia	100 mg standardized extract (70 mg kavalactones) t.i.d.	GI, allergic skin, photo-sensitivity, headache Occasional: drowsiness, tremor, restlessness, dystonia, hepatitis, fatigue, liver failure, ↓ effects of levodopa D/C: pregnancy Toxic dose > 240 mg kavalactones/day

TABLE 3.1 *Continued*

CAM	Clinical Uses	Daily Dose	Side Effects, Drug Interactions,* Contraindications
7-keto DHEA	PTSD, dissociative symptoms	25–200 mg	Bipolar patients may become agitated, irritable, anxious. Contraindication: estrogen-sensitive cancer or prostate cancer
Lemon balm (*Melissa officinalis*)	anxiety, herpes (cold sore)	600 mg	No serious side effects
Melatonin	insomnia, jet lag, REM sleep behavior disorder	1–12 mg h.s.	Occasional agitation, depression, abdominal cramps, fatigue, dizziness, headache, vivid dreams. D/C: pregnancy
Omega-3 fatty acids	anxiety, agression	3–6 g	Belching, loose stools
Passionflower (*Passiflora incarnata*)	anxiety	90 mg	Minimal
Rhodiola rosea	PTSD, combat stress, jet lag	50–900 mg	Agitation, insomnia, anxiety, headache Rarely: palpitations, chest pain Caution: bipolars
Theanine Green tea *Camellia sinenis*	mild anxiety	200 mg 1–4	Minimal Contraindication: anticoagulants
St. John's Wort (*Hypericum perforatum*)	mild–moderate anxiety	300–600 mg t.i.d.	Nausea, heartburn, loose bowels, jitteriness, insomnia, fatigue, bruxism, phototoxic rash, mania in bipolar,

			blocks CYP 3A4, 1A2 and P-glycoproteins. Reduces digoxin, warfarin, indivir, cyclosporine, theophyline, birth control pills D/C: 2 weeks prior to surgery, pregnancy
Valerian (*Valeriana officianalis*)	insomnia, anxiety	450–900 mg h.s. 50–100 mg	Occasional GI, headaches, minimal hangover on high doses > 600 mg. D/C: pregnancy, hepatic disease
Bio-Strath **B vitamins +** **antioxidants**	stress	1 Tbsp b.i.d. 3 tabs b.i.d.	Keep liquid refrigerated Caution: cardiac stents**
ADAPT-232 *R. rosea* *E. senticosus* *S. chinensis*	mild to extreme stress, combat stress	2–3 tabs/day	Rare: overactivation, anxiety, insomnia Caution: bipolars
Easy Energy *R. rosea* 70 mg *E. senticocus* *S. chinensis* *A. Mandshurica* *R. carthamoides*	mild to extreme stress, physical strength, calms patients who become agitated on activating herbs	2–4 pills/day	Minimal: side effects of component herbs Caution: bipolars

D/C = discontinue; GI = gastrointestinal; ↓ = decrease.

*Common side effects are listed. There are additional rare side effects. Individuals with high blood pressure, diabetes, pregnancy (or during breast-feeding), or any chronic or serious medical condition should check with their physician before taking supplements. Patients taking anticoagulants should consult their physician before using supplements.

**May increase risk of restenosis of cardiac stents in men only with baseline homocysteine less than 15 µmol/liter.

CHAPTER 4 OUTLINE

1. **Key Concepts:** Effects of CAM treatments on brain function

2. **Neurodevelopment and Neuroprotection**
   a. omega-3 fatty acids, vitamins, S-adenosylmethionine, picamilon

3. **Mitochondrial Energy Production and Antioxidant Protection**
   a. coenzyme Q10, idebenone, ubiquinol, acetyl-L-carnitine

4. **Cholinergic Enhancing Agents**
   a. galantamine, citicholine, huperzine-A

5. **Adaptogens**
   a. *Rhodiola rosea, Schizandra chinensis, Eleutherococcus senticosus, Panax ginseng, Withania somnifera (Ashwaganda), Lepidium meyenii (Maca)*
   b. adaptogen combinations for complex cases

6. **Other Herbs for Cognitive Enhancement**
   a. lemon balm, sage, vinpocetine, ginkgo, bacopa

7. **Nootropics**
   a. centrophenoxine (Meclofenoxate), BCE-001, racetams (pyrrolidinones), selegiline, alpha-lipoic acid, phosphatidyl serine

8. **Ergot Derivatives**
   a. hydergine and nicergoline

9. **Cognitive Enhancing Hormones**
   a. DHEA, melatonin

10. **Neurotherapy**

Disorders of Cognition and Memory

Disorders of cognition and memory can been viewed as stemming from any combination of processes in which the impairment or accumulated damage to neurons exceeds the capacity for self-maintenance and repair. Complementary and alternative medicine (CAM) includes nutrients, neuroprotective supplements, and methods to enhance cellular repair and neuroplasticity. Ideally, cognitive enhancement should include maternal nutrition, supplements for fetal brain development, infant nutrition, a nurturing environment with physical and psychological support to minimize damage by excess stress (high levels of excitatory neurotransmitters and cortisol that can damage developing neural structures), avoidance of neurotoxic substances (tobacco, excess alcohol, substances of abuse, and environmental toxins), and the use of supplements and mind–body practices that support the growing and aging brain while counteracting neurodegenerative forces throughout adulthood.

TEN KEY CONCEPTS TO UNDERSTANDING THE EFFECTS OF CAM TREATMENTS ON BRAIN FUNCTION

1. *The membrane hypothesis* of aging proposes that free radicals damage cell membranes, nuclear membranes, and organelles

through lipid peroxidation and that this contributes to brain aging and neurodegenerative disorders such as Alzheimer's and Parkinson's disease (Zs-Nagy, 2002). Free radical endothelial damage and arteriosclerosis also lead to cerebrovascular disease, including multi-infarct dementia and stroke.

2. *Membrane fluidity*, which tends to decrease with age, is essential for neurotransmitter receptor function. It enables receptors to fold and unfold for the optimal opening and closing of membrane ion channels. The flow of ions in and out of cells through these channels creates the membrane potentials necessary for electrical transmission. Oxidative damage, aging, and loss of membrane omega-3 fatty acids lead to loss of fluidity and increased rigidity of membranes.

3. *Mitochondrial energy enhancers* improve the ability of mitochondria (organelles that generate energy) to produce and maintain high-energy molecules, such as adenosine triphosphate, for energy transport within cells. A greater supply of energy sustains the production of all the molecules necessary for optimal cellular functioning. In addition, this energy is needed to maintain cellular repair mechanisms such as repairing breaks in DNA and damage to cell membranes by free radicals. When energy is depleted due to stress, age, illness, or other factors, repair mechanisms cannot keep up with cellular injury, resulting in cumulative damage. Cellular function is compromised and with excess damage, apoptosis (cell death) occurs.

4. *Oxidative damage* is a key factor in neurodegeneration. Brain cells have a very high metabolic rate and therefore produce more free radicals as byproducts of metabolism than other tissues. Furthermore, the high concentration of polyunsaturated fatty acids in nerve cell membranes makes them vulnerable to lipid peroxidation (damage by free radicals). Damage from oxygen free radicals causes loss of membrane permeability, increased intracellular density, accumulation of cross-linked proteins and lipofuscin (waste products), slowing of RNA synthesis, and decreased protein turnover and repair. When oxidative damage to mitochondria exceeds the rate of repair, the ability of the cell to maintain energy production declines. In addition to internally generated free radicals, the human body is exposed to numerous

environmental free radicals including smoke (cigarettes and marijuana), pollution, pesticides, and radiation. Antioxidant supplements and substances that increase the ability of cells to produce more antioxidants help to prevent damage by neutralizing free radicals before they strike.

5. *Inflammation* plays an important role in brain aging. Evidence suggests that sustained brain inflammation might be an essential cofactor in Alzheimer's disease and other neurodegenerative disorders such as Parkinson's disease.

6. *The cholinergic hypothesis:* The pathological changes associated with Alzheimer's disease are extracellular deposition of amyloid beta-peptide in senile plaques, intracellular neurofibrillary tangles, and the loss of cholinergic neurons with extensive synaptic changes in cerebral cortex, hippocampus, and other brain areas involved in cognitive functions (Loizzo, Tundis, Menichini, & Menichini, 2008). The decline in cholinergic function underlies the neurodegeneration seen in Alzheimer's. Agents that enhance cholinergic function, such as cholinesterase inhibitors, have been shown to improve cognitive function in some studies. In traumatic brain injury, damage to cholinergic afferent pathways to the hippocampus may contribute to cognitive impairment (Arciniegas, 2001; Arciniegas, Topkoff, Rojas, Sheeder, Teale et al., 2001)

7. *Neuroplasticity*, a process by which synaptic connectivity changes, has been divided into fast, slow, and stable forms (Peled, 2005). Fast plasticity involves changes in coherence synchrony and phase-locking membrane potentials in cortically spread neuronal assemblies. Slow plasticity refers to synaptic and neurogenic processes, for example, brain-derived neurotrophic factor–dependent processes. Stable plasticity connotes those synaptic and neuronal pathways that have been consolidated into long-lasting circuits.

8. *Brain-derived neurotrophic factor* and its receptor, tropomyosin receptor-related kinase B, modulate numerous neuronal functions that reduce the likelihood of cell death. In addition to neuroprotection, BDNF promotes the growth of neurons, neurogenesis.

9. *Long-term potentiation* (LTP) is a form of neuroplasticity based on an increase in interneuronal connectivity. *Long-term depres-*

sion (LTD) is associated with a decrease in connectivity. N-methyl-D-aspartate (NMDA) excitatory amino acid receptors, modulated by brain-derived neurotrophic factor, are involved in rapid connectivity changes (LTP and LTD) that last at least three weeks .

10. *Nootropics* are manufactured cognitive enhancing and neuroprotective agents. While nootropics have been widely studied and used in Europe, most American health care professionals are not familiar with them. Evidence suggest that nootropics act through a variety of mechanisms, including improving antioxidant status, membrane fluidity, mitochondrial function, neurotransmitter levels, messenger RNA protein synthesis, cerebral blood flow, neuroplasticity, and long-term potentiation.

NEURODEVELOPMENT AND NEUROPROTECTION: OMEGA-3 FATTY ACIDS AND VITAMINS

Of the many macronutrients and micronutrients that are essential for the structure and function of the nervous system, the omega-3 fatty acids and vitamins are foremost in clinical practice.

Omega-3 Fatty Acids

Polyunsaturated fatty acids, including the omega-3 fatty acids (FAs) alpha-lipoic acid (ALA), docosahexanoic acid (DHA), eicosapentanoic acid (EPA), and arachidonic acid (ARA) are necessary to maintain membrane fluidity, membrane enzyme activities, and production of molecules involved in inflammatory modulation (e.g., prostaglandins). DHA is one of the building blocks of cell membranes. Omega-3 FAs are also involved in gene expression and antioxidant defense against neuronal damage from free radicals. The need for adequate supplies of polyunsaturated fatty acids is most critical during fetal development, infancy, pregnancy, and later adulthood as the brain ages.

Research has established the importance of omega-3 FAs, especially DHA in neuronal development (Bourre, 2006, 2007; Crawford, 1993). In double-blind placebo-controlled studies, infants given omega-3 enriched formula showed improved brain and eye development (Jensen, Voigt, Prager, Zou, Fraley et al., 2005), better problem solving at 10 months (Willatts, Forsyth, Dimodgno, Varma, & Colvin, 1998), and higher scores on the mental development index (Birch, Garfield, Hoffman, Uauy, & Birch, 2000; Helland, Smith, Saarem, Saugstad, & Drevon, 2003). Although more long-term, large-scale studies with measures of development are needed, there is no question that omega-3 FAs provide key structural elements for neuronal development in the fetus and newborn and that particular attention should be given to them in nutritional counseling.

Early in pregnancy, maternal DHA plasma concentration increases regardless of diet in order to supply the rapidly proliferating fetal brain cells. However, the overall maternal DHA level falls during pregnancy, especially in the third trimester as the mother's reserves are depleted. This puts the mother at greater risk for postpartum depression and bipolar depression (Hibbeln, 2002). Therefore, it is vital to ensure adequate levels of dietary DHA for women during pregnancy and breast-feeding and in infant formulas, particularly in premature infants.

Fish oil supplements high in DHA but low in EPA may adversely affect omega-3FA balance. It is preferable to take a 1,000 mg/day blend of DHA and EPA. Fatty acids in breast milk come from two sources: the mother's diet and the mother's adipose tissue. Fish oil supplements increase the concentration of DHA and EPA in maternal adipose tissue and breast milk both directly and indirectly.

Low levels of omega-3FAs have been found in patients with dementia and Alzheimer's disease (Conquer, Tierney, Zecevic, Bettger, & Fisher, 2000). In an eight-year prospective study of 1,200 elderly subjects, those with low serum DHA had a 67% greater chance of developing Alzheimer's disease than those with high DHA (Kyle & Arterburn, 1998). DHA supplementation improved neurological symptoms in Alzheimer's patients (Nidecker, 1997; Soderberg, Edlund, Kristensson, & Dallner, 1991). In a double-blind randomized placebo-controlled (DBRPC) study of 174 very mildly impaired Alzheimer's disease patients, 600 mg EPA slowed cognitive decline over a six-month period (Freund-Levi et al., 2006). More studies are needed to confirm the neuroprotective effects of antioxidants and omega-3FAs in patients with neurodegenerative processes (Youdim, Martin, & Joseph, 2000).

Dietary studies have found significant deficiencies in omega-3FAs (30–90% below recommended dietary allowances) in many countries, including the United States, Canada, Europe, and Australia. Wild fatty fish (salmon and trout) are the best sources of EPA and DHA. High omega-3FA eggs have become a new source. Feeding omega-3FAs increases the level in chickens only two-fold, but in their eggs it increases 20-fold (Bourre & Galea, 2006). Nuts (particularly walnuts), flaxseed, and dark green vegetables are good sources. Patients unwilling to eat fish regularly can be encouraged to take fish oil or flaxseed oil capsules. Because some people have low levels of the enzymes necessary to convert linoleic acid from flaxseed into DHA, fish oils are preferable. Credible evidence suggests that polyunsaturated fatty acids enhance cognitive development and protect against neurodegeneration. While increasing consumption of unsaturated, nonhydrogenated fats may lower the risk of Alzheimer's, the high consumption of saturated or trans fats increases the risk of Alzheimer's (Morris, Evans, Bienias, Tangney, Bennett et al., 2003). A recent epidemiologic study found a reduced risk of Alzheimer's in individuals who eat a Mediterranean type of diet (Scarmeas, Stern, Tang, Mayeux, & Luchsinger, 2006). Beneficial components of this diet may include polyunsaturated fats, fish, fresh vegetables, red grape skin, and red wine. Polyphenols (i.e., resveratrol) have neuroprotective and cardiovascular protective properties. They are found in grape leaves, red grape skin and red wine, pomegranates, blueberries (most other berries), green tea, ginkgo, *Rhodiola rosea*, pycnogenol (extract of French maritime pine bark), and other plants.

Vitamins

Vitamins and trace elements are necessary for the production of energy and the modulation of cognitive function in the elderly (vitamin B_1, thiamine; B_{12}, cobalamin), brain development and memory during aging (B_9, folate), membrane protections (vitamin E, alpha-tocopherol), and frontal lobe and language function (B_{12}). Specific brain functions have been associated with certain vitamins: B_1, B_2 (riboflavin), B_3 (niacin), and B_9 (folate) for abstract thinking; vitamin C for visuospatial performance; B_6, B_{12}, A, and E for visuospatial memory (Bourre, 2006).

A three-year cross-sectional prospective study of 4,740 elderly subjects found that a combination of vitamin C □□500 mg/day plus E □□400 IU/day (but not either alone, nor B complex) reduced the prevalence and incidence of Alzheimer's (Zandi et al., 2004). Other studies support this finding (Sano, 2003).

B Vitamins, Folate, and Homocysteine

The synthesis of cellular proteins, the maintenance of cell membranes, and the production of antioxidants occur through methylation (donation of methyl groups) pathways that depend on B vitamins as cofactors. Abnormalities of mood, memory, and cognitive function have been associated with B vitamin deficiencies (Bottiglieri, 1996; Hassing, Wahlin, Winblad, & Backman, 1999). The concentration of homocysteine and its cofactors, folate, B_6 (pyridoxine) and B_{12}, were analyzed in 812 adults (mean age 61) who had no evidence of dementia or stroke. Homocysteine levels were inversely related to cognitive performance, with adjustment for age, gender, and cardiovascular disease. Folate, B_6, and B_{12} levels were positively related to cognitive performance, but after adjustment for cardiovascular disease and cardiovascular risk factors, the relationship persisted for B_6 only (Elias, Robbins, Budge, Elias, Brehman et al., 2006). Higher folate (B_9), B_6, and B_{12} concentrations have been associated with better cognitive performance. Supplementation with B vitamins improves mood and cognitive function in healthy subjects (Benton, Griffiths, & Haller, 1997). In a three-month DBRPC trial, Bio-Strath, a supplement containing B vitamins and antioxidants, was given at double the usual dose to 75 patients (55–85 years of age) with mild dementia. While the placebo group deteriorated, the Bio-Strath group showed improvement in short-term memory and in physical and emotional well-being (Pelka & Leuchtgens, 1995). It is probably worthwhile to treat geriatric and brain-injured patients with B vitamins in combination with vitamins C and E.

S-Adenosyl-L-Methionine

SAMe (S-adenosyl-L-methionine) is the most active methyl donor driving the methylation pathways (see Figure 2.1). It is crucial for maintenance of neuronal membrane integrity and fluidity, neurotransmitter synthesis, and energy metabolism. SAMe is formed by the condensation of the amino acid methionine and adenosine triphosphate (see Chapter 2 for biochemistry of SAMe). The many applications of SAMe in psychiatry, neurology, and internal medicine have been reviewed (Brown et al., 2000). SAMe reduced impairments and enabled recovery from reserpine-induced lesions in motor cortex and dorsolateral prefrontal cortex in primates. SAMe was found to enhance the migration of macrophages engaged in tissue repair (Takahashi, Nishino, & Ono, 1986; 1987). In aged rats, SAMe improved cholinergic function and reduced learning deficits (Pavia, Martos, Gonzales-Correa, Garcia, Rius et al., 1997). In the brain tissues of rats given 10 mg/kg/day subcutaneous SAMe, free radical production decreased by about 50%, glutathione increased 50%, and both glutathione peroxidase and transferase increased nearly 100% (De La Cruz, Pavia, Gonzales-Correa, Ortiz, Sanchez de la Cuesta et al., 2000). Glutathione is one of the most important antioxidants, particularly in protection of nerve cell membranes.

Forty-one patients were enrolled in a DBRPC pilot study within 24 hours of ischemia or hemorrhagic stroke. Subjects were given either SAMe 2,400 mg/day IV, SAMe 3,200 mg/day IV, or placebo for 14 days. SAMe significantly improved survival and was well tolerated (Monaco, Pastore, Rizzo, et al., 1996). A less rigorous single-blind study of 40 elderly subjects with mild to moderate organic brain syndromes given SAMe for two months found improvement in 13 of 19 items on the Sandoz Clinical Assessment Geriatric Scale. Scales of energy, drive, confusion, and self-care indicated improvements of 25–40% (Fontanari, DiPalma, Giorgetti et al., 1994). In a DBRPC one-month study, 30 patients with postconcussion syndrome received either SAMe 150 mg/day IV or placebo. Mean clinical scores of postconcussion symptoms decreased 77% in those given SAMe versus 49% in those on placebo. On average, the SAMe group had shortened hospital stays (Bacci Ballerini, Lopez, Anguera, Alcaraz, & Hernandez Reyes, 1983).

Increasing evidence indicates the importance of SAMe for healthy brain function, prevention and treatment in the aging brain, and in Alzheimer's disease (Chan & Shea, 2007). Sidebar 4.1 reviews some pathways believed to be involved in neurodegenerative processes.

Neurodegenerative disorders often require many layers of treatment to obtain improvements. Taking the time to offer elderly

SIDEBAR 4.1 **NEUROPROTECTIVE EFFECTS OF SAMe**

Folate deficiency leads to a decline in SAMe with decreased DNA methylation and increased DNA breakage during aging and Alzheimer's disease (see Figure 2.1). The reduction in folate and SAMe potentiates Alzheimer's risk factors: increased neurotoxicity from elevated homocysteine; presenilin-1 overexpression; reduced use of glutathione to counter oxidative stress; and increased beta-amyloid deposits. The C677T polymorphism of 5,10-methylene tetrahydrofolate reductase (MTHFR) uses folate to regenerate methionine from homocysteine. SAMe is produced from the condensation of adenosine triphosphate and methionine. MTHFR is an ApoE4-dependent risk factor for Alzheimer's. In Alzheimer's, as SAMe decreases, S-adenosylhomocysteine increases, further inhibiting methylation. In their studies of rodents, Chan and Shea (2007) showed differential effects of SAMe supplements on cognitive impairment and aggressive behavior. In a study of adult and aged mice with genetic variants of murine ApoE, human ApoE, with and without normal and heterozygously lacking MTHFR, supplementation with SAMe improved cognitive performance in all genotypes, and SAMe indirectly contributed to acetylcholine synthesis.

patients sequential layers of CAM can be quite rewarding. The following complex case illustrates the role of SAMe as a first-line treatment in Parkinson's disease (see Chapter 2) and the complementary effects of *Rhodiola rosea* (see section Herbal Alternative Treatments), dihydroepiandosterone (DHEA; see Chapter 6), and huperzine-A (see Cholinergic Enhancing Agents).

Case 1—Parkinson's Disease: SAMe, R. rosea, DHEA, Huperzine-A, and Neurotherapy

Dr. P. was a successful writer. At the age of 81, having published many books on political science, she was still teaching privately but was frustrated with writing, able to work only two to three hours a day. She had developed Parkinson's disease in her early 70s, which had become increasingly severe with memory loss and depression. During the day she was having "sleep attacks," episodes of suddenly falling into deep sleep that occur in patients treated with dopamine agonist drugs such as ropinirole (Requip) and levodopa. Also, her osteoarthritis had become increasingly painful and she was able to walk only with difficulty using a cane. Consequently, she could no longer use public transportation.

In order to improve her energy level and memory, Dr. P. was started on Rosavin (Ameriden brand of *R. rosea*) at 300 mg a.m. and gradually increased to 400 mg b.i.d. over the next two years. To further enhance her energy and to alleviate depression and osteoarthritis, she was started on SAMe 400 mg b.i.d. and increased to 800 mg b.i.d. The net result was significant improvement in energy, physical strength, bradykinesia, tremulousness, handwriting, and arthritis pain. The sleep attacks ceased. A trial of huperzine-A for memory was discontinued due to gastrointestinal distress. Dr. P. was found to have low levels of DHEA (44) and free testosterone, which were treated with DHEA 25 mg/day. This further improved her energy level. She left her cane in the closet and resumed many of her formerly abandoned activities, including attending concerts and lectures, riding the subway, and enjoying her sex life. However, she still complained of some inattentiveness and a tendency to mentally drift during lectures. She was referred for 10 neurotherapy treatments. She then reported subjective improvements in attention and concentration, enabling her to lecture effectively and increase her daily hours of productive work.

Picamilon

Picamilon contains the inhibitory neurotransmitter gamma-aminobutyric acid (GABA) and vitamin B_3 (niacin). It increases cerebral blood flow by decreasing cerebral blood vessel tone. In a double-blind, controlled study, picamilon was more effective than vinpocetine in improving cerebral blood flow (Mirzoian, Gan'shina, Kosoi, Aleksandrin, & Aleksandrin, 1989). Picamilon has both a mild tranquilizing action (decreasing aggressive behavior) and mild stimu-lative properties, improving alertness and cognition. Picamilon was found to cross the blood–brain barrier rapidly (Dorofeev & Kholodov, 1991) and to have low toxicity in animal experiments (median lethal oral dose is more than 10 g/kg of body weight). Russian researchers using picamilon 20 to 50 mg two to three times a day in therapies ranging from two weeks to three months, found the best results in patients with organic brain syndromes due to head trauma, cerebral atherosclerosis, and toxic brain lesions (Kruglikova, 1997). Picamilon can be beneficial in patients with cerebral vascular impairment, particularly with decreased alertness, anxiety, and depression. Further studies are warranted.

The following case of multi-infarct dementia shows how picamilon can be combined with other CAM treatments to improve energy, cognitive function, mood, and social behavior.

Case 2—Multi-Infarct Dementia

George was a prominent figure in the entertainment industry, who began having personality changes, impaired cognitive function and memory, poor judgment, and social withdrawal at the age of 60. While he was being evaluated, he had sev-eral motor vehicle accidents due to seizures. All brain scans appeared normal for the next two years. He was eventually diagnosed as having progressive multi-infarct dementia. Unable to work, George became apathetic and depressed, and could not participate in any social activities because of agitation and extremely inappropriate behavior. His wife bore the burden of caring for him because he could not communi-cate with other caregivers.

First, George was treated with lamotrigine (Lamictal) 400 mg/day to control the seizures. Then he was started on SAMe 400 mg b.i.d. to improve apathy and brain function. The addition of Rosavin Plus (Ameriden brand *R. rosea*) 300 mg/day and picamilon 300 mg/day significantly improved his energy, cognitive function, and mood. He became socially more appropriate and was able to participate in family gath-erings and public events, including receiving an award for his work in film.

George did well for eight years but then began to decline with memory loss and catatonic-like depressions. He stopped talking altogether. The depression was aggressively treated with Effexor XR 300 mg/day. He had been chain smoking. Wellbutrin 200 mg/day was used to help him stop smoking. The memory problem was first treated with galantamine with increases to 48 mg/day, bringing some improvement in short-term memory. When 30 mg/day memantine (Namenda) was added, he became less agitated, less anxious, more appropriate, and he resumed speaking to his wife and others. His wife was able to take breaks as he became able to accept and relate to caregivers. This relative improvement in a progressive degenerative process provided important relief for the patient and his family.

ENHANCEMENT OF MITOCHONDRIAL ENERGY PRODUCTION AND ANTIOXIDANT PROTECTION

Maintaining energy supplies supports optimal brain function and repair mechanisma.

Coenzyme Q10, Idebenone, Ubiquinol

Coenzyme Q10 (CoQ10) and its variants enhance the adenosine triphosphate-producing mitochondrial electron transport chain responsible for providing the energy needed for cellular functions (Gillis, Benefield, & McTavish, 1994; Matsumoto et al., 1998; Mordente, Martorana, Minotti, & Giardina, 1998; Rego, Santos, & Oliveira, 1999). Ubiquinol, the reduced form of CoQ10, is an important antioxidant protecting membrane lipids from peroxidation. CoQ10 variants are of interest for prevention in neurodegenerative and cardiovascular diseases because of their essential roles in both cellular energy production and antioxidant defense.

In animal studies Idebenone, a variant of CoQ10, has been shown to improve cognitive function following lesions in the basal forebrain cholinergic system and cerebral ischemia, protect cultured astrocytes against reperfusion damage, augment the action of vinpocetine (see below for information on this semisynthetic vasodilator used to treat

---

CLINICAL PEARL

In patients who are overstimulated by prescription cholinesterase inhibitors (e.g., donepezil, Aricept), idebenone provides a less stimulating alternative.

---

cerebrovascular disorders), enhance long-term potentiation (necessary for learning and memory), and improve transcallosal response (interhemispheric communication). Although two studies of idebenone in mild-to-moderate Alzheimer's patients showed some improvements on measures of efficacy similar to cholinesterase inhibitors (Gutzmann & Hadler, 1998; Okuyama & Aihara, 1988), a one-year multicenter DBRPC trial of 536 patients with mild-to-moderate Alzheimer's found that those on idebenone did better on ADAS-Log (measure of activities of daily living) but not on CGI-change (Clinical Global Impression), indicating that the effects were not clinically significant (Thal, Grundman, Berg, Ernstrom, Margolin et al., 2003).

In clinical practice, the authors find that idebenone is especially beneficial for cerebrovascular disease (e.g., multi-infarct dementia) and disorders of mitochondrial function (e.g., Friedreich's ataxia). Idebenone tends to improve alertness.

Newer modifications of CoQ10 such as ubiquinol have greater potency in animals. Antioxidants that target mitochondria are being developed to pass easily through the blood–brain barrier and cell membranes and become highly concentrated inside the mitochondria (Murphy & Smith, 2007). The next generation of CoQ10 derivatives may prove to be even more effective for neuroprotection in clinical trials.

Acetyl-l-Carnitine

Acetyl-l-carnitine (Alcar) facilitates the uptake of acetyl coenzyme A into mitochondria during fatty acid oxidation and increases energy production via the oxidative phosphorylation chain (Di Donato, Frerman, Rimoldi, Rinaldo, Taroni et al., 1986; Pettegrew, Levine, & McClure, 2000). Neuroprotection and enhanced recovery have been demonstrated in rat models of stroke (Lolic, Fiskum, & Rosenthal,

1997). Oxidative stress is important in the pathogenesis of Alzheimer's disease. In a model of oxidative toxicity using 4-hydroxy-2-nonenal, Alcar combined with alpha-lipoic acid protected cortical neurons from protein oxidation, lipid peroxidation, antioxidant depletion, and apoptosis (Abdul & Butterfield, 2007). Animal studies suggest that Alcar may be more effective in delaying age-related deterioration of mitochondria when combined with alpha-lipoic acid, CoQ10, and essential fatty acids (Di Donato et al., 1986; Lolic et al., 1997).

In clinical studies of mild Alzheimer's, Alcar showed minimal effects, though it slowed progression of the disease in those subjects who were 60 years of age or younger (Brooks, Yesavage, Carta, & Bravi, 1998). In a double-blind placebo-controlled study of 12 elderly subjects with cerebral vascular disease, Alcar improved reaction time, memory, and cognitive performance (Arrigo, Casale, Buonpcore & Ciano, 1990). Alcar 1,500 mg IV increased regional cerebral blood flow in eight out of ten men with cerebral ischemia (Rosadini, Marenco, Nobili, Novellone, & Rodriguez, 1990). Although studies of Alcar in Alzheimer's disease are weak, it may prove useful in prevention or as an augmentation to cholinesterase inhibitors in mild Alzheimer's (Bianchetti, Rozzini, & Trabucchi, 2003; Hudson & Tabet, 2003; Montgomery, Thal, & Amrein, 2003). In patients with traumatic brain injury and cerebrovascular disease, the authors have found that Alcar 1,500 mg b.i.d. often improves energy and cognitive function within two weeks. Alcar is a low-risk augmentation with few side effects. Rarely, it may cause mania in bipolar patients.

CHOLINERGIC ENHANCING AGENTS

Cholinergic deficits underlie the main symptoms of Alzheimer's disease and are the most consistent pathophysiological findings. Cholinergic agents have been found to improve cognitive function and delay deterioration in some studies of Alzheimer's.

Galantamine: Snowdrop
For hundreds of years, an alkaloid extract of snowdrop (*Galanthus nivalis*) was used in folk medicine of Russia and Eastern Europe to enhance memory as people aged. Galantamine (Razadyne) is an

allosteric modulator of nicotinic receptors and a weak inhibitor of acetylcholinesterase. It was FDA approved for treatment of Alzheimer's disease (Giacobini, 1998; Raskind, Peskind, Wessel, & Yuan, 2000; Tariot, Solomon, Morris, Kershaw, Lilienfeld, 2000). Many patients do not tolerate prescription galantamine because it causes gastrointestinal disturbances. The herbal extract of *Galanthus nivalis* combined with *R. rosea* can be as effective and more tolerable in some cases. The cognition-enhancing effects of galantamine, donepezil (Aricept), huperzine, nefiracetam, and aniracetam (see section on learning disabilities in Chapter 5 for more information on racetams, nootropics that enhance membrane fluidity and improve interhemispheric transmission) may be due to their potentiation of cholinergic and N-methyl-D-aspartate (NMDA) activity (Narahashi, Moriguchi, Zhao, Marszalec, & Yeh, 2004).

Citicholine, CDP-choline

Cytidine 5'-diphosphocholine (CDP-choline), a phospholipid cholinergic precursor, has been used to treat stroke, dementia, and brain injury in Europe and Japan (Alvarez, Mouzo, Pichel, Perez, Laredo et al., 1999). CDP-choline is well absorbed, crosses the blood–brain barrier, and breaks down into choline (a precursor of acetylcholine) and cytidine (a ribonucleoside). Choline is incorporated into the membrane phospholipid structure, improves mitochondrial metabolism and synthesis of phospholipids, and elevates norepinephrine, dopamine, and serotonin. In animal models, it has been shown to alleviate cerebral hypoxia and protect against ischemia, edema, and neuronal death in the cerebral cortex, forebrain, and hippocampus, in part by reducing glutamate release and increasing adenosine triphosphate levels (Baskaya, Dogan, Rao & Dempsey, 2000; Hurtado, Moro, Cardenas, Sanchez, Fernandez-Tome et al., 2005; Rao, Hatcher, & Dempsey, 1999). In rat brain injury and aging models, CDP-choline improved memory and cognitive performance and potentiated neuroplasticity mechanisms (Dixon, Ma, & Marion, 1997).

In a six-week study of 214 patients with acute middle cerebral artery ischemic stroke, those given CDP-choline within the first 24 hours showed significantly less enlargement in lesion volume on repeat MRI 12 weeks after the stroke (Mitka, 2002). A meta-analysis of controlled trials of CDP-choline by the Cochrane Stroke Review Group concluded that there is some evidence that CDP-choline has positive effects on memory and behavior in the short to medium term in cerebral disorders in the elderly. The evidence for improved global impression was stronger. It warrants more long-term studies, particularly for vascular cognitive impairment, vascular dementia, and age-related memory decline (Fioravanti & Yanagi, 2005). It may be necessary to start CDP-choline within 24 hours of stroke onset for benefits to occur (Parnetti, Mignini, Tomassoni, Traini, & Amenta, 2007).

CDP-choline treatment has been associated with earlier recovery of consciousness, clinical and EEG improvements, accelerated motor rehabilitation, and shortened hospital stays in studies of head-injured patients, including three DBRPC and two comparative studies (Calatayud Maldonado, Calatayud Perez, & Aso Escario, 1991; Levin, 1991; Lozano, 1991). According to toxicity studies, CDP-choline is quite safe and causes virtually no side effects.

Huperzine-A

Huperzine-A, an alkaloid derived from the Chinese club moss (*Huperzia serrata*), is a strong, specific, reversible acetylcholinesterase (AChE) inhibitor with additional neuroprotective properties, including cell protection against hydrogen peroxide free radicals, beta-amyloid protein formation, glutamate, and ischemia. It protects mitochondria, reduces oxidative stress, and upregulates nerve growth factor. Huperzine-A is rapidly absorbed, readily penetrates the blood–brain barrier, and has a relatively long duration of AChE inhibitory action. In animal and primate studies it improves learning and memory (Tang, 1996; Xu, Zhao, Xu, Shao, & Qin, 1996). Three double-blind controlled trials with more than 450 people and one open trial done in China showed significant benefits in Alzheimer's disease. Four trials in vascular dementia and Alzheimer's using huperzine-A in combination with other medicines, nicergoline (a nootropic that protects neurons by inhibition of inflammatory mediators and upregulation of neurotrophic factors by glial cells), and estrogen compounds or mental training showed favorable outcomes. Other trials showed positive outcomes in vascular dementia, traumatic brain injury, age-related memory decline, and schizophrenia (Akhondzadeh & Abbasi, 2006; Wang et al., 2006). Huperzine-A is well tolerated with few side effects and minimal peripheral cholinergic effects.

Case 3—Traumatic Brain Injury

Linda, a successful corporate financial advisor, was found unconscious at the age of 35, having been struck by a motor vehicle while jogging. After 12 hours of observation in an emergency room, she was sent home thinking she was fine. However, she developed problems with memory and lost her ability to think clearly. Unable to continue as a financial analyst, she was losing her career, but she appeared to be unconcerned. Sometimes she was depressed and other times she seemed inappropriately giddy. She had no prior history of depression or mood swings. Finally, after six years of deterioration, her friends convinced her to seek treatment with a psychiatrist who treated her with Zoloft. She became manic and was referred for consultation. Neuropsychological testing revealed major cognitive and memory impairments. The consultant's diagnosis was traumatic brain injury with secondary mixed dysphoric mania.

The first layer of treatment was directed at improving neuronal repair and function including the mitochondrial, antioxidant, and cholinergic systems. She was treated with *R. rosea* (Arctic Root SHR-5 by ProActive BioProducts) 450 mg/day. As her mind began to work better during the first three months, she was able to absorb information and to recognize her problems. The second layer, addition of CDP-choline 1,000 mg b.i.d. over the next eight months led to further improvements in her abilities to think clearly, remember, write coherently, resume working, socialize appropriately, and resume educational activities.

The third layer of treatment addressed her mood using SAMe 1,200 mg/day with improvement in depression. Note that the patient was not given SAMe initially because it could have triggered mania, as the other antidepressants had done. However, after the overall improvement in neuronal repair from the *R. rosea* and CDP-choline, it was considered safe to add SAMe.

Although she had recovered about 60% of her cognitive ability, she complained of difficulty focusing and concentrating. The fourth layer of treatment was directed to the residual problems with mental focus and memory. Although Aricept 2.5 mg helped a bit, Linda could not tolerate the side effects of nausea and diarrhea. She was started on huperzine-A 50 mcg b.i.d. for three months and then increased to 100 mcg b.i.d. This led to marked improvement in her memory and mental focus. With renewed confidence, she has been restored to full functioning in her career.

This case illustrates the benefits of combining agents that target more than one aspect of neuronal dysfunction. Most research studies focus on the effects of only one intervention and are therefore of limited use in exploring the full potential impact of layered treatments. However, layered treatments may be necessary for return to full or optimal functioning.

HERBAL ALTERNATIVE TREATMENTS

Medicinal herbs have been used to enhance memory and cognitive function for thousands of years.

Adaptogens: *Rhodiola rosea, Schizandra chinensis, Eleutherococcus senticosus, Panax ginseng*, Ashwaganda (*Withania somnifera*), and Maca (*Lepidium meyenii*)

Adaptogens are plants containing bioactive compounds that act as metabolic regulators. In their extensive review of the effects of adaptogens on the central nervous system, Panossian and Wagner (2005) suggested that extracts from several adaptogenic herbs have synergistic effects on stress response when combined, for example, *Rhodiola rosea, Schizandra chinesis,* and *Eleutherococcus senticosus.* An adaptogen is a substance that increases resistance against multiple stressors (biological, chemical, or physical), normalizes physiology (whether a body parameter is too high or too low, the adaptogen should bring it towards normal), and does not disturb normal body functions more than necessary to improve stress resistance (Brekhman & Dardymov, 1969). A 1994 report on extensive studies done on Soviet cosmonauts and military personnel found that ADAPT, a combination of *R. rosea, E. senticosus,* and *S. chinesis* sig-

CLINICAL PEARL

Adaptogens can be used to enhance mood, energy, and physical and mental performance under stress in healthy individuals as well as those with fatigue, cognitive impairment, or memory disorders.

nificantly improved intellectual and physical performance and endurance under conditions of stress (Baranov, 1994).

Rhodiola rosea (Golden Root, Arctic Root, or Roseroot)

Rhodiola rosea, an ancient medicinal herb, grows at high altitudes (8,000–10,000 feet) in the Caucasus, Siberia, Scandinavia, northern Canada, and Alaska. For thousands of years it was used in folk medicines to enhance physical endurance and preserve memory in old age. Through trade routes it became known to Chinese emperors as the golden root. It was described by the Greek physician Dioscorides in *De Materia Medica* in 77 a.d. (Gunther, 1968). It was also used by the Vikings. Analysis of the root by high-pressure liquid chromatography has identified species-specific marker compounds, cinnamyl alcohol betavicianidines, called rosavin, rosin, and rosarin. *R. rosea* extracts contain bioactive alkaloids, polyphenols, and phenylpropanoids including tyrosol and salidroside (Bikov, Zapesochnaya, & Kurkin, 1999; Dubichev, Kurkin, Zapesochnaya, & Vornotzov, 1991; Kurkin & Zapesochnaya, 1986). The whole root extract has greater physiological activity than individual compounds. *R. rosea* extracts are standardized to contain at least 1% salidroside and 3% rosavin and should be free of drying agents (e.g., maltodextrin) or other carriers. The history, research, and clinical uses of *R. rosea* have been thoroughly presented in *The Rhodiola Revolution* by Brown and Gerbarg (2004).

Two flavonoid glycosides (gossypetin-7-O-1-rhamnopyranoside and rhodio-flavonoside) isolated from the alcohol extract of *R. rosea* were shown to cause 58 ± 15% and 38 ± 4% AChE inhibition respectively when tested at 5 g/L. This AChE inhibition may account in part for mental and memory-enhancing properties. Active guided fractionation revealed a multitude of components that may be responsible for AChE inhibition (Hill-House, Ming, French, & Towers, 2004).

R. *rosea* enhances energy metabolism and increases the capacity of mitochondria to produce energy-rich compounds, adenosyl triphosphate and creatine phosphate, in the brain (including the brain stem reticular formation and cerebral hemispheres) as well as in muscle, liver, and blood (Furmanowa, Skopinska-Rozewska, Rogala, & Malgorzata, 1998; Kurkin & Zapesochnaya, 1986). In cerebral cortex and brain stem, R. *rosea* increases norepinephrine (NE), dopamine (DA), and serotonin (5-HT) and, in the hypothalamus, NE and DA (Petkov, Yonkov, Mosharoff, Kambourova, Alova et al., 1986; Stancheva & Mosharrof, 1987). R. *rosea* has antiarrhythmic and positive inotropic effects on the heart. It prevents catecholamine release and adenosine 3', 5'-cyclic monophosphate elevation in the myocardium and stress-related depletion of adrenal catecholamines (Maslova, Kondrat'ev, Maslov & Lishmanov, 1994).

In the 1960s, the Department of Defense of the Soviet Union began extensive animal and human studies of R. *rosea* and other adaptogens for enhancement of mental and physical performance under stress in Olympic athletes, scientists, military personnel, and cosmonauts (Saratikov & Krasnov, 1987a). This strategic research, kept in classified files until after the collapse of the Soviet Union in 1992, was translated into English by Dr. Zakir Ramazanov (July 2001, personal communication). Reviews of more recent research are available (Brown & Gerbarg, 2004; Brown, Gerbarg, & Ramazanov, 2002; Furmanowa, Oledzka, Michalska, Sokolnicka & Radomska, 1995; Germano, Ramazanov, & Bernal Suarez, 1999; Kelly, 2001). Epidemiologic studies found that the high percentage of centenarians and of mentally and physically well elderly among mountain dwellers in the Republic of Georgia was based on environmental and dietary (rather than genetic) factors (Agakishiev, 1962; Ferrell et al., 1985). These studies have been challenged on the basis that birth records were not available to verify the ages of many of the subjects. R. *rosea* is believed to contribute to the longevity of Georgians living at high altitudes who use R. *rosea* root extract to brew their daily tea.

Soviet scientists found R. *rosea* extracts to have the following effects on brain function: cognitive stimulation with emotional calming; enhanced learning and memory; and increased accuracy in men-

tal performance for prolonged periods of time. The plant was classified as an adaptogen because it protected every organism tested,
from snails to humans, against physical and mental stresses, fatigue,
heat, cold, toxins, and radiation.

Studies found that *R. rosea* enhanced intellectual work capacity,
abstract thinking, and reaction time in healthy subjects (Saratikov &
Krasnov, 1987c; Spasov, Mandrikov & Mionova, 2000; Spasov, Wikman, Mandrikev, Mironova, & Neumoin, 2000). Benefits of *R. rosea*
have been described in patients with organic brain syndrome, most
dramatically in posttraumatic and vascular brain lesions, especially
in the early postinjury stages. However, most of this is based on older
open studies using outdated classification systems. Piracetam can be
used to augment *R. rosea* for improvement of cognitive function. *R.
rosea* was reported to exacerbate the condition in patients described
as "volatile or euphoric" (Saratikov & Krasnov, 1987c; Ramazanov,
July 2001, personal communication). There may be some risk of
inducing mania in bipolar patients. However, in the authors' experience, *R. rosea* can be quite helpful in bipolar patients on mood stabilizers whose mood swings are primarily depressive with only
occasional mild hypomanic symptoms.

R. rosea improved short- and long-term memory in rat experiments. After 10 days, the levels of NE, DA, and 5-HT rose significantly in the brain stem. However, in the cerebral cortex, NE and DA
decreased while 5-HT increased markedly. In the hypothalamus, NE
and DA increased to three times the level in untreated controls. *R.
rosea* also increased blood–brain barrier permeability to DA and 5-
HT precursors. These findings are consistent with activation of the
cerebral cortex and limbic systems. *R. rosea* extracts also reversed the
blockage of acetylcholine in pathways (ascending from limbic system
to cortex) involved in memory storage (Brown et al., 2002).

Vigodana (Dr. Loges GmbH & Co. Kg, Winsen, Germany) contains *R. rosea* (100 mg Rosenwurzwurzel-Extract, Wirstaff), magnesium 60 mg, and small amounts of vitamins B_6, B_{12}, and folate. It
was found to be safe in an open 12-week study of 120 adults (ages
50–89 years) with complaints of physical (exhaustion, decreased
motivation, daytime sleepiness, loss of libido, and sleep disturbance)
and cognitive deficits (decreased concentration, forgetfulness,
decreased memory, susceptibility to stress, and irritability). No

adverse events occurred. Tolerability was rated as "good" or "very good" by 99% of the patients and their physicians (Fintelmann & Gruenwald, 2007). Although this was an uncontrolled trial, differences in efficacy between two dosing schedules were suggested. Group 1 took two capsules of Vigodana in the morning and group 2 took one capsule in the morning and after lunch. In group 1, 90% reported improved cognitive functions versus 64.4% in group 2. Scores on digit connection tests improved an average of 30% in group 1 and 16% in group 2. A weakness of this study was that the measures of physical and cognitive deficits were largely based on the patients' subjective ratings on a 4-point scale. The deficits were not well characterized. The only objective measure was the digit connection test. Nevertheless, there was a very high rate of satisfaction, global improvement, safety, and tolerability. Vigodana contains 100 mg *R. rosea* extract, but the standardization was not specified.

In patients with brain injury, *R. rosea* exerts a mild cognitive stimulant effect while it is also emotionally calming. However, very anxious patients may not tolerate higher doses because the activating effects sometimes exacerbate their anxiety. *R. rosea* can be even more effective in improving memory and cognitive functions when combined with *E. senticosus, S. chinensis, Panax ginseng, Ginkgo biloba*, or *Withania somnifera* (Ashwaganda). *R. rosea* has no reported adverse interactions with drugs. However, caffeine and other stimulants can have additive effects. In clinical practice, the authors use *R. rosea* in a wide range of disorders of memory, cognition, and fatigue with generally good results. Further research on the use of this herb would be highly beneficial.

Case 4—Cognitive Decline and Memory Impairment Due to Lyme Disease

Lyme disease has become epidemic in many areas of the United States and other countries. When deer ticks feed on animals and humans, borrelia organisms transfer from the stomach of the tick to the bloodstream of the victim. These spirochetes can lodge in any tissues of the body, including the walls of cerebral blood vessels, reducing the blood supply to vital areas of the brain and causing a confusing array of neurological and psychological symptoms: cognitive slowing, progressive memory impairment, word-finding difficulties, ataxia, reduced concentration, pain, headache, chronic fatigue, Bell's palsy, and secondary anxiety and depression. Patients with cerebral Lyme may not receive correct diagnosis and treatment for many years. While rigorous courses of antibiotics may eradicate Lyme organisms, patients are often left with significant impairments due to neuronal damage. CAM treatments that enhance neuronal repair by increasing cellular energy, neuroplasticity, and antioxidant defense are critical for recovery.

Leah was a 30-year-old writer who spent weekends on a small farm in Dutchess County, New York, an area with a high rate of Lyme disease. When she developed joint pains, her Lyme tests were read as negative. Over the next few years she became increasingly forgetful, with severe fatigue and poor concentration. She lost her ability to write and had difficulty even reading because by the time she reached the end of a sentence, she had forgotten its beginning. Brain scans and neurological workups were inconclusive. When one neurologist conveyed to her that her symptoms were hysterical and without organic basis, Leah began to doubt the validity of the disabling illness she was experiencing. When she developed Bell's palsy (paralysis of the right side of her face), the diagnosis of Lyme disease was made. She was treated with intravenous antibiotics. Fortunately, the Bell's palsy resolved, but her cognitive functions and memory did not recover. One year later, after reading *The Rhodiola Revolution*, she contacted Dr. Gerbarg for a consultation.

During the first visit, Leah was given a thorough evaluation, including blood tests. The patient was given information about the potential risks and benefits of CAM treatments. She was started on vitamins, nutrients, and antioxidants including a daily multivitamin, omega-3 fish oil 1,000 mg b.i.d., and Bio-Strath (B vitamin complex with antioxidants). At the next visit, *Rhodiola rosea* was added (Rosavin Plus) 150 mg 20 minutes before breakfast with instructions that if she had no side effects (anxiety, jitteriness, insomnia) for four days, she could increase it to twice a day. Once she began the *R. rosea*, Leah noticed an immediate improvement in her energy level followed by an increase in physical stamina. Over the next two weeks, her dose was increased to two tablets in the morning and one tablet taken 20 minutes before lunch. After four weeks on 450 mg/day, her memory and concentration began to improve. Gradually over the following five months, her concentration and cognitive functions returned to normal. Her memory recovered to nearly normal except for some residual delay in retrieval time, particularly when she was tired. What was most important to Leah was recovering her ability to write and live the life she had known before her encounter with Lyme.

Schizandra chinensis

Schizandra is a Chinese medicinal herb (Bei Wu Wei Zi or Chosen-Gomishi) found to improve concentration and physical endurance. It was used by Chinese emperors to enhance energy. This adaptogen has antidepressant, emotional calming, and anti-inflammatory effects. Extracts of the fruit of Schizandra chinensis were found to show significant inhibition of the activity of AChE (Hung, Na, Min, Ngoc, Lee et al., 2007). Because S. chinensis is emotionally calming, it is useful to counterbalance the stimulating effect of R. rosea in patients who tend to become anxious or jittery.

Eleutherococcus senticosus

Eleutherococcus senticosus (Acanthopanax senticosus, Asian ginseng, Oriental ginseng, or Siberian ginseng) is a thorny shrub that grows in Siberia and northern China. It has a long history of use as an adaptogen to enhance nonspecific resistance to stress and fatigue in Russia, China, Korea, and Japan. Depending on the method of extraction, bioactive compounds from E. senticosus, including eleutherosides and isoflaxidin, reduced fatigue and improved recovery of natural killer cell activity and corticosterone levels following stress induced by swimming in mice. Extracts have been used by athletes to enhance physical strength and endurance, but so far, human studies have been equivocal. As an immune modulator, E. senticosus has been used for anti-inflammatory effects in rheumatic diseases in Eastern Europe and the Russian Federation. E. senticosus extracts were found to downregulate inflammatory inducible nitric oxide synthase expression (Jung, Jung, Shin, Park, Jun et al., 2007). While human studies of *E. senticosus* monotherapy are limited, it has been shown to contribute to the antifatigue and mental stimulatory effects of adaptogen combination formulas (Panossian & Wagner, 2005).

Ginseng (*Panax*, Korean)

Panax ginseng root has been used as a traditional medicine in China, Korea, and Japan for thousands of years and is now used worldwide. The active ingredients of ginseng are ginsenosides or ginseng saponins. Studies have shown ginseng's beneficial effects in cardio-vascular diseases, cancer, immune deficiency, and hepatotoxicity. Research suggests that some of ginseng's active ingredients also exert beneficial effects on central nervous system disorders and neurode-generative diseases. Protective mechanisms attributed to ginseng, based mainly on cell cultures and rodent studies, include antioxi-dant, anti-inflammatory, antiapoptotic, and immune-stimulatory activities (Radad, Gille, Liu, & Rausch 2006). These mechanisms involve increasing nitric oxide production by endothelial cells (essen-tial for blood flow and oxygen delivery (Kang, Kim, Schini & Kim, 1995), scavenging of free radicals, counteracting excitotoxicity, and glucoregulatory properties.

A double-blind placebo-controlled eight-week study of 36 dia-betic patients found that ginseng improved psychomotor perform-ance but not memory (Sotaniemi, Haapakoski, & Rautio, 1995). In an eight-week double-blind placebo-controlled study of 49 geriatric patients, 80 mg/day of ginseng did not improve cognitive perform-ance compared to placebo. However, 80 mg of ginseng was an inef-fectively low dose (Thommessen & Laake, 1996). An eight-week DBRPC study of healthy volunteers over 40 years of age showed that ginseng 400 mg/day significantly improved abstract thinking and reaction time, but not memory or concentration in comparison to placebo (Sorensen & Sonne, 1996). Combining ginkgo and ginseng may yield greater cognitive enhancement (Wesnes, Faleni, Heft, Hoogsteen, Houben et al., 1997). Evidence suggest *ginseng* may improve cognitive performance d- tally demanding tasks in healthy individuals, b study (Reay, Kennedy & Scholey, 2006).

A review of the use of herbs in Alzheimer's

studies of herbal combinations with preliminary positive effects. One, a four-week single-blind randomized placebo-controlled study in 52 Alzheimer's patients given Yi-Gan-San, showed cognitive improvement and gentle sedation (Iwasake, Sato, Kakagawa, Maruyama, Monma et al., 2005). The other was a study of eight herbal extracts, Ba Wei Di Huang Wan (BDW), also known in the United States as Rehmannia 8. In a two-month DBRPC study of 50 Alzheimer's patients, BDW improved cognition and reduced agitation. Cholinergic enhancement, NMDA receptor antagonism, and other actions are possible mechanisms (Dos Santos-Neto, de Vilhena Toledo, Medeiros-Souza, & de Souza, 2006).

Ashwaganda (Withania somnifera)

Ashwaganda has antistress (calming and mildly sedating) effects and may protect against Alzheimer's (*Withania somnifera*, 2004). This adaptogen, used in traditional medicines for centuries, has been studied extensively in animals. Data suggest that ashwagandha is a cholinesterase inhibitor (Hawkins, 2000).

The "Student Rasayana"

The "Student Rasayana," another Ayurvedic preparation, is occasionally useful in patients of Asian Indian cultures who are more receptive to traditional preparations. A five-month DBRPC study in 34 third grade students showed that those given Rasayana had a 10-point increase in IQ compared to five points in the placebo group with 78% of the student Rasayana group showing improvement in IQ compared with 50% of the placebo group (more than would be expected from test–retest practice effects) (Nidich, Morehead, Nidich, Sands, & Sharma, 1993). In vitro models show that Rasayana decreases lipid peroxidation and enhances long-term potentiation in the hippocampus (Sharma, Hanna, Kauffman, & Newman, 1995). Additional clinical studies are needed.

Maca (Lepidium meyenii)

The Peruvian adaptogen maca (*Lepidium peruvianum myenii* Chacon) has been used for thousands of years by Andean peoples to ¯mprove energy, sexual activity, fertility at high altitudes, stress toler- ¯e, nutritional status, and menopausal symptoms (Quiros & Cardenas, 1997). Sterols, glucosinolates, or alkaloid components increased follicle-stimulating hormone, estrogen, and testosterone levels in female rats and increased testosterone levels in male rats (Chacon, 1997; Quiros & Cardenas, 1997). However, elevated hormone levels have not been found in humans. Small double-blind placebo-controlled studies suggest that maca may have positive effects on stress reduction, mood, cognition, and exercise capacity in humans. No toxicity or side effects were found in human and animal studies (Aguilar, 1999, personal communication). Maca may be contraindicated in patients with fibroids, estrogen receptor–related cancer risk, endometriosis, or prostate cancer (for more information, see Chapter 6 and http://www.Maca750.com).

Adaptogen Combinations for Complex Cases: Cognitive Impairment and Fatigue

Although studies of adaptogen combinations are limited, the authors find that integrating layers of treatment can lead to significant improvements in severe and complex cases involving neurological and medical conditions. The following 10 guidelines are based on the authors' clinical experience.

1. In general, for patients with cognitive impairment or fatigue, CAM treatment begins with a trial of *R. rosea* starting at 150 mg a.m. and increasing to a maximum of 750 mg/day as needed in divided doses (a.m. and midday).
2. If the patient improves but has residual fatigue or cognitive impairment, *E. senticosus* is started at 500 mg b.i.d. and increased to 1,000 mg b.i.d. if needed.
3. If fatigue or cognitive impairment persist, *S. chinensis* is added in doses of 100 mg a.m. and may be increased to 200 mg b.i.d. It may be more convenient to use a combination capsule of *S. chinensis* 100 mg + *E. senticosus* 100 mg (Kare-n-Liver—see Appendix Table A3 on where to obtain quality products). Another option is Adapt-232 (ProActive BioProducts) containing *R. rosea*, *S. chinensis*, and *E. senticosis* in unspecified amounts.
4. For patients who appear to need further improvement in mental energy, Korean ginseng 250 or 500 mg a.m. can help. Rarely, the patient requires 1,000 mg/day Korean ginseng.

5. For patients whose physical energy is low, adding *E. senticosus* 500–1,000 mg/day is often beneficial.

6. When patients need a more calming effect along with physical strengthening, ashwaganda *(Withania somnifera)* works well given in doses of 200–400 mg at night (helps insomnia) with 200–400 mg a.m. as needed.

7. In nonanxious patients whose energy and cognitive functions improve partially on *R. rosea* but who need more physical, cognitive, and sexual energy, maca *(Lepidium myenii)* 750 mg two to eight capsules per day can be effective, particularly in patients who are physically debilitated due to medical or neurological conditions. Maca should not be given to patients with a history of hormone-sensitive cancer (e.g., prostate, breast, ovarian, uterine).

8. Some patients become too stimulated physically (agitation, jitteriness) or mentally (anxiety, insomnia) on *R. rosea.* In such patients with physical weakness due to medical illness, inactivity, or neurological conditions, an adaptogen combination with a lower dose of *R. rosea* can work well, for example, Easy Energy (Ameriden) containing *R. rosea* 70 mg, *S. chinesis, E. senticosus, Aralia mandshurica* (improves physical strength and has antioxidant activity), and *Rhaponticum carthamoides* (increases protein synthesis and physical strength).

9. Patients who have difficulty following complex medication regimens and who have had partial improvement on *R. rosea* but who need further improvement in physical energy or mental clarity can be switched to ADAPT 232 (ProActive BioProducts, Swedish Herbal Institute). ADAPT contains a proprietary combination of *R. rosea, E. senticosus,* and *S. chinesis.* SHI will not reveal the exact proportions of each herb in its proprietary product. In the original ADAPT formula that was used in studies by the Department of Defense of the Soviet Union, two tablets contained *R. rosea* 360 mg (1% salidrosides and 3% rosavins), *S. chinensis* 100 mg, and *E. senticosus* 100 mg. Although the amount of each herb is not listed in the ADAPT232 packaging, this preparation has been shown to be effective in research studies and in the author's experience.

10. Although, in general, we do not recommend products containing small amounts of an excess number of ingredients, there are

some useful proprietary supplements that combine substances with synergistic effects. One example, Cognitex with NeuroProtection Complex (Life Extension Foundation), contains pharmaceutical-grade nutrients. Three capsules of Cognitex contain cerebral blood flow promoters (vinpocetine 20 mg and phosphatidylcholine-grape seed extract 150 mg), an acetylcholine booster (alpha-glyceryl phosphorylcholine 600 mg), an AChE inhibitor (ashwaganda 125 mg), enhancers of neuronal cell membrane function (conjugated phosphatydylserine-DHA 1 mg and uridine-5'-monophosphate 50 mg, a phosphatide building block of RNA-DNA), antioxidants (wild blueberry), and anti-inflammatories (hops, ginger, rosemary).

The following cases are used as clinical illustrations of the decision-making process in a layered approach to the use of adaptogens in complex cases.

Case 5—Poststroke With Seizure Disorder, Cognitive Dysfunction, Verbal Expressive Disorder, Apathy, Insomnia, and Pseudobulbar Palsy

Irving was a prominent music critic until he suffered a right temporal lobe stroke from a ruptured cerebral aneurysm at the age of 60. He developed hydrocephalus (enlargement of the cerebral ventricles). Following the placement of a shunt, he began having grand mal seizures and was treated with an anticonvulsant, leviracetam (Keppra). Three years later, when his wife brought him for a consultation, Irving had severe cognitive slowing, difficulty speaking, apathy, daytime napping, insomnia, depression, complete sexual dysfunction, and emotional incontinence with sudden outbursts of crying for no reason (pseudobulbar palsy). He was unable to work or engage in social activities, could not organize his thoughts, stuttered when he became anxious, and had to give up skiing and bicycling.

Irving's neurologist was advised to slowly discontinue his anticonvulsant medication. Once the leviracetam was removed, his cognitive functions improved about 50%. The first layer of treatment, *R. rosea* (Energy-Kare by Kare-n-

Herbs), led to further improvements in cognition and apathy, but Irving could not tolerate more than one tablet in the morning because of insomnia. Next, the emotional incontinence resolved on sertraline 50 mg/day, but he could not tolerate higher doses. He had frequent daily episodes of sitting and staring, which were somewhat relieved with methylphenidate (Ritalin) 7.5 mg/day plus selegiline 5 mg three times a week, the third layer of treatment. However, on higher doses he became unable to sleep. Donepezil (Aricept) 5 mg/day was given with some improvement in memory.

A two-year course of 40 neurotherapy sessions (see section Neurotherapy), the fourth treatment layer, improved cognitive processing time and the ability to perform complex motor sequences. Irving was able to resume skiing and biking at a reduced level. One year after completing neurotherapy, Irving was driving on a highway when his car was rear-ended by a truck. The concussion caused reoccurrence of his cognitive problems, fatigue, stuttering, insomnia, anxiety, and symptoms of PTSD. A second course of 10 neurotherapy sessions restored him to his preaccident level of functioning.

The fifth layer of treatment targeted Irving's residual symptoms of low physical energy, no libido or sexual function, daytime sleeping, and cognitive impairment. To stimulate his system, Irving was given four tablets of maca 750 mg in the morning. He responded with increased physical energy and activity. The daytime naps and the staring episodes ceased entirely. His libido and sexual function began to improve in response to the R. rosea and maca, but he could not tolerate higher doses of maca because it caused jitteriness and insomnia. His DHEA-sulfate level was found to be low. Augmentation with DHEA 50 mg/day further improved erectile function.

The sixth layer added to the treatment was a nootropic, aniracetam. Racetams interact with phospholipids to restore membrane fluidity, improve interhemispheric transmission, and preferentially activate the left hemisphere verbal processing areas (see the section on racetams [p. 178] and Chapter 5 for more information). Aniracetam is generally well tolerated with no adverse effects. On aniracetam 750 mg b.i.d., Irving's verbal expression improved to the point where he was able to write a few hours a day and to resume his participation on several community boards. Although he recovered about 80% of his cognitive ability, he could not write at the high level his former career required. Nevertheless, he was able to write for less prestigious publications and was well enough to teach courses in music history and criticism at a small local college.

Case 6—Advanced Parkinson's Disease

Simon was a university professor who was diagnosed with Parkinson's disease at the age of 60. By the age of 70, his levodopa (Sinemet) had stopped working. He required constant supervision because of extreme memory loss and helplessness. For example, he could no longer feed or dress himself. Simon was deeply depressed and his wife was in despair. Antidepressants were ineffective and caused agitation.

For the first treatment layer, SAMe was started and increased to 400 mg five times a day, resulting in improvements in initiative, energy, and mental focus. When the second treatment layer, *R. rosea* was overstimulating, Simon was switched to Neurogen A/P Formula (Ameriden), a combination of low-dose *R. rosea* 70 mg with *Galanthus wornorii*. For further cognitive enhancement, the patient received Cognitex (Life Extension Foundation's combination of phosphatidylcholine, phosphatidylserine, alpha-glyceryl phosphorylcholine, vinpocetine, grapeseed extract polyphenols, blueberry extract polyphenols and anthocyanins, uridine-5-monophosphate, hops, ginger, and rosemary), cytidine 5'-diphosphate choline 600 mg b.i.d., and huperzine 100 mg b.i.d. When maca 750 mg b.i.d. was added, he experienced increased energy, alertness, mental focus, memory, and capacity for physical activity. He became interested in visiting his family and going on trips. He regained the ability to feed and dress himself. Simon and his wife enjoyed eight good years before he began to deteriorate again. Although in his final years he again had periods of mental confusion, the treatment provided a much better quality of life for Simon and his wife.

OTHER HERBS FOR COGNITIVE ENHANCEMENT

Evidence indicates that herbs can enhance cognition and memory through a variety of mechanisms, including effects on ion channels, membrane fluidity, and antioxident defenses.

Lemon balm (*Melissa officinalis*), Sage (*Salvia officinalis*), and *Salvia lavandulaefolia*

Preliminary randomized controlled trials suggested that lemon balm and sage may have cognitive benefits and reduce agitation in patients with dementia (Akhondzadeh & Abbasi, 2006; Akhondzadeh, Noroozian, Mohammadi, Ohadinia, Jamshidi et al., 2003). A four-week DBRPC trial of *M. officinalis* aromatherapy in 71 severely demented patients showed decreased agitation and withdrawal with improvements in activities of daily living. A DBRPC trial of lemon balm (300 mg or 600 mg) in 18 healthy volunteers found that the higher dose reduced the effects of stress and improved ratings of calmness. The 300 mg/day dose improved math processing speed while maintaining accuracy (Kennedy et al., 2004). A DBRPC crossover study of 24 healthy undergraduates (ages 18–37) given either placebo or 25 or 50 µl *Salvia lavandulaefolia* found that those given the herb, particularly the higher dose, had significant improvements in speed of memory and secondary memory factors, alertness, calmness, and contentedness compared to those on placebo as indicated by the Cognitive Drug Research Battery and mood ratings. *S. lavandulaefolia* was used instead of *S. officinalis* because it contains the same bioactive compounds as *S. officinalis* but has a lower concentration of thujone, a terpenoid ketone that can be toxic in high doses (Tildesley, Kennedy, Perry, Ballard, Wesnes et al., 2005). The cognitive effects of these herbs warrant further study.

Vinpocetine: Periwinkle (*Vinca minor*)

Periwinkle (*Vinca minor*) is the source of vinpocetine, a semisynthetic alkaloid used in Eastern Europe as a vasodilator to treat cerebral vascular disorders. When cells are injured, activation of phosphodiesterases and aberrant expression of cell cycle proteins can induce cell programmed death. In vitro studies of phosphodiesterase inhibitors (PDEIs) indicate that vinpocetine protected rat neuronal cells (55–77%) from destruction by four neurotoxic mechanisms, hypoxia/hypoglycemia, veratridine, staurosporine, or glutamate. PDEIs also suppressed upregulation of cyclin D1 and proapoptotic caspase-3 activity (Chen, Williams, Liao, Yao, Tortella et al., 2007). One of the mechanisms for seizure control by antiepileptic drugs is reduction in cerebral presynaptic voltage-sensitive Na$^+$ channel permeability and, consequently, reduction in glutamate (excitatory neurotransmitter) release. In a study of hippocampal nerve endings preloaded with labeled glutamate, vinpocetine inhibited the veratridine (Na$^+$ channel opener) release of glutamate at lower concentrations than carbamazepine (Tegretol), phenytoin (Dilontin), lamotrigine (Lamictal), and topiramate (Topomax) (Sitges, Chiu, Guarneros, & Nekrassov, 2007).

Vinpocetine inhibits the molecular cascade precipitated by increases in intracellular calcium. Neuroprotective effects include inhibition of calcium/calmodulin-dependent cyclic GMP-phosphodiesterase 1; enhancement of intracellular cyclic guanidine monophosphate GMP levels in vascular smooth muscle; reduction in resistance of cerebral blood vessels; and increased blood flow. A review of DBRPC trials in a total of 731 patients with chronic cerebral vascular disease, including PET scan studies of 12 patients with middle cerebral artery infarcts, concluded that vinpocetine improves cerebral glucose kinetics and blood flow in the peristroke area (Bonoczk, Gulyas, Adam-Vizi, Nemes, Karpati et al., 2000). In clinical practice, the authors find it also helps patients with ischemia secondary to traumatic brain injury or SPECT scan evidence of reduced cerebrovascular blood flow. Vinpocetine can be beneficial in patients with early symptoms or risk factors of multi-infarct dementia. While in vitro studies indicate substantial neuroprotection with vinpocetine, more clinical trials are needed. The development of solid lipid nanoparticles that enhance vinpocetine oral bioavailability may lead to more effective preparations (Luo, Chen, Ren, Zhou, & Quin 2006).

Ginkgo biloba

Ginkgo biloba improves membrane fluidity and resistance to oxidative damage (Drieu, Vranckx, Benassayad, Haourigi, Hassid et al., 2000). Ginkgo extracts from the leaves of the maidenhair tree, used in traditional Chinese medicine to treat cognitive and memory impairment as well as other disorders, are being studied to treat Alzheimer's and cerebral vascular diseases. The mechanisms of action thought to underlie the effects of several components of the extract include increasing blood supply by dilating blood vessels and reducing blood viscosity, modifying neurotransmitter systems, and reducing oxygen free radicals. An excellent review including DBRPC studies was done by Wong (Wong, Smith, & Boon, 1998). Memory improvements with ginkgo are slight at best and are dose related. Side effects are rare and can be minimized by starting at 60 mg/day and increasing gradually to 120 mg b.i.d. Occasionally, nausea, headaches, and skin rashes occur. Although ginkgo somewhat decreases platelet aggregation, it does not appear to affect coagulation or bleeding time (Cott, 2002), fibrinogen, prothrombin time, or partial thromboplastin time (Halil, Cankurtaran, Yavuz, Ozkayar, Ulger et al. 2005). Nevertheless, caution should be exercised when using ginkgo in patients on anticoagulants, and gingko should be discontinued two weeks prior to surgery.

G. *biloba* extract has neuroprotective effects and benefits for memory, age-associated memory impairment, vascular dementia, and Alzheimer's. In a DBRPC multicenter 52-week study of 236 patients with Alzheimer's, G. *biloba* extract (EGb 761) 120 mg/day improved cognitive performance in patients with mild to moderate cognitive impairment and also slowed the deterioration in patients with severe impairment (Le Bars, Velasco, Ferguson, Dessain, Kieser, et al., 2002). A DBRPC comparison study of 109 schizophrenic patients found that patients given Haldol plus EGb 360 mg/day had significant reductions in Scales for Assessment of Negative Symptoms and Positive Symptoms compared to patients treated with haloperidol only. In addition, the EGb-treated group had fewer extrapyramidal side effects. These benefits were hypothetically attributed to EGb scavenging of free radicals (Zhang, Zhou, Zhang, Wu, Su et al., 2001). Ginkgo potentiates other nootropics, such as centrophenoxine and piracetam (see section on Pyrrolidinones; Diamond, Shiflett, Feiwel, Matheis, Noskin et al., 2000; Wong, Smith, & Boon, 1998). The authors' clinical experience is that in traumatic brain injury it is best used as an augmenting agent.

Another review of double-blind placebo-controlled studies of ginkgo concluded that the evidence that ginkgo has predictable and clinically significant benefit for people with dementia or cognitive impairment was neither consistent nor convincing (Birks & Grimley Evans, 2007). Ginkgo is now the subject of the GuidAge five-year DBRPC study of 2,854 elderly subjects with memory complaints enrolled between March 2000 and September 2004 to determine if 450 mg/day ginkgo reduces conversion to Alzheimer's (Vellas, Andrieu, Ousset, Ouzid, & Mathiex-Fortunet, 2006). In the United States, the Gingko Evaluation of Memory study has a similar goal and design. Ginkgo may prove to have a stronger role in prevention than in treatment of Alzheimer's. Green or black tea, blueberries, resveratrol, and curcumin contain polyphenols similar to ginkgo that have potential benefits in Alzheimer's prevention (Ramassamy, 2006).

Bacopa monniera or Brahmi

Bacopa monniera has been used in Ayurvedic medicine for thousands of years to enhance stress resilience, reduce anxiety, and improve cognitive function (probably mediated by saponins and bacosides). Animals and in vitro studies show antioxidant effects in hippocampus, frontal cortex, and striatum (*Bacopa monniera*, 2004; Jyoti & Sharma, 2006).

Acute administration of 300 mg *Bacopa monniera* did not result in changes in neuropsychological tests two hours after ingestion in a DBRPC study of 38 healthy adults (Nathan, Clarke, Lloyd, Hutchison, Downey et al., 2001). However, a DBRPC study of chronic (12-week) administration of 300 mg/day of 55% bacoside extract (*Bacopa monniera* brand Keenmind) showed significantly positive effects on tests of verbal learning, memory, speed of visual information processing, learning rate, memory consolidation ($p < 0.05$), and state anxiety ($p < 0.001$) in 46 healthy subjects compared to placebo. (No effects were seen acutely and maximal effects were found at 12-week testing; Stough, Lloyd, Clarke, Downey, Hutchison et al., 2001). Another DBRPC study of 76 healthy adults (40–65 years of age) found that after three months, subjects on bacopa showed increased retention of new information compared with those on placebo. Six weeks after discontinuation, those who had been on Bacopa showed a decreased rate of forgetting compared with the placebo group (Roodenrys, Booth, Bulzomi, Phipps, Micallef et al., 2002).

Similar to ginseng and *R. rosea*, Bacopa not only shows cognitive enhancing effects, but also antistress or adaptogenic effects (Chowdhuri, Parmar, Kakkar, Shukla, Seth et al., 2002; Dorababu, Prabha, Priyambada, Agrawal, Aryya et al., 2004; Rai, Bhatia, Palit, Pal, Singh et al., 2003). Other medicinal uses of Bacopa included asthma, gastric ulcers, hypothyroidism, sarcoma, cardiovascular disease, opiate toxicity, and opiate withdrawal (see Chapter 5 for use in learning and ADHD). Side effects of Bacopa are negligible.

NOOTROPICS: CENTROPHENOXINE (MECLOFENOXATE, LUCIDRIL), BCE-001, RACETAMS (PYRROLIDINONES), SELEGILINE, ALPHA-LIPOIC ACID, AND PHOSPHATIDYL SERINE

Nootropics are cognitive enhancing and neuroprotective agents whose mechanisms of action are under active investigation. They are believed to exert their effects through several plausible mechanisms: free radical scavenging, increased antioxidants, improved membrane fluidity, mitochondrial function, neurotransmitter levels, messenger RNA protein synthesis, and cerebral blood flow. The following positive effects on neuroplasticity have been noted.

1. Learning and memory involve increased neurotrophin expression as well as synaptic plasticity leading to changes that persist over time. Neurotrophins, such as brain-derived neurotrophic factor (BDNF), promote neuronal growth, neurogenesis. Short- and long-term memory storage involves the strengthening and weakening of synapses. Long-term potentiation occurs when particular pathways become enhanced and long-term depression when particular synapses become inhibited.

2. Glutamate receptors, alpha-amino-3-hydroxy-5-methyl-4-isoxazole-propionate receptors (AMPARs), mediate most excitatory neurotransmission in the central nervous system and participate in synaptic plasticity believed to be involved in memory and learning. Through positive modulation (potentiation) of AMPARs, nootropics may augment excitatory synaptic transmission, enhance GABAergic inhibition, and slow the deactivation of AMPARs, improving short-term memory (Mizuno, Kuno,

Nitta, Nabeshima, Zhang et al., 2005). The pyrrolidinones (piracetam and aniracetam) have been identified as AMPAR potentiators. AMPARs and NMDA-sensitive ionotropic glutamate receptors are important in learning and memory. Modulators that slow deactivation of AMPARs improve short-term memory in humans (Ingvar, Ambros-Ingerson, Davis, Granger, Kessler et al., 1997). Cognitive enhancement by positive allosteric modulators such as aniracetam and CX614 (pyrrolidino-1,3-oxazino-benzo-1,4-dioxan-10-one) may be attributed to slowing the deactivation of AMPARs (Ling & Benardo, 2005).
3. Nootropics provide neuroprotection. AMPARs protect neurons through release of BDNF, activation of the BDNF receptor TrkB-tyrosine phosphorylation, and via the mitogen-activated protein kinase signaling pathway that increases BDNF expression (Wu, Zhu, Jiang, Okagaki, Mearow et al., 2004).

Centrophenoxine (Meclofenoxate, Lucidril) and BCE-001

Centrophenoxine (CPH) is an ester of dimethyl-aminoethanol (DMAE), a component in choline synthesis, and p-chlorophenoxyacetic acid (PCPA), a synthetic form of a plant growth hormone (Nandy, 1978). Elevation of brain acetylcholine (ACh) was thought to be the basis for the therapeutic effects of CPH in cerebral atrophy, dementia, and traumatic brain injury. Although DMAE increases free choline, only a fraction of this is needed for Ach synthesis. The membrane hypothesis of aging proposes that oxygen free radicals, particularly rapidly acting OH-radicals, inflict the highest rate of damage to cell membranes. CPH delivers DMAE rapidly to the brain, where it is incorporated into nerve cell membranes as phosphatidyl-DMAE. Its beneficial neurological effects can be largely attributed to its avid scavenging of OH-radicals in the membranes (Zs-Nagy, 1994). Rat models of cerebral ischemia demonstrate that CPH reduces cognitive deficits, suggesting a preventive role in cerebrovascular disease (Liao, Wang, & Tang, 2004).

The administration of CPH (100 mg/kg body weight per day, injected i.p.) to aged rats for six weeks resulted in increased activity of catalase, superoxide dismutase, glutathione reductase, and glutathione in brain tissues. Lipid peroxidation was significantly decreased (Bhalla & Nehru, 2005).

An eight-week DBRPC trial of CPH in patients with moderate dementia showed increased psychomotor and behavioral performance in about 50% of treated subjects compared to 27% on placebo (Pek, Fulop, & Zs-Nagy, 1989). A three-month DBRPC study involving 62 geriatric patients with mild to moderate Alzheimer's dementia given either Antagonic Stress (a preparation of CPH, vitamins, and nutrients) or nicergoline found that those on the CPH preparation had significant improvements in memory, cognitive function, and behavior compared to those on nicergoline. Data suggest that nootropics work better when combined with vitamins and minerals (Schneider, Popa, Mihalas, Stefaniga, Mihalas et al., 1994). Piracetam and other nootropics may augment the benefits of CPH (Fischer, Schmidt, & Wustmann, 1984).

BCE-001 is a nootropic drug currently in phase IV testing. Similar to CPA, but with a modification of the PCPA moiety, BCE-001 has twice as many loosely bound electrons to neutralize OH-radicals. In vitro and in vivo studies found effects similar to but more rapid than CPH: improved neuronal membrane fluidity, reversal of membrane protein cross-linking in rat brain cortex, and reversal of the neuronal membrane passive potassium permeability with neuronal rehydration. BCE-001 was more effective than CPH in reversing age-related decline in messenger RNA synthesis in rat brain, thus increasing protein synthesis (Zs-Nagy, 1994, 2002).

Pyrrolidinones (Racetams)

Racetams are nootropic compounds (neural metabolic enhancers). Although piracetam has been most frequently studied, aniracetam, oxiracetam, and pramiracetam are more potent. While results in animal studies are intriguing, numerous human studies in mild dementia and age-associated memory impairment have shown only weak support (Flicker & Grimley Evans, 2001; Itil, Menon, Songar, & Itil, 1986). Levetiracetam (keppra) is U.S. FDA approved for the treatment of epilepsy. Unlike other racetams, levetiracetam often causes cognitive side effects as do other antiepileptic medications (a frequent cause of drug discontinuation).

Piracetam increases nerve cell membrane fluidity, activates electroencephalograms (EEGs), improves red cell deformability, and normalizes hyperactive platelet aggregation. In animal learning models

CLINICAL PEARL

The authors find in practice that aniracetam 750 mg b.i.d. is effective in improving cognitive function in adult and child bipolar patients with anticonvulsant-induced cognitive impairment, unipolar depressives on antidepressants, chronic fatigue syndrome, and patients with dyslexia.

and aged rodents, improvements in memory deficits are potentiated by CDP-choline, idebenone, vinpocetine, and deprenyl (Gouliaev & Senning, 1994; Vernon & Sorkin, 1991). Clinical studies combining racetams with CDP-choline and cholinesterase inhibitors would be worthwhile.

Although studies of piracetam for postconcussion syndrome have had methodological limitations (Cicerchia, Santucci, & Palmieri, 1985; Russello, Randazzo, Favetta, Cristaldi, Petino et al., 1990) one DBRPC study of 60 patients with postconcussion syndrome of 2 to 12 months duration found that piracetam 4,800 mg/day for eight weeks reduced the severity of symptoms, especially vertigo and headache (Hakkarainen & Hakamies, 1978). In larger double-blind placebo-controlled studies, piracetam (given within seven hours of stroke) enhanced language recovery in combination with speech therapy (De Deyn, Reuck, Deberdt, Vlietinck, & Orgogozo, 1997) and improved task-related blood flow in left hemisphere speech areas on PET scan (Kessler, Thiel, Karbe, & Heiss, 2000).

A combination of piracetam and ginkgo significantly enhanced cognitive retraining in patients with dyslexia and aphasia: gingko improved attention and perception while piracetam improved learning (Deberdt, 1994; Enderby, Broeckx, Hospers, Schildermans, & Deberdt, 1994). In a DBRPC study of cognitive impairment and ischemic stroke following coronary artery bypass surgery, 98 patients were randomized to either placebo or piracetam intravenously (150 mg/kg/day; 300 mg/kg on the day of surgery) starting one day before surgery to six days after surgery and then 12 mg/day p.o. for up to six weeks. Patients given piracetam showed significant improvement in cognitive function with a statistically significant treatment effect (p = 0.041) versus no treatment effect with placebo (Szalma, Kiss, Kardos, Horvath, Nyitrai et al., 2006).

Selegiline (L-Deprenyl, Eldepryl, Emsam, Jumex)

Selegiline (L-deprenyl, Emsam) has primarily been used as a prescription MAOI (monoamine oxidase inhibitor) antidepressant in the United States. However, it can also be used as a neuroprotective agent in very low doses that do not cause clinically significant MAO inhibition. As an enhancer regulator, L-deprenyl has a bimodal effect (Denes, Szilagyi, Gal, Bori, & Nagy, 2006). In the ultra-low-concentration range, L-deprenyl exerts neuroprotective effects separate from its MAOI action. In animal studies, L-deprenyl protects catecholaminergic and cholinergic neurons by increasing antioxidants (Kitani, Minami, Maruyama, Kanai, Ivy et al., 2000; Maruyama & Naoi, 1999). Evidence suggests that it improves brain mitochondrial function by reducing production of free radicals. In a model of rat traumatic brain injury, L-deprenyl improved cognitive function and neuroplasticity, particularly in the hippocampus (Zhu, Hamm, Reeves, Povlishock, & Phillips, 2000). L-deprenyl was discovered by Joseph Knoll, who described a mechanism of action at a receptor site for an endogenous enhancer, which selectively improved impulse propagation-mediated release of catecholamines and serotonin. Enhancer effects on catecholamine and serotonin systems are strongest in the hippocampus. In response to stimulation of this receptor, glial cells and astrocytes secrete greater amounts of nerve growth factors. Higher activity levels in enhancer-sensitive neurons are associated with delay in age-related neurodegenerative changes and significantly increase longevity in six different animal species. L-deprenyl may slow the progression of Parkinson's and Alzheimer's diseases (Knoll, 2000, 2003). Several human studies show slight improvements in cognitive function in early Alzheimer's disease (Mangoni, Grassi, Frattola-Piolti, Bassi et al., 1991), but more long-term studies are needed (Ebadi, Brown-Borg, Ren, Sharma, Shavali et al., 2006).

Selegiline (L-deprenyl), given in ultra-low doses using 5 mg tablets (half a pill five days of the week) may help slow neurodegenerative changes of aging, neurological diseases, and traumatic brain injury. At these low doses, it is not necessary to maintain a low-tyramine diet as is warranted with higher doses to prevent hypertensive reactions. The authors use it to enhance neuronal repair and to complement other treatments. Liquid L-deprenyl citrate may be more effective, but no comparative studies have been done. L-deprenyl deserves further study for its neuroprotective effects. In higher doses, used to treat depression, L-deprenyl (selegiline) confers the same neuroprotective effects as it does in lower doses.

Alpha-Lipoic Acid

Alpha-lipoic acid (ALA) is a simple metabolic antioxidant, which has been used as a prescription drug in Europe for the treatment of cardiac autonomic problems related to diabetic neuropathy as well as other consequences of diabetes. ALA has shown neuroprotective effects in cerebral ischemia and reperfusion animal models, excitotoxic amino acid brain injury, mitochondrial dysfunction, diabetic neuropathy, inborn errors of metabolism, and other causes of acute or chronic damage to nerve tissue including excess levels of iron, copper, or other metals. The significance of preliminary data will depend on further clinical research (Packer & Colman, 1999). ALA and CoQ10 may be helpful in poststroke recovery and ischemic heart disease. ALA generates large amounts of glutathione in animal brain models (similar to SAMe). For patients who cannot afford SAMe, ALA in combination with vinpocetine can be helpful when ischemia is a major factor, as well as in other brain injuries. A dose of ALA 300 mg t.i.d. may be useful in traumatic brain injury.

Phosphatidyl Serine

Bovine-derived phosphatidyl serine (Ptd Ser) has been studied for age-associated memory impairment (AAMI; Caffarra & Santamaria, 1987; Cenacchi, Bertoldin, & Palin, 1987), Alzheimer's disease (Amaducci, 1988), and related conditions. Double-blind placebo-controlled studies have shown modest memory improvement in these conditions (Crook, Tinklenberg, Yesavage, Petrie, Nunzi et al., 1991). AAMI includes normal healthy individuals over age 40, who notice some memory problems. Crook et al. found that in AAMI Ptd Ser 300 mg/day for one month followed by 100 mg/day improved memory such that subjects performed on average as though they were 10 years younger (for a review, see Pepeu, Pepeu, & Amaducci, 1996). Ptd Ser, a small component of the inner phospholipid layer, may make the nerve cell membrane more fluid (as discussed in the section on SAMe).

Bovine brain-derived Ptd Ser, rich in docosahexanoic acid (DHA) increased brain dopamine, norepinephrine, and epinephrine levels in animals (Salem, 1989; Salem, Kim, & Yergey, 1986). In contrast, Ptd Ser from soy, which is low in DHA, did not alter catecholamine levels (Toffano, Leon, Benvegnu, Boarato, & Azzone, 1976). There is little research data to show that soy Ptd Ser improves memory. The apparent benefits of bovine Ptd Ser may be enhanced by effects of omega-3FAs (Hibbeln & Salem, 1995).

Although no cases of mad cow disease (bovine spongiform encephalopathy, Jakob-Creutzfeldt Disease) have been reported in association with the use of bovine cortex-derived phosphatidyl serine (BC-PS), the risk of acquiring prions from bovine neural tissue should not be ignored. Prions have also been found concentrated in the adrenals, pancreas, neural tissue, and tongue of cows and other ungulates, including sheep, deer, and moose. The fact that there can be a delay of five or more years from the time of prion exposure to the appearance of symptoms makes in difficult to trace the cause of this untreatable, fatal illness. Despite governmental attempts to protect consumers, animals with mad cow disease are periodically identified in North America. At this time, we advise limiting the use of phosphatidyl serine to products made from soybeans or from animals raised in New Zealand or Australia where surveillance for prion-related diseases is highly regulated.

Soy-derived phosphatidyl serine (S-PS) is a promising and safer alternative to bovine-cortex-derived phosphatidyl serine (BC-PS). Although S-PS has not been studied as extensively, data suggest that it may be effective. One study comparing BC-PS with S-PS in middle-aged rates showed comparable improvements in cognitive performance in the two-way active avoidance test. In contrast, egg-derived phosphatidyl serine showed no effect (Blokland, Honig, Brouns, & Jolles, 1999). Administration of soybean lecithin transphosphatidylated phosphatidyl serine (SB-tPS) ameliorated scopolamine-induced memory impairment in rodents (Suzuki, Kataoka, & Furushiro, 2000), improved spatial memory in aged rats

CLINICAL PEARL

In clinical practice, soy-derived phosphatidyl serine is a useful complementary treatment for age-associated memory impairment. In more severe disorders of memory, stronger treatments are advised.

(Suzuki, Yamatoya, Sakai, Kataoka, Furushiro et al., 2001), prevented ischemic brain damage in gerbils (Suzuki, Furushiro, Takahashi, Sakai, & Kudo, 1999), and enhanced learning ability in normal adult rodents (Kataoka-Kato, Ukai, Sakai, Kudo, & Kameyama, 2005).

One double-blind, randomized, placebo-controlled study of S-PS in 120 elderly subjects (older than 57 years) with age-associated memory impairment (some also had age-associated cognitive decline) found no effect on tests of learning, memory, and attention in doses of 300 mg daily or 600 mg daily compared to placebo. There were no effects on hematologic parameters, blood pressure, or heart rate. The absence of adverse effects indicated that S-PS in doses up to 200 mg t.i.d. is safe in people over the age of 57 (Jorissen, Brouns, Van Boxtel, Ponds, & Verhey, 2001).

In a double-blind, placebo-controlled crossover study of 28 health adults given 120 mg ginkgo biloba extract (GBE), 120 mg GBE complexed with S-PS (Virtiva), or 120 mg GBE complexed with phosphatidyl choline, only those given the GBE complexed with S-PS showed improved secondary memory performance and increased speed on memory tasks (Kennedy, Haskell, Mauri, & Scholey, 2007).

How do we account for the seemingly contradictory findings? First, the molecular composition of phosphatidyl serine preparations varies, dpending on the source and method of synthesis. Molecular species of S-PS are rich in linoleic and palmitic acids in comparison to BC-PS which contain stearic and oleic acids (Sakai, Yamatoy, & Kudo, 1996). For example, in their rodent studies, Kataoka-Kato and colleagues (2005) used phosphatidyl serine produced from soybean lecithin and L-serine by the transphosphatidylation reaction of phospholipase D. Furthermore, the measured effects of phosphatidyl serine also depend upon the age and neurological status of the sub-jects, the dosages and length of administration, and the specific types of memory tests utilized.

ERGOT DERIVATIVES

The authors no longer advise using ergot derivatives because of adverse side effects. However, consumers who have read about these products may ask their health care provider for information.

Hydergine and Nicergoline

Readers interested in ergot derivatives should refer to reviews of hydergine and nicergoline in Alzheimer's and other organic brain syndromes (Fioravanti & Flicker, 2001; Olin, Schneider, Novit, & Luczak, 2001; Pantoni, 2004). In more than 47 trials of hydergine in Alzheimer's, the effect has been slight at best, although there is a suggestion that higher doses may be somewhat effective. Nicergo-line, used to treat subarachnoid hemorrhage, shows more significant though modest effects.

Nicergoline enhances glutamate reuptake, protects against ischemic damage in rats, improves brain blood flow, helps brain cholinergic systems, increases nerve growth factor in aged rat brains, blocks calcium channels and alpha-1-adrenergic receptors in aged rats (Nishio, Sunohara, Furukawa, Akiguchi, & Kudo, 1998), inhibits inflammation, upregulates BDNF (Mizuno, Kuno, Nitta, Nabeshima, Zhang, et al., 2005), protects against amyloid toxicity (Caraci, Chisari, Frasca, Canonico, Battaglia et al., 2005), and increases antioxidant defense enzymes reduced by haloperidol (Vairetti, Ferrigno, Canonico, Battaglia, Berte et al., 2004). Human data showed that nicergoline improves cognitive function by 15% under hypoxic conditions compared to placebo (Saletu, Grun-berger, Linzmayer, & Anderer, 1990). Nicergoline 60 mg/day was compared to placebo in a six-week double-blind parallel group study of 56 patients with multi-infarct dementia and 56 patients with Alzheimer's. In both groups, nicergoline significantly improved cognitive measures and vigilance on EEG mapping. Adverse effects of nicergoline include hot flushes, malaise, agitation, hyperacidity, nausea, diarrhea, dizziness, somnolence, and enhancement of the cardiac depressant action of propranolol.

COGNITIVE ENHANCING HORMONES

A decline in certain hormones, dehydroepiandrosterone and melatonin, has been associated with changes in memory, mood, cognition, and brain activiation. Supplementation may provide improved neuroprotection and brain function.

Dehydroepiandrosterone

DHEA is produced primarily in the adrenal glands and secondarily in the ovaries and testes. Among its neurological effects, DHEA has been reported to improve memory, brain activation on EEG, and mood (Wolkowitz, Reus, Keebler, Nelson, Friedland et al., 1999). A three-month study of normal older men found no change in cognition or well-being with DHEA (van Niekerk, Huppert, & Herbert, 2001). Patients whose DHEA is low for their age, particularly menopausal women who have had ovaries and adrenal glands removed (Gurnell & Chatterjee, 2001; Yen, 2001) and debilitated geriatric patients with medical or neurological diseases (the authors' clinical experience) are more likely to show improved memory and mood when given DHEA. Side effects include insomnia, irritability, hirsutism, acne, slight increases in estrogen, and potential interactions with steroids. Concerns about effects on prostate can be addressed by serial testing of prostate-specific antigen. DHEA is contraindicated in patients with estrogen sensitive cancer or prostate cancer. In general, only pharmaceutical-grade DHEA in doses sufficient to restore physiological levels (25–50 mg/day) should be administered. In most patients, energy improves on 25–50 mg/day. For treatment of depression, 75–100 mg/day and occasionally higher doses may be needed.

Melatonin

Melatonin is a methoxyindole neurohormone secreted primarily, but not exclusively, by the pineal gland that diffuses readily through

CLINICAL PEARL

In elderly patients, including those with Alzheimer's and Parkinson's disease, melatonin in doses of 3–9 mg at bedtime can help to improve sleep, mood, memory, and sundowning. It may slow progression of cognitive decline in patients with early Alzheimer's disease. Melatonin may have a role in long-term prevention of neurodegeneration, particularly if it is started at the age of 40 or 45.

membranes and enters cell organelles. It has numerous neuroprotective properties and regulates circadian rhythms (Srinivasan, Pandi-Perumal, Cardinali, Poeggeler, & Hardeland, 2006). Melatonin is an extremely effective scavenger of free radicals, particularly reactive hydroxyl radicals, carbonate radicals, and reactive nitrogen species. In addition, melatonin exerts anti-excitotoxic effects (preventing excitation-dependent generation of free radicals), suppresses lipid peroxidation, upregulates antioxidant enzymes, and potentiates the effects of other antioxidants such as ascorbate (vitamin C), trolox (vitamin E derivative), glutathione, and others. Melatonin may improve cognitive function to some extent in long-term use, with its strongest effects being preventative.

Secretion of melatonin declines with age and has been found to be abnormal in Alzheimer's and Parkinson's disease. In those diseases, melatonin's primary protective role has been attributed to protection of mitochondrial membranes and mitochondrial DNA from oxidative damage, enhancement of glutathione production and regeneration, and improvement of electron transport capacity. Anti-amyloid-beta and antifibrillogenic effects have also been observed. Several small studies in elderly patients, including some with early Alzheimer's and mild cognitive impairment, have demonstrated that melatonin can improve sleep, mood, and memory, reduce sundowning, and possibly slow the progression of cognitive decline. In a double-blind placebo-controlled study of 20 patients with Alzheimer's those given melatonin 3 mg at bedtime showed significantly greater improvements on the Alzheimer's Disease Assessment

Scale, evaluated for both cognitive (p = 0.017) and noncognitive (p = 0.002) behavioral scores, compared to the placebo group. However, no significant differences were found between groups on Mini Mental Status Exam (Asayama, Yamadera, Ito, Suzuki, Kudo et al., 2003). Epidemiological studies are needed to determine long-term benefits of melatonin on disease progression in Alzheimer's.

NEUROTHERAPY

Traditional neurotherapy (neurofeedback or EEG biofeedback) trains patients to become aware of and influence their state of alertness based on EEG-driven feedback. For this method of operant conditioning, the patient must follow instructions and actively cooperate during many treatments over a period of months. A modern innovation of neurotherapy uses the International 10–20 system of brain mapping and therapeutic procedures based on changing the frequency or amplitude of brain waves at specific sites on that system (Robbins, 2000).

Protocols have been developed for seizure disorders using the sensorimotor rhythm (SMR, 12–15 Hz) formerly called lo-Beta (Lubar & Bahler, 1976; Sterman & Macdonald, 1978), ADHD (Lubar & Lubar, 1984), traumatic brain injury (Ayers, 1987), PTSD combined with alpha training (alpha-theta protocol) to reduce the risks of retraumatization during recall (Ochs, 1994), and in depressed alcoholics (Peniston & Kulkosky, 1989). Quantitative EEGs (QEEGs), measuring frequencies and amplitudes over the entire brain, have improved the quality of diagnostic and treatment protocols. Inhibition of theta and reinforcement of SMR (immobile attention, still, but alert) have been postulated to explain the therapeutic effects of biofeedback. EEG-driven stimulation uses the patients' brain waves to provide feedback to the brain via light-emitting diodes.

Commercial light and sound machines have been used to entrain brain waves to a fixed frequency. However, light flashing at the brain's own frequency can amplify existing instabilities, causing adverse reactions (e.g., seizures) in people with central nervous system damage. Len Ochs developed the low-frequency neurotherapy system (LENS), using "offsets" to decrease rather than increase such amplitudes, producing disentrainment rather than entrainment (Glieck, 1988; Ochs, 2006). Weak signals derived from the patient's own EEG are modified with an offset and then delivered back to the patient using low-energy radio waves at a level of intensity far below those of a cell phone. This short, painless procedure requires minimal cooperation and can be readily tolerated even by young children.

LENS has been successful in significantly reducing symptoms of attention-deficit disorder (ADD), PTSD, affective disorders, pain syndromes, chronic fatigue, and fibromyalgia (Larsen, 2006). Some of the best responses have been in traumatic brain injury (TBI); including patients with seizures (Ochs, 1994). A preliminary, randomized study of 12 mild to moderately severe TBI patients with substantial cognitive impairment given 25 LENS (previously called Flexyx) treatments found significant improvements in Beck Depression Inventory, mental fatigue, digit span backwards, delayed recall on the auditory verbal learning test, ability to function at work and at school, and other measures when compared to a wait-list control group (Schoenberger, Shif, Esty, Ochs, & Matheis, 2001).

LENS neurotherapy is a promising treatment with few adverse effects when administered by an experienced clinician. Side effects include temporary reexperiencing of symptoms related to trauma. Excess treatment can cause fatigue and restlessness. Some biofeedback practitioners use other systems to reduce theta and enhance alpha or beta frequencies for ADD/learning disabled children (Beauregard & Levesque, 2006; Becerra et al., 2006; Monastra, Monastra, & George, 2002).

In the authors' clinical practice, many patients with complex treatment-resistant disorders report synergistic benefits when given LENS neurotherapy (minimum of 10 sessions) followed by Sudarshan Kriya Yoga. Among the responders were patients with diagnoses of anxiety and panic disorders, depression, PTSD, ADD, schizoaffective disorders, obsessive-compulsive disorder, substance abuse, neurodegenerative diseases, and traumatic brain injury. Improvements included general reduction of symptoms on reduced levels of medication as well as improvements in daily function at work and at home, mood, anxiety, mental focus, mental clarity, self-esteem, self-actualization, and quality of life.

TABLE 4.1 Treatment Guidelines for Cognition and Memory

■ **Vitamins, Nutrients, Nootropics, Hormones**

CAM	Clinical Uses	Daily Dose	Side Effects, Drug Interactions,* Contraindications
Acetyl-L-carnitine ALCAR	Alzheimer's disease (AD), traumatic brain injury (TBI), stroke, fatigue	500–1,500 mg	Mild gastric upset Take with food
Alpha-lipoic acid	ischemia, stroke, TBI	300 mg t.i.d.	Minimal
B vitamins B complex B₁₂ folate	TBI, stroke, dementia	1 tab/day 1,000 mcg/day 800 mcg/day	Caution: cardiac stents**
Centro-phenoxine	AD, TBI	500–2,000 mg/day	Minimal when combined with other cholinergic agents: headache, muscle tension, insomnia, irritability, agitation, facial tics
CDP-choline	TBI, stroke, ischemia	1,000–3,000 mg/day	None significant
DHEA	memory, mood	25–200 mg/day	Irritability, insomnia, acne, hirsutism, possible increase in prostate-specific antigen, interaction with steroids Caution: bipolars Contraindication: estrogen-sensitive cancers, prostate cancer

TABLE 4.1 *Continued*

CAM	Clinical Uses	Daily Dose	Side Effects, Drug Interactions,* Contraindications
Galantamine	AD, TBI, cerebrovascular disease (CVD)	8–32 mg/day	Mild nausea, GI upset
Huperzine	AD, TBI, CVD	100–400 mcg/day	Rare: mild nausea, diarrhea, dizziness
Idebenone (CoQ10)	CVD, AD, TBI	270–900 mg/day	None
L-deprenyl	AD, Parkinson's disease (PD), CVD, TBI	10–15 mg/week 0.7–1.5 mg/day	Take 2.5 mg 5 days a week. Higher doses > 10 mg/day may cause MAOI effects (hypertension)
Melatonin	In dementia: sleep, memory, mood	3–9 mg h.s.	Occasional agitation, abdominal cramps, fatigue, dizziness, headache, vivid dreams
N-acetylcys-teine	CVD, stroke	1,200 mg b.i.d.	No significant side effects reported in appropriate doses
Omega-3 fatty acid EPA/DHA ~2:1	Neuroprotection	2,000–3,000 mg/day	GI distress, belching, loose stools, may affect glucose metabolism in diabetics
Picamilon	TBI, PD, CVD, stroke, toxic brain lesions	50 mg b.i.d. up to 100 mg t.i.d.	High dose: hypotension
Racetams, pyrrolidinone	poststroke aphasia, dyslexia, medication-related cognitive impairment	aniracetam 750 mg b.i.d.	Minimal. Rarely: anxiety, insomnia, agitation, irritability, headache

S-adenosyl methionine (SAMe)	AD, TBI, PD, dementia, depression, stroke	400–4,000 mg/day Give in divided doses	Occasional GI symptoms, agitation, anxiety, insomnia; rare palpitations. Mania in bipolars.

■ Herbs

Ashwaganda (*Withania somnifera*)	anxiety insomnia	100–400 b.i.d. of withanolides	Mild sedation. Combined effects with other sedatives
Ginkgo (*Ginkgo biloba*)	age-associated memory impairment, mild cognitive impairment AD, CVD	120–240 mg/day	Minimal: headache, reduced platelet aggregation Rare agitation. D/C 2 weeks prior to surgery. Contraindication: Anticoagulants.
Ginseng (*Panax ginseng*)	dementia, neurasthenia	300–800 mg/day	Overstimulation, GI symptoms, anxiety, insomnia, headache, tachycardia, reduced platelet aggregation. Contraindication: anticoagulants
Kava (*Piper methysticum*)	anxiety	70–140 mg/day kavalactones	Sedation, dependency, hepatitis, liver failure, dystonia, extrapyramidal symptoms. Can be toxic at doses > 240 mg/day
Lemon balm (*melissa officianalis*)	agitation in dementia	800 mg/day	None significant
Rhodiola rosea	cognitive enhancement, memory, TBI, PD, AD, CVD	100–600 mg/day	Activation, agitation, insomnia, jitteriness Rare: increased BP, angina, bruising. Contraindications: bipolar I, anticoagulants

TABLE 4.1 *Continued*

CAM	Clinical Uses	Daily Dose	Side Effects, Drug Interactions,* Contraindications
Sage (*Salvia officinalis Salvia lavendu- laefolia*)	agitation, memory, alertness in dementia	50 drops, 1.5% tincture	Minimal
Vinpocetine (*Vinca minor*)	CVD, TBI	10 mg t.i.d.	Rare: nausea, low BP

◼ **Combination Products**

CAM	Clinical Uses	Daily Dose	Side Effects, Drug Interactions,* Contraindications
ADAPT 232 *R. rosea* *E. senticosus* *S. chinensis*	cognition, memory, mental focus, mental accuracy and endurance, neural fatigue	2–3 tabs/day	Rare: overactivation, anxiety, insomnia Caution: bipolars
Bio-Strath **B vitamins** **Antioxidants**	TBI, stroke, dementia	1 Tbsp b.i.d 3 tabs b.i.d.	Caution: cardiac stents**
Cerefolin **600 mg NAC** **2 mg methyl-cobalamine** **5.6 mg methyl-folate**	CVD, AD, vascular dementia, stroke, mild cognitive impairment	1–2 tabs/day	Caution: cardiac stents**
Easy Energy *R. rosea* **70 mg** *E. senticocus* *S. chinensis* *Aralia mandshurica* *R. carthemoides*	cognition, memory, increased phys-cal strength, calms patients who tend to get agitated on activating herbs	1–2 tabs/day	Minimal: side effects of component herbs Caution: bipolars

Mentat (BR16-A) Many herbs, including ba-copa, gotu kola, ashwaganda, triphala, morning glory, arjuna	AAMI age-associated memory impairment, AD, CVD, TBI, medication-induced cognitive impairment	1–2 pills once or twice a day with food	Minimal: side effects of component herbs. May raise levels of carba-mazepine and phenytoin. Caution: bipolars
Neurogen A/P *R. rosea* **Galanthus**	AD, PD, CVD, AAMI	1–2 pills/day or as directed	Minimal: side effects of component herbs Caution: bipolars

AD = Alzheimer's disease; PD = Parkinson's disease; TBI = traumatic brain injury; CVD = cerebrovascular disease; AAMI = age-associated memory impairment; MAOI = monoamine oxidase inhibitor; BP = blood pressure; GI = gastrointestinal; D/C = discontinue.

*Common side effects are listed. There are additional rare side effects. Individuals with high blood pressure, diabetes, pregnancy (or during breast-feeding), or any chronic or serious medical condition should check with their physician before taking supplements. Patients taking anticoagulants should consult their physician before using supplements.

**May increase risk of restenosis of cardiac stents in men only with baseline homocysteine <15 μmol/liter.

CHAPTER 5 OUTLINE

1. **Dietary Treatments, Vitamins, Minerals, and Nutrients**
   a. food additives, vitamins, zinc, iron, S-adenosylmethionine, amino acids, acetyl-l-carnitine, omega-3 fatty acids, dimethylaminoethanol

2. **Cognitive Activators**
   a. picamilon, ginseng, ginkgo, pycnogenol, bacopa, Chinese herbs

3. **Biofeedback and Neurotherapy**

4. **Mind–Body Practices: Meditation and Yoga**

5. **Dyslexia and Learning Disabilities:** Racetams

6. **Integrative Approaches for Treating ADD/ADHD and Learning Disabilities**

Attention-Deficit Disorder and Learning Disabilities

A ttention-deficit disorder (ADD) with or without hyperactivity is comprised of a constellation of symptoms that appears by age seven years and frequently persists into adult life. These symptoms derive from inability to inhibit impulsiveness or to focus attention. Although the etiology is not well understood, theories involve dopamine (DA), norepinephrine (NE), and acetylcholine (Ach) neurotransmitter systems combined with underarousal of the brain. Genetic and imaging studies support the belief that the disorder has a biological basis. Attention-deficit disorder (ADD) is frequently associated with comorbid conditions that complicate treatment including learning disabilities, oppositional behavior, depression, anxiety, bipolar, tics, obsessive-compulsive behavior, and the high risk of later substance abuse and antisocial behavior. Studies show that treating ADD reduces the risk of substance abuse in later years.

Although pharmacological interventions for ADD can be effective, many patients experience incomplete benefits, nonresponse to treatment, or adverse reactions such as growth delays, overstimulation, insomnia, and withdrawal symptoms (e.g., fatigue, depression). Another problem is that as the prescription stimulant wears off, the patient may experience a crash with loss of energy, amotivation, or depressed mood. Conventional approaches rely on psychostimulants such as methylphenidate (Ritalin, Concerta), dextroamphetamine (Dexadrine), atomoxetine (Strattera), and mixed amphetamine salts (Adderall). Many parents avidly seek alternatives for their children because of concerns about side effects and the potential for abuse. A study found that 54% of parents used complementary and alternative therapies for their children with ADHD (Chan, Rappaport & Kemper, 2003). Only 11% of the parents discussed this with their physicians. In animal studies, psychostimulants (e.g., methamphetamine) have been shown to cause neurotoxicity by depleting dopamine, its metabolites, and tyrosine hydroxylase activity in the striatum (Volkow, Chang, Wang, Fowler, Leonido-Yee et al., 2001). Methamphetamine also reduced serum and liver levels of S-adenasylmethionine (SAMe) in animal studies (Cooney, Wise, Poirier, & Ali, 1998). Dextroamphetamine depleted energy in rat striatum, reducing the high-energy compound ATP/ADP ratio (adenosine triphosphate/adenosine diphosphate) (Wan, Lin, Kang, Tseng, & Tung, 1999). Mice treated with methylphenidate have increased risk of liver cancer (Dunnick & Hailey, 1995; Ernst, 2001). Although these studies have not been done in human subjects, many parents and health care professionals are concerned about possible long-term side effects.

This discussion is limited to CAM treatments that the authors find to be helpful in clinical practice, those for which there is credible evidence of efficacy, and those that are frequently requested by parents: dietary elimination, vitamins, minerals, omega-3 fatty acids (omega-3FAs), SAMe, acetyl-l-carnitine, dimethylaminoethanol, centrophenoxine, pyrrolidinones, picamilon, *Rhodiola rosea*, ginkgo, ginseng, pcynogenol, yoga, and neurotherapy (for excellent reviews of CAM for ADHD, see Arnold, 2001; Kidd, 2000). Many of the herbs, nutrients, and nootropics shown to improve memory, attention, verbal processing, and cognitive function in adults have potential benefits in children. For more detailed discussion of research and clinical effects, see Chapter 4. Although not all of the CAM treatments in this chapter have been studied in children, they are all low in risk, particularly when compared with stimulants, and they have been used clinically.

Misuse of prescription stimulants is increasingly prevalent among students. A survey of middle school and high school students treated with stimulants found that 23.3% reported being approached to sell, give, or trade their medication (McCabe, Teter, & Boyd, 2004). In a random Internet survey of more than 9,000 undergraduate college students, 8.1% reported lifetime illicit use of prescription stimulants (Teter, McCabe, Cranford, Boyd, & Guthrie, 2005). The availability of prescription stimulants is a growing problem that can have serious consequences, as the following case illustrates.

Case 1—One-Time Adderall Abuse, Panic Disorder

Samantha, a 14-year-old high school freshman, was brought to the emergency room because of tachycardia and chest pain. Examination revealed a heart rate of 170 in an otherwise healthy teenager. Samantha had no prior history of medical illness, anxiety, panic, or substance abuse. After medical clearance she was sent home with a diagnosis of panic attack and referred to a psychotherapist. Over the next six weeks she remained in a constant state of panic, preoccupied with somatic sensations and the belief that there was something wrong with her heart. She was unable to sleep, attend school, socialize, or engage in any sports activities. Samantha's psychologist referred her for psychiatric evaluation. The history and mental status were unremarkable except for her state of near panic and somatic worries. Her legs shook continuously and she was unable to make eye contact. Mirtazepine (Remeron) in a dose of 15 mg hs was started at the first visit to improve sleep and anxiety with rapid response. Samantha's sleep improved and she felt a bit less anxious.

At the second visit, Samantha expressed reluctance to take more medication. As an alternative, she chose to learn a form of yoga breathing called Ujjayi (Victory Breath or Ocean Breath) which enabled her to feel deeply relaxed for the first time since the problem began (see Chapter 3 for a discussion of the effects of yoga breathing on the stress response systems). She was instructed to practice Ujjayi for 10 minutes twice a day in conjunction with Coherence Breathing (using the Respire 1 CD) and to do additional breathing as needed.

Coherence breathing is a program of paced respiration at 5 breaths per minute that optimizes oxygenation and synchronizes heart and brain rhythms (Elliott & Edmonson, 2006). Samantha enjoyed yoga breathing, which gave her a sense of mastery and control over the anxiety. She learned to direct her thoughts away from the somatic worries. She continued psychotherapy sessions once a week.

In the third session, Samantha appeared embarrassed. She reported remembering an important fact that she had forgotten to tell anyone: On the day of her first panic attack she had taken one Adderall from a friend to help her concentrate better on a test that day. Two hours after taking the Adderall, she had purchased a large soft drink containing caffeine and ginseng. Shortly after finishing the drink she developed rapid heartbeat, panic, and chest pain. Evidently, the combination of Adderall with the caffeine and ginseng in the soft drink had triggered her symptoms. While ginseng and caffeine may improve some symptoms of ADD such as mental focus, they can cause overstimulation, particularly when combined with prescription stimulants.

In Samatha's case, the symptoms persisted long after the stimulating substances had left her body. The initial experience of tachycardia and chest pain was accompanied by feelings of panic and fear of dying. This became a traumatic experience that continued through many hours of medical testing in the hospital. Samantha developed a form of PTSD in which her anxiety was triggered by any slight increase in heart rate or any mild (even normal) sensation in her chest. Consequently, whenever she walked quickly or climbed stiars, the increase in heart rate triggered panic and the panic further accelerated her heart, creating a self-perpetuating cycle. Her solution was to completely avoid even mild physical exertion. Secondarily, she developed a fear of having panic attacks and she became mentally preoccupied with her physical sensations.

After two months of steady improvement, Samantha reduced the frequency of her psychotherapy and stopped doing the Ujjayi regularly. Her symptoms began to worsen.

Once she realized the importance of maintaining the yoga breath practices and therapy sessions, she restabilized and was able to discontinue mirtazepine. Samantha resumed all of her former social, educational, and athletic activities.

DIETARY TREATMENTS, VITAMINS, MINERALS, AND NUTRIENTS

Although the role of foods or additives in causing behavioral disorders in children, particularly ADHD, has been controversial, some acceptable scientific evidence supports the use of dietary elimination strategies in subgroups, such as those with specific food allergies. The typical responder (a minority of ADD children) is a preschooler with insomnia, irritability, atopy (allergic tendencies), physical symptoms, behavioral problems, and sometimes high copper levels. Few families are able to maintain the limited diet. Eliminating the more suspicious items (artificial food colorings, benzoate preservatives, sugars, and artificial sweeteners) may help in about 50% of children. A DBRPC (double-blind, randomized, placebo-controlled) study of 277 children found a general adverse effect of artificial food coloring and benzoate preservatives on hyperactive behavior in three-year-old children. However, this effect was detectable by parents, but not by a simple clinic assessment (Bateman, Warner, Hutchinson, Dean, Rowlandson et al., 2004). Methodological problems and investigator bias in sugar elimination studies have left this issue unresolved (Kidd, 2000). More research is needed on the toxic effects of heavy metals (lead, aluminum) and organic chemical pollutants (pesticides, dioxin, polychlorinated biphenols, hydrocarbons, etc.).

Moderate levels of vitamin and mineral supplementation (not megavitamins) have been beneficial in studies of normal children, retarded children, and teen delinquents. A DBRPC three-month trial (n = 245) found that among children whose pretest showed low serum levels of B vitamins or C vitamins, those treated with vitamin supplements manifested reduced levels of aggression and antisocial behavior as well as improved cognitive performance (IQ increased 2.5 points). In 20% of subjects, mean IQ scores increased 16 points (Schoenthaler & Bier, 1999). The authors use Bio-Strath, a preparation derived from brewer's yeast grown on antioxidant herbs that is high in antioxidants, minerals, and vitamins, particularly B vitamins. It does not contain any whole yeast. The liquid form of Bio-Strath can be used as a vitamin supplement for normal children and in those with ADD. Tablets or liquid Bio-Strath can be beneficial in adults with or without ADD. (Bio-Strath comes in liquid and tablet form. The dose is 1 teaspoon of liquid twice a day or 3 tablets twice a day. Most people prefer the liquid rather than take 3 large pills twice daily.)

Zinc

Zinc (15 mg elemental) augmented the effects of methylphenidate better than placebo in a six-week DBRPC trial of 44 ADHD children (Akhondzadeh, Mohammadi, & Khademi, 2004). In a 12-week DBRPC study of 328 boys and 72 girls with ADHD, zinc sulfate 40 mg/day significantly reduced ADHD symptoms compared with placebo (Bilici, Yildirim, Kandil, Bekaroglu, Yildirmis et al., 2004). The results of these two studies may have been influenced by the greater prevalence of zinc deficiency in Turkey and Iran where they were performed. Nevertheless, in a study of middle-class American children, low serum zinc levels correlated with inattention but not hyperactivity-impulsivity (Arnold & DiSilvestro, 2005). The use of supplements for deficiencies of magnesium, iron, and zinc warrants further study (Arnold, 2001; Kidd, 2000).

Iron

Iron is necessary for dopamine synthesis. Enhanced dopamine transmission is a feature of most drugs found to be effective in treating ADD. In one study, ferritin levels (a measure of iron stores) were low in 84% of 53 ADHD children versus 18% of 27 matched controls. The low ferritin levels correlated with worse cognitive deficits and more severe ADHD ratings (Konofal, Lecendreux, Arnulf, & Mouren, 2004). Studies of iron supplementation in ADHD children with low ferratin levels have shown mixed results (Millichap, Yee, & Davidson, 2006). Improvements have been shown in learning and memory in iron-deficient adolescents given iron supplements (Bruner, Joffe, Duggan, Casella, & Brandt, 1996). The role of iron in ADHD remains to be clarified. Low iron levels and low folate have been associated with restless leg syndrome (Patrick, 2007). In chil-

---

CLINICAL PEARL

Children with ADHD or symptoms of restless leg syndrome should be
tested for deficiencies of iron and folate.

---

dren, restless leg syndrome can be mistaken for hyperactivity. Children with ADHD or symptoms of restless leg syndrome should be
tested for iron and folate deficiencies.

S-adenosylmethionine (SAMe)

SAMe potentiates amphetamine response and stimulates dopamine
transmission, a feature of most drugs found to be effective in ADD.
Also, ADD has been associated with abnormal increases in slow
alpha and theta frequencies. SAMe, at doses of 400 mg/day and
1,600 mg/day, showed beneficial effects on electroencephalogram
(EEG) compared with placebo. SAMe treatment increased alpha-2
and beta frequencies in elderly subjects (57–73-year-olds). Some
improvements in critical flicker fusion frequency was found in subjects given SAMe 1,600 mg/day at Day 15 (Arnold, Saletu, Anderer,
Assandri, di Padova et al., 2005). These results are consistent with a
nootropic effect. Although SAMe is generally well tolerated, some
subjects experienced transient sleepiness several hours after taking
SAMe. The authors find that SAMe can enhance and accelerate
response to biofeedback.

A four-week open study of eight men with adult ADHD, residual
type, found that SAMe 2,400 mg/day improved ratings on measures
of ADHD and mood in six out of the eight. Side effects were not significant (Shekim, Antun, Hanna, McCracken, & Hess, 1990).
Longer term trials are needed to explore the use of SAMe in children
and adults with ADHD. The importance of SAMe as a methyl donor
for the synthesis of dopamine and its central role in maintaining the
methionine cycle are discussed in Chapters 2 and 3. At this time,
SAMe may be worth trying in cases with incomplete response, habituation, intolerance of prescription stimulants, or to minimize the
risks of medication side effects.

Amino Acids: Tryptophan, Phenylalanine, Levodopa, And L-Tyrosine

Amino acid supplements, including tryptophan, phenylalanine, levodopa, and L-tyrosine have shown only short-term benefits in ADHD with loss of effect after a few weeks. At this time there is insufficient evidence of sustained efficacy to recommend them. Out of three open trials of glyconutritional supplements (saccharides needed for synthesis of glycoproteins and glycolipids) in children with ADHD, two showed reductions in some symptoms, and one found none. Further study is needed (Arnold, 2001).

Acetyl-L-Carnitine

Acetyl-L-carnitine, a small, water-soluble molecule, easily diffuses in the extracellular space and enters neurons through specific transporters. Studies show that it improves cell membrane function, energy metabolism, synthesis of ATP and neurotransmitters, essential fatty acid (EFA) utilization, and possibly the attention component of the cholinergic system (Pettegrew et al., 2000). Fragile X is the most common inherited disease causing mental retardation. In a DBRPC study of 20 fragile X boys with hyperactivity, acetyl-L-carnitine significantly reduced hyperactive behavior as tested by the Conners Abbreviated Parent-Teacher Questionnaire (Torrioli, Vernacotola, Mariotti, Bianchi, Calvani et al., 1999). Studies of acetyl-L-carnitine in combination with EFAs may be worthwhile.

Omega-3 Fatty Acids

Omega-3FA deficiencies have been found in a subgroup of boys with ADHD (Antalis, Stevens, Campbell, Pazdro, Ericson et al., 2006). In a study of children with developmental coordination disorder (ADHD is often part of the syndrome), omega-3FAs improved behavior and cognitive functions (Richardson, 2006). Studies of EFA supplementation in ADHD children who were not selected for EFA deficiencies have found no significant effects. Further studies of EFAs, particularly in patients with low serum levels of specific EFAs, are needed in ADHD before recommendations can be offered.

Dimethylaminoethanol and Meclofenoxate

Dimethylaminoethanol (DMAE), commonly found in over-the-counter (OTC) supplements used in ADHD, was studied in numerous double-blind placebo-controlled trials with outdated methodology. One more recent rigorous trial suggested a modest effect of 0.2 to 0.5 in doses of 500 mg/day or more (less than methylphenidate's effect size of 0.8 to 1.3; Arnold, 2001).

Centrophenoxine, a combination of DMAE and PCPA (p-chlorophenoxyacetic acid), is well studied, inexpensive, and low in side effects. It is potentiated by ginkgo and caffeine. Pyrrolidinones (racetams including piracetam and aniracetam) are nootropic agents that improve learning and cognitive functions. The authors have found the combination of centrophenoxine and aniracetam to be particularly effective in a small number of children and adults with ADD and learning disabilities. Different cerebral areas use this molecule to metabolize glucose and lipids to provide for ATP and neurotransmitter synthesis. DMAE may be useful for mild symptoms of ADD in patients who do not want prescription medication (see Chapter 4 for more detailed discussion of nootropics).

COGNITIVE ACTIVATORS

Cognitive activators, antioxidants, nutrients, nootropics, and cell membrane enhancers may be beneficial in ADD. Picamilon (gamma-aminobutyric acid, GABA, plus niacin) improves cerebral blood flow and has mild stimulative effects, such as improving alertness and attention (see Chapter 4). At the same time, it tends to reduce aggressive behavior. Although there have been no studies of picamilon for adult ADHD, Dr. Richard Brown has found it to be extremely beneficial in several adult patients using doses of 100–300 mg/day. Controlled studies in ADD treatment using these compounds are needed.

Herbs: Ginkgo, Asian Ginseng, American Ginseng, *Rhodiola Rosea*, Passionflower, Huperzine

Herbal treatments for ADHD may cause cognitive activation, calming, or both. Ginkgo and ginseng improve learning in animals and humans. They are known to affect the neurotransmitter systems and they are cognitive activators (Itil, 2001; Petkov et al., 1986). While controlled studies are needed, some preliminary data are promising. Compared to Asian ginseng (*Panax ginseng*), American ginseng (*Panax quinquefolius*) is gentler, less stimulating, and less likely to cause agitation or headaches. Therefore, although American ginseng is less studied than Asian ginseng, it may be more suitable for children. An open study of 36 children with ADHD given American ginseng 400 mg/day plus *Ginkgo biloba* 100 mg/day for four weeks found that 74% improved significantly on Conner's ADHD scale and 44% improved on a social problems measure. Only two children experienced mild side effects (agitation; Lyon, Cline, Totosy de Zepetnek, Shan, Pang et al., 2001). *R. rosea* has a similar profile of cognitive activation and may be used in ADHD. It tends to improve accuracy, alertness, and attention, particularly for tasks such as schoolwork or tedious computer work that require prolonged periods of mental focus. It can be very stimulating in children. *R. rosea* is occasionally beneficial in children ages 8 to 12. However, it is most useful in students in junior high, high school, and college who have to complete longer papers and spend many hours reading. Although Passionflower is a frequent ingredient in OTC preparations for ADD, no studies have been done in ADD. Side effects and toxicity have not been investigated. Huperzine (see cholinergic agents) is of interest because it has minimal side effects (unlike prescription cholinesterase inhibitors; Arnold, 2001).

Pycnogenol

In a DBRPC study of 61 children with ADHD, an extract from French maritime pine bark called Pycnogenol was superior to placebo. Standardized measures and teacher and parent ratings after one month showed that students on Pcynogenol had significantly greater improvements in hyperactivity, attention, concentration, and visual-motor coordination (Trebaticka et al., 2006). Larger randomized controlled trials are needed to explore these interesting findings.

Bacopa monniera (Brahmi)

Bacopa monniera or Brahmi, is an Ayurvedic medicine containing saponins and bacosides. In a DBRPC trial in 36 children with ADHD given either Bacopa or placebo for 12 weeks followed by four-week washout, those given Bacopa performed better on tests of sentence repetition, logical memory, and paired associate learning. Improvements persisted four weeks after Bacopa was discontinued (Negi, Singh, Kushwaha, et al., 2000). In a 12-week randomized placebo-controlled study of 40 normal children, those given Bacopa had greater improvements in maze learning, perceptual organization, and reasoning compared to controls. This study is limited in that it was a nonblinded trial (Sharma, Chaturvedi, & Tewari, 1987).

Open trials of preparations containing Chinese herbal combinations have shown significant improvements in ADHD symptoms using 80 S (Zhang & Huang, 1990), Tiaoshen liquor (Wang, Li, & Li, 1995), Yizhi wit-increasing syrup (Sun, Wang, Qu, Wang, Fang et al., 1994), and others (Shen & Wang, 1984). While these open studies warrant further investigation, caution should be exercised in using Chinese herbal preparations because they may contain stimulants. Also, supplements manufactured in China sometimes contain heavy metals and other contaminants.

BIOFEEDBACK AND NEUROTHERAPY

In a randomized controlled trial of 18 children with ADD/ADHD, those given EEG biofeedback once a week for 40 weeks showed a nine-point increase in IQ compared to less than one point in the wait-list group ($P < 0.05$). The biofeedback group also had a 28% decrease in inattention compared to a 4% increase in the wait-list group ($p < 0.05$; Linden, Habib, & Radojevic, 1996). In an open pilot study of 19 ADHD children, ages 6 to 13, autonomic nervous system biofeedback modality, using heart rate variability (HRV) biofeedback, led to significant improvements in ADHD in all subjects. Students with high pretreatment HRV (n = 10) showed more significant improvements on test measures than those with low HRV (n = 9). Overall improvement correlated with increased parasympathetic nervous system activity on HRV measures (Eisenberg, Ben-Daniel, Mei-Tal, & Wertman, 2004). Larger studies are needed to extend these interesting findings.

Excess theta and reduced beta or alpha rhythms have been noted on EEGs of ADHD children. Promising results have been reported using neurotherapy to enhance alpha or beta rhythms, but further studies are needed (Larsen, 2006; Lubar & Lubar, 1984; Nash, 2000; Ramirez, Desantis, & Opler, 2001). In a 12-week nonrandomized study of children with ADHD between the ages of 8 and 12 years, 22 children were given neurotherapy and 12 were treated with methylphenidate. Children whose parents preferred an alternative to medication were assigned to neurotherapy treatment. Both treatments significantly improved scores on all subscales of the Test of Variables of Attention (TOVA) and on both the parent and teacher Conners Behavior Rating Scales (Fuchs, Birbaumer, Lutzenberger, Gruzelier, & Kaiser, 2003).

One hundred children with ADD and ADHD, 6 to 19 years old, were treated for one year in an outpatient program where they all received methylphenidate (Ritalin), parent counseling, and academic support at school. EEG biofeedback therapy was also given to 51 of the participants. Posttreatment testing while using Ritalin showed significant improvement on the TOVA and the Attention-Deficit Disorders Evaluation Scale. However, at one-year follow-up, only those children whose parents employed consistent reinforcement strategies at home and who had received EEG biofeedback sustained these gains when tested without Ritalin. Quantitative electroencephalographic scanning process revealed significant reduction in cortical slowing only in patients who had received EEG biofeedback (Monastra, Monastra, & George, 2002).

To achieve long-term sustained improvement, patients with ADHD may require 20 to 60 neurotherapy sessions. In clinical practice, the authors have found a more recent modification of neurotherapy called disentrainment neurotherapy (see section on neurotherapy in Chapter 4) to be helpful in alleviating inattentive and hyperactive symptoms of ADHD.

DYSLEXIA AND LEARNING DISABILITIES

Racetams are nootropics with several documented effects that may underlie their capacity to help dyslexics. Racetams interact with phospholipids to restore membrane fluidity and improve interhemispheric transmission.

Racetams: Piracetam, Aniracetam

In dyslexics, piracetam preferentially activates the left hemisphere (verbal processing areas) (Ackerman, Dykman, Holloway, Paal, & Gocio, 1991; Helfgott, Rudel, & Kairam, 1986; Tallal, Chase, Russell, & Schmitt, 1986). Early studies of racetams in dyslexic children showed mixed results, probably due to heterogeneity of subjects, use of low doses, and inadequate duration of trials. A DBRPC multicenter study of 225 dyslexic children (ages 7–12 years) using piracetam 3,600 mg/day demonstrated significant improvements in reading ability and comprehension evident at 12 weeks and sustained for the 36 weeks of the trial (Wilsher, Bennett, Chase, Conners, DiIanni, et al., 1987). Piracetam was well tolerated with no adverse effects. In clinical practice, the authors find aniracetam 750 mg b.i.d. to be more effective and well tolerated.

MIND–BODY PRACTICES FOR ADHD AND LEARNING DISABILITIES

Yoga education is being introduced into schools to help children learn how to calm down, focus their minds, and improve body awareness, balance, and flexibility.

Meditation

Meditation has effects on EEG rhythms similar to theta/beta biofeedback training. Two promising controlled studies in ADHD children found improvements in attention, particularly in the classroom (Arnold, 2001).

A study of autonomic dysregulation comparing adolescents, ages

---

CLINICAL PEARL

The authors have found that most ADD children and adults cannot sit still or concentrate long enough to meditate. It is usually necessary for them to proctice yoga breathing for some time to quiet their mind before attempting meditation.

12 to 17 years, 17 with ADHD, 20 with aggressive conduct disorder (CD), and 22 controls, found that reduced RSA (respiratory sinus arrhythmia) in those with ADHD and CD indicated reduced baseline cardiac vagal tone (Beauchaine, Katkin, Strassberg, & Snarr, 2001). These subjects also had lower thresholds for fight-flight reactions and were at increased risk for aggressive behavior. Interventions that enhance parasympathetic activity may be beneficial for individuals with ADHD. In the study of autonomic nervous system biofeedback mentioned above, improvements in symptoms of ADHD correlated with increases in parasympathetic nervous system (PNS) tone. Mind–body practices such as yoga breathing combined with yoga postures and relaxation have the potential to calm the mind and improve mental focus. Such practices are also associated with increased PNS activity and autonomic balance (see Chapter 3).

In a pilot study of 19 boys with hyperactive-impulsive ADHD, ages 8–13, a program of yoga postures, yoga breathing, and relaxation led to significant improvements on standardized ADHD tests such as the Conners. The degree of improvement correlated with the number of yoga sessions attended and with the amount of home practice each student performed (Jensen & Kenny, 2004). Nineteen children with ADHD were randomized to a yoga program or conventional motor exercises. For all outcome measures, including scores of attention and parent ratings of ADHD symptoms, the yoga training was superior, with a medium-to-high-range effect size (0.60–0.97; Haffner, Roos, Goldstein, Parzer, & Resch, 2006).

The authors refer children to a program of yoga postures, breathing, and meditation combined with games to improve life skills and self-esteem called ART-Excel taught by the Art of Living Foundation that seems to calm the children and improve their attention and behavior (see section on yoga breathing in Chapter 3). While additional studies are needed, encouraging preliminary data support the use of yoga, a low-risk intervention, as an adjunctive treatment for ADHD. In an open pilot study, 53 high school students, ages 15–19, participated in the six-day, 18-hour intensive Youth Empowerment Seminar (YES!) and subsequent weekly follow-up session for six months (Schaenfield, in process). Each day of the seminar, students learn stress management techniques and yoga, and participate in interactive discussions, educational games, and group processes. Stress management techniques include yoga breathing (Ujjayi, Bhastrika, and Sudarshan Kriya), yoga postures, and meditation. Students were recruited from three New York City schools including an alternative school for high school dropouts, a public high school, and a performing arts high school. Pre- and postintervention assessments showed significant improvements on Identity Conflict Resolution (Rosenthal, Gurney & Moore, 1981), Rosenberg Self-Esteem Inventory (Rosenberg, Schooler & Schoenbach, 1989), Modified Anger Coping, Planning and Concentration Scale, Distractibility Scale, and Irritability Scale (Ridenour, Ferrer-Wreder, Gottschall, in review).

Massage, Vestibular Stimulation, and Channel-Specific Perceptual Training

Other promising nonpharmacological approaches include massage, vestibular stimulation, and channel-specific perceptual training. One open trial and three single-blind studies of vestibular stimulation, a technique of rotational stimulation (which enhances vagal input to the brain), yielded promising results (Arnold, 2001). Further research is needed, particularly to establish how long treatment effects last.

INTEGRATIVE APPROACHES TO TREATING ADHD AND LEARNING DISABILITIES

The symptoms and functional effects of ADD and learning disabilities can be extremely varied and are often confounded by comorbid disorders. The following complex cases illustrate how a layered approach to integrative treatment can improve behavior, cognitive function, work performance, and quality of life. In the first case, a highly articulate patient was able to describe the subtle changes in cognitive function that he experienced with each treatment.

Case 2—Adult ADD With Explosive Behavior and Learning Disabilities

George, a 41-year-old lawyer, found out he had been adopted in infancy when he was 17 years old. As a child, he had been misdiagnosed as having conduct disorder when, in retrospect, he probably had ADHD and learning disabilities. During law school, George responded to Ritalin with improvement in his academic performance. His girlfriend convinced him to seek further consultation because of his explosive anger. An attempt to switch him to Adderall did not help. Once he habituated to both Ritalin and Adderall, he would crash in the evening and become explosive. For the first layer of treatment, George was given Adderall-XR 20 mg t.i.d. to prevent the evening crash. He described improvements in his cognitive functions: "It's like going from DOS to Windows XP." Unfortunately, the Adderall-XR caused heart palpitations.

The next layers of treatment were aimed at reducing the dose of Adderall-XR to relieve palpitations and further enhance cognitive functions. When George started 385 mg *Rhodiola rosea* (brand Rhodax) in the morning, he noticed enhancement of his mental clarity, "like going from color TV to high-definition TV." He was better able to organize and prioritize his work. It became possible to reduce the Adderall-XR from 20 mg t.i.d. to 10 mg a.m. plus 15 mg midday with alleviation of the palpitations. However, George had persistent concerns about long-term effects of Adderall (possible depletion of norepinephrine and cardiomyopathy) and wanted additional CAM trials to minimize prescription drugs. The third layer, 16 sessions of neurotherapy over a period of 10 months, reduced anxiety and further improved his ability to organize and prioritize. The fourth layer, *Eleutherococcus senticosus* (Siberian ginseng) 500 mg a.m. further boosted his productivity. The combined productivity effect of his CAM treatments was a threefold increase in his income. For the fifth layer, SAMe starting with 400 mg b.i.d. and increasing to 800 mg b.i.d., gave George a "greater depth of focus." He was also able to take weekend holidays off the Adderall-XR with no violent episodes.

George believed he had writing and reading disabilities that had not been formally diagnosed. Aniracetam is beneficial for verbal disabilities. In the sixth layer of treatment, he was given aniracetam 750 mg b.i.d. for two months. George reported improvements in his abilities to read, write, and communicate verbally, particularly in presenting cases in court. As his talents became evident, he was courted by prominent law firms. The consistent improvement in his behavior along with greater cognitive and communicative skills solidified the relationship with his girlfriend. They are now happily married.

Case 3—Treatment-Resistant ADD and Bipolar II Disorder

At age 33, Jim had never been able to support himself because of treatment-resistant ADHD and bipolar II disorder. He was too disorganized, inattentive, emotionally labile, and insecure to hold a job. As a child he had been extremely hyperactive with both verbal and mathematical learning disabilities. Adderall 60 mg/day stopped his explosive outbursts, but the improvement in his mental focus was modest at best. He said that without the Adderall he felt paralyzed. Valproate (depakote) significantly reduced his anger but caused such severe acne that he stopped taking it. On buproprion (Wellbutrin) he developed hepatitis, and worse aggression. After trials of gabapentin (Neurontin), provigil (Modafanil), and St. John's Wort had destabilized his moods resulting in mixed dysphoric manic states, Jim was sent for a consultation.

For mood stabilization, lamotragine (Lamictal) was tried in doses up to 400 mg/day with no clear benefit. A switch from Adderall to Concerta reduced aggression but left the patient with no energy, no motivation, and no concentration. Aricept (donepezil) had no effect. However, when he started taking *Rhodiola rosea* 360 mg/day (Arctic Root SHR-5 by ProActive BioProducts) there were marked improvements in his energy, mood, concentration, organization, and ability to get things done. Jim got a job coach and a computer tutor. For the first time, he developed the necessary confidence and motivation to look for a job and to start dating. At the time of this writing, the excellent response to *R. rosea* had persisted for over four years. He is now happily married with two children and is progressing well in his work at a new company.

Integrative Treatment Approach for ADD/ADHD

1. History and physical exam to identify specific treatable causes: thyroid dysfunction, allergies, dietary deficiencies, exposure to lead or other heavy metals, other medical problems, concurrent psychiatric diagnoses, and use of other medications that may affect attention, cognition, and arousal. Careful assessment for psychological trauma, abuse, and neglect are essential because these are contributory causes of inattention, hyperactivity, and behavioral problems.

2. Laboratory studies: blood count, chemistry profile. If there is a question of dietary deficiency, malabsorption, or lead exposure, check vitamin, lead, iron, and zinc levels.

3. Correction of nutritional deficiencies with supplementation.

4. Discussion of treatment options with the patient and family including risks and benefits of prescription medications and CAM. Development of a treatment plan including behavioral approaches and family counseling.

5. If the patient is already taking a prescription stimulant that is showing some benefit, it should be maintained unless it is causing unacceptable side effects.

6. When faced with incomplete response to prescription medication or unacceptable side effects, one should try to optimize response by switching to a different prescription medication before starting CAM. If the patient does not have a good response or encounters too many side effects, begin CAM trials as described above.

7. When there is strong motivation to discontinue prescriptions due to concerns about potential long-term risks or philosophical objections, CAM trials may be indicated.

8. Prescription medications should not be discontinued until there is a positive response to CAM. At that point, the stimulant can be gradually tapered while the patient is monitored.

9. All patients with ADD or ADHD should be given trials of biofeedback if possible. Patients whose ADD/ADHD symptoms improve on prescription medications can benefit further by the addition of CAM and should be referred for biofeedback. Depending on what treatments are available, the authors recommend:
   a. Low-energy neurotherapy (LENS; www.ochslabs.com)

    b. Theta-beta training (neurotherapy)

    c. HeartMath (www.HeartMath.com) is a biofeedback program that can be practiced on a home computer.

    d. After the patient becomes proficient in HeartMath, progress to a biofeedback training based on heart rate variability and galvanic skin response called Journey to the Wild Divine (www.wilddivine.com).

    e. Delayed auditory processing often causes academic problems. For delayed auditory or visual processing, use interactive metronome training (www.InteractiveMetronome.com).

10. In cases where the family wants to avoid prescription medications or the patient has had side effects or insufficient response to prescription medications, choose CAM treatments depending on the age of the patient, the target symptoms, and the presence of other learning disabilities, psychiatric diagnoses (e.g., anxiety, OCD, depression, bipolar disorder, PTSD, abuse, or neglect), or medical conditions (e.g., seizures).

Children Under the Age of 12

1. Careful diagnostic workup is needed to establish whether the child has ADD/ADHD and other comorbid conditions.

2. A child psychiatrist or psychopharmacologist should be consulted if one is available, and psychological testing should be completed.

3. Mild regimens are preferable and can be layered. If minor side effects occur, stop the increases and maintain on a lower, tolerable dose. If significant side effects occur, discontinue. Patients and families should be informed that these treatments have shown benefits in clinical practice, but they have not been formally studied in children under the age of six. The clinician must use discretion, lower doses, and careful monitoring, particularly in younger children.

    a. Begin with Pycnogenol 50 mg b.i.d. If no response occurs after two weeks, discontinue. If positive response, then maintain and add the next layers of CAM.

    b. Add picamilon 50 mg b.i.d., increasing every five to seven days up to 100 mg t.i.d.

    c. Add ginkgo 60 mg, increasing every five to seven days up to 120 mg b.i.d.

d. Add centrophenoxine (meclofenoxate) starting with 1 tablet per day and increasing by 1 tablet every seven days up to 4 tablets per day maximum.

e. If there has been no response to steps a–d above, then try *R. rosea* 25 mg (one quarter of a 100 mg capsule) and increase by 25–50 mg every three to seven days to a maximum of 300 mg/day as long as it does not cause agitation or insomnia.

f. Alternatively, one can try SAMe starting with 200 mg/day and increasing by 200 mg every five to seven days to a maximum of 1,200 mg/day with physician monitoring for side effects, including agitation, anxiety, nausea, diarrhea, and insomnia. SAMe tablets will lose their effectiveness if they are broken. For younger children or those with sensitive stomachs, SAMe may be taken with food to reduce the amount absorbed and to lessen any nausea.

Adolescents 12–18 Years Old

1. Begin with *R. rosea* 50 mg/day and increase in 50 mg increments up to a maximum of 500 mg/day as long as it does not cause anxiety, agitation, or insomnia.

2. Next try SAMe 200 mg/day with increases of 200 mg/day every three to seven days until response occurs up to a maximum of 2,400 mg/day as tolerated. SAMe should not be given after 3:00 p.m. as it may cause insomnia.

3. Add picamilon beginning with 100 mg/day and increase every five to seven days up to 100 mg t.i.d.

Adult ADD/ADHD

Although dosing CAM treatments twice a day (morning and midday) may be more effective, most adults with ADD have difficulty remembering to take the second dose. Therefore, the authors suggest starting with morning doses until the patient is able to comply with a more complex schedule.

Yoga breathing is very helpful in ADD. However, most patients lack the discipline to comply with daily practice. The authors find that is best to wait until the patient has shown some improvements on other CAM regimens and is better able to benefit from yoga practices.

1. Start all patients on biofeedback training.
2. Begin with *R. rosea* 400 mg a.m. (30 minutes before breakfast) and increase to 600 mg a.m. If no response occurs after four weeks, discontinue *R. rosea*.
3. Add Action Labs PowerMax 4X (combination of Korean, Chinese, Siberian, and American ginseng) 1 tablet in am for one week and then add 1 tablet midday as needed. Alternatively, try Hsu Korean (*Panax*) ginseng 1 a.m. for one week and then add 1 midday (www.Hsuginseng.com).
4. If the patient can afford SAMe, start 400 mg a.m. (30 minutes before breakfast) and increase by 400 mg every three to five days up to 2,400 mg/day, as tolerated.
5. Add picamilon 100 mg a.m., increasing every three to seven days up to 300 mg/day.
6. For reading, writing, and other learning disabilities, give aniracetam 750 mg/day and increase to 750 mg b.i.d.
7. Add centrophenoxine 1 tablet a.m., increasing up to 2 tabs b.i.d.
8. Treat comorbid conditions with appropriate integrative regimens.

TABLE 5.1 Attention-Deficit Disorder (ADD) and Learning Disabilities Treatment Guidelines

CAM	Clinical Uses	Daily Dose	Side Effects, Interactions* Contraindications
B vitamins	ADD		Minimal
B12		1,000 mcg	Caution: cardiac stents**
folate		800 mcg	
B complex			
Bio-Strath			
Omega-3 fatty acids (PUFA)	ADD	1,200–2,400 mg b.i.d.	Minimal GI distress, belching
Picamilon	ADD	50 mg b.i.d. up to 100 mg t.i.d.	High dose: hypotension
Pycnogenol	ADD	50 mg b.i.d.	Minimal
Racetams	learning disabilities, dyslexia, medicine-related cognitive impairment	aniracetam 750 mg b.i.d.	Minimal Rare: anxiety, insomnia, agitation, irritability, headache
S-adenosyl-methionine (SAMe)	ADD	400–4,000 mg/day give in divided doses	GI, agitation, anxiety, insomnia; rare palpitations Mania in bipolars.
Ashwaganda (*Withania somnifera*)	anxiety, agitation, insomnia	1–2 tabs b.i.d.	Mild sedation, combined effects with other sedatives
Ginkgo biloba	ADD	120–240 mg	Minimal: headache, reduced platelet aggregation contraindications: anticoagulants Rare: agitation. D/C 2 weeks prior to surgery

Panax ginseng American ginseng *Panax quinquefolios*	adult ADD child ADD	300–800 mg depends on age, weight, and diagnosis	Activation, GI, anxiety, insomnia, headache, tachycardia, reduced platelet aggregation Caution: anticoagulants
Rhodiola rosea	Mental focus, attention, memory, alertness, cognitive function	100–600 mg	Activation, agitation, insomnia, jitteriness, mania. Rare: rise in BP, angina, bruising. Contraindication: bipolar I. Caution: bipolar II
Brahmi (*Bacopa monniera*)	ADD	1–3 tabs	Minimal
Mentat BR16-A Many herbs including bacopa, gotu kola, ashwaganda, triphala, morning glory, arjuna	ADD, attention, medication-induced cognitive impairment	1–2 pills once or twice a day with food	Minimal: side effects of component herbs may raise levels of carbamazepine and phenytoin.

PUFA = polyunsaturated fatty acid; BP = blood pressure; GI = gastrointestinal side effects; D/C = discontinue

*Common side effects are listed. There are additional rare side effects. Individuals with high blood pressure, diabetes, pregnancy (or during breast-feeding), or any other chronic or serious condition should check with their physician before taking supplements. Patients taking anticoagulants should consult their physician before taking supplements.

**May increase risk of restenosis of cardiac stents in men only with baseline homocysteine < 15 μmol / liter.

CHAPTER 6 OUTLINE

1. **Life Stage Issues for Women**
   a. **premenstrual syndrome, premenstrual dysphoric disorder**
      i. vitamins, minerals, nutrients
      ii. vitex, pycnogenol, St. John's Wort, *Rhodiola rosea*, light therapy
   b. **pregnancy, postpartum and breast-feeding**
      i. omega-3 fatty acids, choline, SAMe
      ii. acupuncture, mind–body practices, self-hypnosis, light therapy
   c. **menopause**
      i. hot flushes: phytoestrogens, St. John's Wort, flaxseed, wheat germ, mind–body practices, exercise, sleep
      ii. cognition, memory, energy, mood: ginkgo, DHEA, and *R. rosea*

2. **Female Sexual Enhancement and Fertility**
   a. sexual enhancement: arginmax, maca, *R. rosea*, herb-vX (Muira puama + ginkgo), DHEA or 7-Keto-DHEA, mind–body practices, exercise
   b. fertility: vitamins, minerals, nutrients, combination products, *R. rosea*, maca, vitex, mind–body practices

3. **Male Sexual Enhancement and Fertility**
   a. sexual enhancement: *Panax ginseng*, DHEA, muira puama, maca, *R. rosea*, yohimbine, ginkgo, arginine, carnitines, exercise, mind–body practices
   b. prostatic enlargement and sexual dysfunction: saw palmetto, pygeum, stinging nettle
   c. fertility: folate, zinc, carnitines, exercise, mind–body practices

Sexual Enhancement and Other
Life Stage Issues

LIFE STAGE ISSUES FOR WOMEN

Complementary and alternative medicine (CAM) approaches may have better safety profiles than prescription medications and may provide substantial relief for somatic and neuropsychological symptoms related to the menstrual cycle, pregnancy, breast-feeding, and menopause. A review of 45 CAM studies in pregnancy-related conditions, 33 trials for premenstrual syndrome (PMS), and 13 for dysmenorrhea (Fugh-Berman & Kronenberg, 2003) found that most studies were small, inadequately reported, and lacked controls. Although demographic and animal studies support the safety of many herbs and supplements, the dearth of long-term safety studies in humans should be made known to patients as part of informed consent. Low-risk CAM approaches, particularly omega-3 fatty acids and mind–body techniques, are particularly beneficial during pregnancy and breast-feeding when medications ought to be minimized. Hormonal changes with aging affect cognition, memory, mood, and energy. Older patients often have difficulty tolerating medication side effects. Moreover, they are likely to have medical problems and be taking multiple medications that complicate the use of psychotropics.

Premenstrual Syndrome and Premenstrual Dysphoric Disorder

CAM treatments are widely used by women to ameliorate menstrual symptoms due to the physical and psychological effects of the changes in hormone levels. Premenstrual syndrome (PMS) refers to a range of transient emotional and physical changes that many women experience during the week prior to menstruation. Symptoms include depression, irritability, insomnia, hypersomnia, fatigue, decreased concentration, changes in appetite, weight gain, water retention, headache, breast tenderness, and pain in the abdomen, pelvis, back, joints, or legs. While 11–32% of women have emotional and physical changes associated with menses, only 3–9% meet criteria for premenstrual dysphoric disorder (PMDD).

The understanding and diagnosis of changes in mood and behaviors prior to menstruation continues to evolve. For example, "paradoxical insanity" related to PMS was used as a legal defense in the medical testimony during an 1865 murder trial (Spiegel, 1988). By 1930, the term *premenstrual tension syndrome* was being used. In 1987, the *DSM-III-R* of the American Psychiatric Association (APA) defined late luteal phase dysphoric disorder to include women who do not menstruate (e.g., posthysterectomy), but who have cyclic changes in mood and behavior. However, in 1994, the APA renamed it premenstrual dysphoric disorder to emphasize mood changes over physical symptoms and to further distinguish it from PMS.

PMDD is defined as the occurrence of five or more specific symptoms for most of the late luteal phase, with remission starting within a few days after the onset of the follicular phase. The symptoms must be absent during the week postmenses. The five symptoms must include at least one of the following: markedly depressed mood, marked anxiety, marked affective lability, persistent and marked anger or irritability or increased interpersonal conflicts, decreased interest in usual activities (American Psychiatric Association, 1994). It is important, but often difficult, to differentiate PMDD from a premenstrual exacerbation of an underlying unipolar or bipolar mood disorder.

The menstrual cycle has two phases: the follicular phase (development of the ovarian follicle to prepare for release of the egg) precedes ovulation (release of the egg), whereas the luteal phase (development of the corpus luteum after the follicle ruptures) follows ovulation. During the second week of the menstrual cycle, as the follicles grow, they release more estradiol, reaching a peak at about 72 hours before ovulation. The early luteal phase begins on the day of ovulation. During the midluteal phase, progesterone and estrogen increase and reach a plateau around Day 22. If implantation does not occur, the levels of estrogen and progesterone decline during the late luteal phase, which ends the day prior to the next menses. PMS and PMDD are associated with the drop in hormone levels during the last week of the menstrual cycle, the late luteal phase (see Sidebar 6.1).

Vitamins, Minerals, and Nutrients

A reduction in intracellular magnesium has been found in some women with PMS. In a double-blind randomized placebo-controlled trial (DBRPC), 32 women were given 360 mg/day of magnesium or placebo started on Day 15 of menses. The group given magnesium

---

SIDEBAR 6.1 **THE MENSTRUAL CYCLE: THE EFFECTS OF HORMONES ON MOOD**

The biological clock that drives the menstrual cycle is set by the release of gonadotropin-releasing hormone (GnRH) by the hypothalamus. The timed release of GnRH is affected by external events such as psychological factors (via the cerebral cortex ⟶ limbic system ⟶ hypothalamus) and the rhythmic shifts from day to night. Release of GnRH is also influenced by feedback from sexual steroids produced by the ovaries.

GnRH ⟶ pituitary ⟶ follicle-stimulating hormone (FSH) ⟶ ovarian follicle development ⟶ estrogen

GnRH ⟶ pituitary ⟶ luteinizing hormone (LH) ⟶ follicle ruptures and sustains corpus luteum ⟶ progesterone

Estrogen and progesterone ⟶ Regulate secretion of GnRH, FSH, LH
Induce uterine endometrium to proliferate and prepare for implantation

showed significant improvement in negative affect and arousal by the second month, followed by improvements in pain and water retention by the fourth month. Intracellular magnesium increased, but serum magnesium levels did not (Facchinetti, Borella, Sances, Fioroni, Nappi et al., 1991). Magnesium may be beneficial for PMS.

The benefits of calcium in reducing PMS have been demonstrated in DBRPC studies. A study of 497 women with PMS demonstrated that calcium (1,200 mg/day) reduced PMS symptoms by 48% versus 30% with placebo. Side effects included mild nausea, stomach distress, and headache (Thys-Jacobs, Starkey, Bernstein, & Tian, 1998). To avoid renal stone formation, calcium should be taken with meals.

A study comparing differences in calcium and vitamin D metabolism between women with and without PMDD (Thys-Jacobs, McMahon, & Bilezikian, 2007) found that women with PMDD showed a lack of compensatory responsiveness in vitamin D during the late luteal phase with significantly lower levels of ionized calcium at Phase I (menses), urine calcium at late follicular, midcycle, and early luteal phases, and 1,25-dihydroxyvitamin D [1,25(OH)2D] at luteal phase. This relative vitamin D and calcium deficiency may contribute to some of the symptoms of PMDD.

Limited evidence supports the use of B vitamins and minerals in PMS. In a six-month DBRPC study, 40 women were given either a nutritional supplement (containing magnesium, B_6, vitamin E, folic acid, iron, and copper) or placebo. The supplement reduced PMS symptoms to 18% of baseline versus 73% in the placebo group. No side effects occurred (Facchinetti, Nappi, Sances, Neri, Grandinetti et al., 1997).

B_6 (pyridoxine) is a cofactor in the metabolism of tryptophan, a precursor to serotonin and dopamine. A review of 12 double-blind placebo-controlled (DBPC) studies of PMS treatment with B_6 found three with positive results, five with ambiguous results, and four with negative results. The usefulness of vitamin B_6 for PMS is questionable (Kleijnen, Ter Riet, & Knipschild, 1990). High doses of B_6 (>200 mg/day) can cause sensory neuropathy.

L-tryptophan outperformed placebo in a DBPC three-month study of women with PMDD. Those treated with tryptophan 2,000 mg t.i.d. during the 17 days from ovulation until the third day of menses showed a 35% decrease in dysphoria, tension, and irritability versus a 10% decrease with placebo (Steinberg, Annable, Young, & Liyanage, 1999). Tryptophan fell out of favor when impurities caused serious side effects. However, safe, pharmaceutical grade L-tryptophan is available in the United States by prescription.

Carbohydrate treatment has been used to increase the ratio of tryptophan (indirectly increasing serotonin) to other amino acids. In a DBPC crossover study in 24 women with PMS, a balanced carbohydrate-rich drink (PMS Escape) decreased anger and depression 3.5 hours after the drink and improved memory. It also reduced carbohydrate craving 1.5 hours after the drink (Sayegh et al., 1995). A second DBPC study of 53 women with mild to moderate PMS showed that PMS Escape relieved mood symptoms in one third of the subjects versus 5% on placebo (Freeman, Stout, Endicott, & Spiers, 2002).

Several small studies suggest that omega-3 fatty acids, polyunsaturated fatty acids (eicosapentanoic acid, EPA, and docosahexanoic acid, DHA) may ameliorate dysmenorrhea, possibly by reducing sensitivity to steroids and prolactin. The popular concept that evening primrose oil (*Oneothera biennes*) normalizes fatty acid levels is dubious because it contains predominantly omega-6FAs, which are sufficient in most modern diets. A meta-analysis identified seven placebo-controlled studies but only in five trials was randomization clearly indicated (Budeiri, Li Wan Po, & Dornan, 1996). Inconsistent scoring and response criteria precluded statistical pooling and rigorous meta-analysis. The two most well-controlled studies failed to show any beneficial effects for evening primrose oil, although because the trials were relatively small, modest effects cannot be excluded (Khoo, Munro, & Battistutta, 1990; Collins, Cerin, Coleman, & Landgren, 1993). While current evidence does not indicate

---

CLINICAL PEARL

In practice, the authors find that PMS Escape not only alleviates anger and depression but also reduces bloating and carbohydrate craving in many women with PMS.

evening primrose oil to be of value in the management of PMS, it does not cause side effects and some patients feel that it is helpful.

Herbs and Plant Extracts

Herbs can be combined with other CAM treatments to address a wide range of symptoms associate with PMS and PMDD.

Vitex agnus-castus

Chaste tree or chasteberry (*Vitex agnus-castus*), used for 70 years in Germany to treat PMS and menopause, contains diterpines that bind to dopamine receptors, inhibit prolactin release, and reduce lactation (Klepser & Nisly, 1999). These actions are the likely basis for the relief of mastodynia (mastalgia; Wuttke, Jarry, Christoffel, Spengler, & Seidlova-Wuttke, 2003). Estrogenic flavonoids (penduletin and apigenin) bind to estrogen receptors selectively (Jarry, Spengler, Porzel, Schmidt, Wuttke et al., 2003). In a DBPC study conducted over three menstrual cycles, 52% of 86 women given vitex 20 mg/day (ZE440 standardized for castecin) had significant improvement on five out of six self-assessment measures of mood and physical symptoms versus 24% of 84 women on placebo (Schellenberg, 2001). Four subjects had mild transient side effects similar to those reported by the placebo group.

In a small randomized comparison study of women with PMS symptoms, there was no statistically significant difference in the rate of response (68.4%, n = 13) with fluoxetine and 57.9% (N = 11) with *Vitex agnus-castus* using the Penn Daily Symptom Report and Hamilton depression scale (Atmaca, Kumru, & Tezcan, 2003). Vitex was more effective for physical symptoms, while fluoxetine was better for psychological symptoms. A review of chasteberry concluded that research supports the use of chasteberry for breast discomfort and PMS (Roemheld-Hamm, 2005).

Pycnogenol (Pine Tree Bark Extract)

In an open trial of 47 women with dysmenorrhea, Pycnogenol (pine tree bark extract) reduced abdominal pain. Improvements were greater in the second cycle than in the first (Kohama, Suzuki, Ohno, & Inoue, 2004). Phenolic acids with spasmolytic activity may account for the relief of dysmenorrhea.

The following case illustrates the use of a combination of three herbs, St. John's Wort, *Rhodiola rosea*, and vitex, to ameliorate the psychological and somatic symptoms of PMS and depression in a patient who was sensitive to side effects of prescription medications. This patient was not given the diagnosis of PMDD based on the history of recurrent major depression with premenstrual exacerbations.

Case 2—St John's Wort, R. rosea, and Vitex for Depression and PMS

Elaine, a 37-year-old high school science teacher, married with three children, had a long history of recurrent major depression, premenstrual exacerbation of depression, and panic disorder. During the 10 days prior to menses, she would become increasingly depressed, suicidal, and irritable. Somatic symptoms included bloating, water retention, weight gain, carbohydrate craving, fatigue, insomnia, and breast tenderness. When she was treated with paroxetine (Paxil), her depression improved, but she gained 20 pounds and developed headaches and anorgasmia (inability to have an orgasm). Similarly, sertraline (Zoloft) caused a 30-pound weight gain and sexual dysfunction, which exacerbated her depression.

In order to avoid side effects of weight gain and sexual dysfunction, for the first layer of treatment, she was started on *R. rosea* (brand Rhodax) increasing to 170 mg four times a day (a very high dose). Elaine felt more resilient with less crying, but was still depressed and overwhelmed with marital stress. (For discussion of *R. rosea*, see section Perimenopausal Disorders and Chapter 3.) Although the *R. rosea* was helping energy and stress resilience, the high dose in this physically small woman caused her to feel anxious. The dose was reduced to 170 mg twice a day, enough to maintain the improvements in energy and stress tolerance without anxiety.

Because the history revealed that the patient's depression had responded to a serotonin reuptake inhibitor, and because she had premenstrual worsening of mood, she was given a trial of St. John's Wort. The dose was limited to 500 mg t.i.d. because it also caused anxiety in higher doses. She became more stable with improvement in depression on *R. rosea* 170 mg b.i.d. and St. John's Wort 300 mg t.i.d. Vitex was added to alleviate the physical symptoms of her PMS.

Benzodiazepines and Ambien had been tried for insomnia, but they made her feel more depressed and cognitively impaired. Trazodone (Desyrel) caused excess sedation. Elaine was too afraid of weight gain to try mirtazepine (Remeron). Her history of agitation in reaction to stimulating herbs (R. rosea and St. John's Wort) and some winter seasonal worsening raised the possibility of a mild bipolar II disorder. Based on these considerations and her intolerance of sedative-hypnotic medications, she was given a low dose of quetiapine (Seroquel) 12.5 mg for sleep, which worked quite well.

In order to resolve the emotional and physical symptoms of PMS in this patient, four layers of treatment were necessary:

1. R. rosea 170 mg b.i.d. improved energy, stress resilience, sexual function, and mood.
2. St. John's Wort 300 mg t.i.d. relieved depression.
3. Vitex reduced physical symptoms of PMS.
4. Quetiapine (Seroquel) in a low dose (12.5 mg) restored sleep.

Mind–Body Interventions

Mind-body practices may ameliorate PMS partly by reducing stress (an important factor in the symptomatology) and possibly thorugh other mechanisms. In a five-month study, 46 women randomly assigned to a relaxation response group, a reading group, or a charting group showed that those doing daily relaxation had significantly greater improvement in PMS symptoms. Subjects who reported more severe symptoms attained the most improvement in emotional symptoms (Goodale, Domar, & Benson, 1990). Moderate exercise has been associated with a reduction in premenstrual symptoms (Stoddard, Dent, Shames, & Bernstein, 2007).

Acupuncture

In a small randomized controlled trial, 43 women were followed for one year in one of four groups: real acupuncture group; placebo acupuncture group given weekly random point acupuncture for three menstrual cycles; standard control group without medical or acupuncture intervention; visitation control group with monthly nonacupuncture visits with the project physician for three cycles. In the real acupuncture group, 10 of 11 (90.9%) women showed improvement in menstrual pain compared with 4 of 11 (36.4%) in the placebo acupuncture group, 2 of 11 (18.2%) in the standard control group, and 1 of 10 (10%) in the visitation control group. There was a 41% reduction in the use of analgesic medication for women in the real acupuncture group versus no change or increased medication use in the comparison groups (Helms, 1987). While this study is small, with only 10 or 11 subjects in each group, it suggests that acupuncture may be beneficial in relieving primary dysmenorrhea.

Light Therapy

Abnormalities in circadian rhythms (biological changes that cycle with changes in daylight) with phase advancement have been found in women with PMDD. Bright light given in the evening was found to delay these abnormally advanced circadian cycles in three well-designed crossover trials and one unblended trial (Krasnik, Montori, Guyatt, Heels-Ansdell, & Busse, 2005; Parry, Mahan, Mostofi, Klauber, Lew et al., 1993; Parry, Hauger, Lin, Le Veau, Mostofi, et al., 1994). Meta-analysis of these three small studies showed a small pooled effect size of 0.2, leaving uncertain the issue of the effectiveness of light therapy for PMDD. Notably, in a study of 96 women, those with winter seasonal affective disorder showed a much higher rate of PMDD than healthy controls (46% vs. 2%; Praschak-Rieder, Willeit, Neumeister, Hilger, Stastny, et al., 2001).

Integrative Approach for Treatment of PMS and PMDD

1. Ascertain physical and psychological symptoms before, during, and outside the time of menstruation. Inquire carefully about symptoms not related to menses. Many women have premenstrual exacerbation of an underlying mood disorder and therefore will not meet *DSM-IV* criteria for PMDD. Only 3–9% of women have PMDD. Clarifying whether the underlying disorder is bipolar or unipolar depression is necessary in order to choose the appropriate treatment.

2. Review diet, sleep, work, and exercise habits. Encourage exercise and healthy diet.

3. If stress and psychological symptoms are contributory factors, daily yoga stretches, yoga breathing, or relaxation techniques are advisable, along with appropriate psychotherapy. Patients usually find it easier to benefit from meditation if they do yoga breathing first.

4. Start multivitamin, multi-B vitamin (B50 or B100), calcium 1,200 mg/day, magnesium 600 mg/day, and omega-3FA 1,000 mg b.i.d. Also give vitamin D_3 2000 mg/day for women living in northern climates with reduced sun exposure nine months of the year or who spend little time outdoors. In warmer climates, D_3 500–1,000 mg/day is sufficient. The dose of vitamin D may be adjusted according to serum levels (vitamin D profile). Try PMS Escape.

5. If psychological symptoms persist and there is no evidence of bipolar disorder, a selective serotonin reuptake inhibitor (SSRI) may be started one week before menses and continued for 7 to 14 days as needed each cycle. Some patients will need uninterrupted daily maintenance. If the patient does not want an SSRI, she could be offered tryptophan, St. John's Wort, or light therapy (10,000 lux 30–45 minutes in p.m.; Facchinetti et al., 1997).

6. For predominantly somatic complaints (pain) do a three-month trial of *Vitex agnus-castus* 20 mg/day. For persistent pain, Pycnogenol, acupuncture, or prescription L-tryptophan (2,000 mg t.i.d.) may be tried.

Pregnancy and Postpartum

Pharmacological treatments in women who are pregnant or breast-feeding are limited due to a lack of safety data for many drugs and proven hazards for others. Adverse effects during pregnancy have been identified for sedative-hypnotics, anxiolytics, antidepressants, mood stabilizers, and antipsychotics. Stressors of pregnancy and discontinuation of psychotropics may destabilize a psychiatric disorder, increasing risks such as self-destructive behavior, poor nutrition, or elevations of cortisol, adrenaline, and excitatory neurotransmitters that may be harmful to fetal development.

Omega-3FA for Perinatal Depression—Pregnancy and Postpartum

The need for safe alternative treatments during pregnancy and post-partum is urgent. Concerns about adverse effects of antidepressants and mood stabilizers on neonates and breast-feeding infants create a bind for mothers and health care providers when trying to manage mood disorders during the perinatal period. Neonatal complications, minor malformations, cardiovascular malformations (especially with paroxetine), pulmonary hypertension, and withdrawal symptoms have been found with SSRIs. Omega-3FAs are necessary for brain and retinal development in utero and during infancy. Supplementation with omega-3FAs protects against preterm delivery, preeclampsia, and cerebral palsy. During pregnancy, maternal omega-3FAs decline (especially in the third trimester) because they are used for fetal growth and are not adequately replaced by dietary intake (Hibbeln, 2002). The decline in maternal omega-3FAs increases the risk of postpartum depression and bipolar depression.

In a flexible-dose open trial, 15 pregnant women with major depressive episodes who did not want antidepressant medication were given 0.93–2.8 g/day of a combination of EPA and DHA for two months. Their mean scores for depression showed significant reductions with a 40.9% drop on the Edinburgh Postnatal Depression Scale (EPDS) and a 34.1% drop on the Hamilton Rating Scale for Depression (HRSD; Freeman, Hibbeln, Wisner, & Watchman,

---

CLINICAL PEARL

During pregnancy, the decrease in maternal stores of omega-3FAs increases the risk of postpartum depression and bipolar depression. It is vital to ensure adequate levels of dietary EPA and DHA for women during pregnancy and breastfeeding and in infant formulas, particularly in premature infants. Although there is no agreed-upon optimal dose, a total of 1,500–2,400 mg/day omega-3 fish oil, containing 1,000–1,600 mg EPA plus 500–800 mg DHA, would probably be sufficient.

2006). Although this was a small trial without a placebo control, it supports the potential benefit of omega-3FAs for depression in pregnant women. The U.S. FDA recognizes 3,000 mg/day omega-3FA as generally safe.

Approximately 10–15% of women experience postpartum depression with potential long-lasting effects on mother and child. An eight-week randomized dose-ranging pilot trial of EPA plus DHA in 16 mothers with postpartum depression found mean percentage decreases of 51.5% on EPDS and 48.8% on HRSD. No adverse events occurred (Freeman, Hibbeln, Wisner, Brumbach, et al., 2006).

Bright Light Therapy During Pregnancy: Antepartum Depression

One open trial of bright light therapy in 16 depressed pregnant women showed significant improvements in depression with no adverse effects (Oren, Wisner, Spinelli, Epperson, Peindl et al., 2002). This work was extended in a 10-week DBRPC study of 10 pregnant women with major depressive disorder. One group received a 7,000 lux light treatment, while the placebo group was given only a 500 lux light box. After five weeks, there was a small group advantage with 7,000 lux, but after 10 weeks, there was a significant improvement in the group treated with 7,000 lux compared to the placebo group (p = 0.001) with an effect size of 0.43. This effect size was comparable to that seen in trials of antidepressant medications (Epperson, Terman, Terman, Hanusa, Oren et al., 2004). Several companies produce light boxes for seasonal affective disorder (SAD) that emit primarily in the blue-green spectrum and minimize exposure to ultraviolet radiation that could be damaging to the eyes. Patients with bipolar disorder may become overly stimulated with

---

CLINICAL PEARL

Evening light therapy using a 7,000–10,000 lux SAD light box for 30 to 60 minutes may alleviate depression during pregnancy. Response may take 5 to 10 weeks.

light exposure. If agitation, irritability, or insomnia occur, reduce the length of light box exposure to 10–20 minutes and if the overstimulation persists, discontinue usage. Portable light boxes can be bought for about $200–$300. Usually, adverse reactions appear during the first week of treatment. Most companies offer full refunds for return of a light box within 30 days.

Perinatal Bipolar Disorder

The management of bipolar episodes during pregnancy and postpartum can be extremely challenging with serious risks for the mother and child. In the absence of clinical studies, we offer our approach based on clinical experience and evidence from studies in nonpregnant bipolar women and in perinatal depression.

When pregnancy occurs in a woman on anticonvulsant mood stabilizers, the medications should be discontinued because of high risk to the fetus unless the bipolar symptoms are so severe as to cause imminent danger to the mother. The risk of neural tube defects is 1–5% with valproate and 0.5–1% with carbamazepine. In the first trimester, lithium carries a risk of 0.05–0.1% for cardiovascular malformations (MacNeil, 2006). Abrupt discontinuation of lithium is associated with a high rate of relapse with rebound mania. To prevent mania, it is often necessary to use low-dose haloperidol (Haldol) because it may be less likely to cause birth defects than other antipsychotics (Cohen & Rosenbaum, 1998). Although a small study did not show an increased rate of malformation on atypical antipsychotics after the first trimester, larger studies are needed before safety can be assumed. Women with bipolar disorder being treated with mood stabilizers should be maintained on a multivitamin with additional folate (800 mcg/day) to reduce the risk of neural tube defects in the event of an unplanned pregnancy.

Omega-3FAs are safe during pregnancy and may help stabilize mood. Omega-3FA (EPA + DHA) 3,000–6,000 mg/day should be started immediately. If tolerated, increase to 8,000–10,000 mg/day. To reduce gastrointestinal symptoms, it is worth trying a more refined fish oil preparation (see Table 6.1 at end of this chapter). Further studies are needed to establish the benefits and optimal doses of omega-3FAs for perinatal depression. See Chapter 2 for discussion of side effects. However, considering the high degree of safety, the additional health benefits for mother and child, and the dearth of proof of the safety of most psychotropic medications, clinicians should not hesitate to offer omega-3FAs during pregnancy and postpartum as a preventive measure or as a treatment for mood disorders.

Acupuncture can be helpful if the acupuncturist is experienced with pregnancy, mood disorders, and hormonal problems.

Pure choline (not phosphatidylcholine) has been shown to reduce mania (Stoll et al., 1996). It can be used safely as a complementary treatment in doses of 3,000–7,000 mg/day pure choline for bipolar symptoms during pregnancy.

S-Adenosyl Methionine (SAMe) during Pregnancy and for Postpartum Depression

In a placebo-controlled study, SAMe 1,600 mg/day was administered to 30 women with postpartum depression. Their depression and anxiety ratings dropped 50% in 10 days and 75% in 30 days. A comparable group of 30 women with postpartum depression given placebo achieved less than 50% improvement by day 30 (Cerutti, Sichel, Perin, et al., 1993).

SAMe has been used to treat gallstones of pregnancy in Europe. In numerous trials, SAMe has been given parenterally and orally to women with cholestasis of pregnancy without adverse effects on the mother, the course of the pregnancy, or fetal development (Frezza et al., 1990; U.S. Department of Health and Human Services, Agency for Healthcare Research and Quality, 2002b). Tests of SAMe in pregnant rodents found no teratogenic potential (Cozens, Barton, Clark, Gibson, Hughes et al., 1988). Although there are no definitive prospective studies of SAMe to rule out teratogenic or neurodevelopmental effects in humans, it should be noted that there are no such studies with standard prescription antidepressants. No mutagenic activity has emerged in studies of SAMe in vitro or in vivo (Pezzoli, Galli-Kienle, & Stramentinoli, 1987).

The amount of SAMe passing to infants through breast milk has not been measured. However, infants normally have high levels of SAMe, three to seven times higher than in adults (Surtees & Hyland, 1989). SAMe is needed for myelination of the developing brain (the myelin sheath that forms around neurons enables transmission of electrical impulses). It is, therefore, unlikely that the amount of SAMe passed to breast-feeding infants would be harmful.

Mind–Body Approaches for Anxiety Disorders, Stress, and PTSD

Anxiety and stress during pregnancy can adversely affect pregnancy outcomes, resulting in problems such as low birth weight and prematurity. The prevalence rate for anxiety and depression during pregnancy is estimated to be 30%. Mind–body techniques offer safer alternatives to the risks of adverse effects from psychotropics. In a randomized controlled trial of 110 primigravid women, the addition of seven weeks of applied relaxation training to standard prenatal care significantly reduced state-trait anxiety (Spielberger State-Trait Anxiety Inventory) and perceived stress (Cohen Perceived Stress Scale) (Bastani, Hidarnia, Kazemnejad, Vafaei, & Kashanian, 2005). The training included progressive relaxation, release-only relaxation (without tensing muscle groups), deep breathing techniques, an exercise focused on breathing with self-instruction to relax just before exhalation, differential relaxation (selective relaxation of different body parts), rapid relaxation, and instruction on anxiety, stress, and relaxation during pregnancy. The following case illustrates the use of several mind–body techniques to treat PTSD in the second trimester of pregnancy.

Case 1—PTSD During Pregnancy

Laura, a 32-year-old elementary school teacher, was five months pregnant with her second child when she was involved in a motor vehicle accident. A drunk driver ran a stoplight and struck the back of her car, sending it into a spin. Laura suffered minor injuries including a mild concussion, but the baby was not injured. After the terrifying accident, she had recurring nightmares of the accident, waking up screaming, trembling, and sweating. Whenever she rode in a car, the sight of approaching vehicles triggered flashbacks and panic reactions. When she came for a consultation, she was distraught, anxious, tearful, and exhausted. Mental status exam revealed problems with memory, wordfinding, and concentration. She complained of difficulty organizing and completing routine tasks.

Laura was suffering from PTSD and postconcussion syndrome. She was afraid to take any medication that might harm her baby. She agreed to a trial of psychotherapy and Ujjayi breathing (see Chapter 3). After five minutes of Ujjayi breathing, she felt mentally and physically relaxed for the first time since the accident. She readily agreed to practice yoga breathing 10 minutes twice a day, at bedtime and as needed. The following week she looked happy and rested. Her anxiety was much improved and she was no longer waking up in a terror. She was having fewer nightmares, but driving was still triggering panic. During the third session, she chose an image to substitute in her mind whenever she noticed herself visualizing the accident. She admitted that when she had tried driving, she kept looking out the side windows checking for oncoming cars. In talking about it, Laura realized that overchecking was not making her safer; quite the opposite. She agreed to keep her eyes on the road ahead except when checking was appropriate and she put a small sticker on the window to remind herself. By the fourth session, Laura's anxiety improved. Her nightmares and fear of driving had resolved completely as she continued her Ujjayi breathing.

Laura complained of recurring residual moderate anxiety and muscle tension. She appeared to worry excessively and to overreact to events and minor stressors. Although acupuncture ameliorated the tension and anxiety, there were still times when she would worry excessively and escalate her state of distress. Laura had been treated with hypnosis during adolescence for abdominal pain. She responded to retraining in self-hypnosis and was able to achieve states of deep relaxation when needed.

In this case, the patient skillfully and creatively integrated mind–body practices into her daily life with the guidance of her therapist. She was able to maintain a better overall level of calmness using yoga breathing, psychotherapy, acupuncture, and imagery. During more stressful times, she could choose to do yoga breathing or self-hypnosis. Laura's pregnancy went well. She and her husband were delighted to deliver a healthy baby boy.

Female Menopause

Concerns among women with perimenopausal symptoms regarding increased cancer risks and disappointing news about the putative long-term benefits of hormone replacement therapy (HRT) have caused many women to seek safer alternatives. Although dietary supplements and herbs are widely used for relief of perimenopausal symptoms, more scientific evidence is needed to support the benefits that have been claimed. Potential long-term risks have not been adequately studied. A review of 29 randomized controlled trials by Fugh-Berman and Kronenberg (2003) concluded that black cohosh and foods containing phytoestrogens, for example whole soy and red clover, are promising treatments for menopause. In reviewing 18 randomized controlled trials, Huntley and Ernst (2003) found no convincing evidence. However, they identified black cohosh and red clover as having potential benefits. It is important to inform women that while there is some evidence of efficacy, it is not conclusive. Similarly, while there is no evidence of harm, long-term safety studies in humans have not been done. Women must weigh this against the known risks of HRT and the severity of the symptoms they are experiencing. For example, if a woman is having intense hot flashes, mental slowing, and memory problems that interfere with her ability to function socially and at work, she may accept the limits of scientific information about the risks of CAM and choose to do trials.

Isoflavones exert estrogenic and antiestrogenic effects. Analysis of studies of soy found a small reduction in breast cancer risk associated with the use of whole soy but not high-dose isoflavone supplements (Trock, Hilakivi-Clarke, & Clarke, 2006). Red clover (*Trifolium pratens*) contains mildly estrogenic isoflavones, similar to soy, that bind to human alpha and beta estrogen receptors (Booth et al., 2006). Hops (*Humulus lupulus*) and red clover extracts upregulate progesterone receptor messenger RNA and interact with transcription factors (NF-KappaB; Overk, Yao, Chadwick, Nikolic, Sun et al., 2005).

During menopause, estrogen and progesterone decrease, while follicle-stimulating hormone (FSH) and luteinizing hormone (LH) increase. Symptoms include hot flashes, vaginal dryness, mood swings, depression, insomnia, fatigue, forgetfulness, and poor concentration (Mayo, J. L., 1997). The 1990 Nurses Health Study (121,700 women followed for 10 years) found a 40% greater risk of breast cancer in women taking HRT versus placebo. Estrogen replacement therapy (ERT) also elevates the risk of uterine cancer. Adding progesterone to ERT reduces but does not eliminate the heightened risk of uterine cancer (Beresford, Weiss, Voigt, & McKnight, 1997; Colditz, Stampfer, Willett, Hennekens, Rosner et al., 1990; Colditz, Hankinson, Hunter, Willett, Manson et al., 1995). The Office of Women's Health Research at the National Institutes of Health reported insufficient evidence of risk versus benefit to support the use of HRT to prevent osteoporosis, cardiovascular disease, or dementia (U.S. Department of Health and Human Services Agency for Healthcare Research and Quality, 2002a). Studies of the relationship between dietary phytoestrogens and risks of cancer have had mixed and confusing results. A prospective study of 15,555 women aged 50–69, a Dutch cohort of the European Prospective Investigation into Cancer and Nutrition, concluded that a high intake of isoflavones or mammalian lignans has no significant relationship to breast cancer risk (Keinan-Boker, van Der Schouw, Grobbee, & Peeters, 2004).

While most research on hot flashes has focused on hormonal treatments, Robert Freedman (2005) proposed that elevated sympathetic and noradrenergic activation contributes to hot flashes. This provides a new paradigm for the benefits of mind–body practices, which is discussed in more detail below.

Women with hot flashes often complain of difficulty sleeping. To better understand the relationship between sleep and hot flashes, 18 postmenopausal women with hot flashes, 6 without hot flashes, and 12 women with menstrual cycling were studied for four nights. During the first half of the night, postmenopausal women had significantly more awakenings and most of their hot flashes preceded arousal and wakening. In the second half of the night, the awakenings were less frequent and preceded the hot flashes. Rapid eye movement sleep (REM) suppressed hot flashes during the second half of the night, reducing arousals and awakenings (Freedman & Roehrs, 2006). Sleep apnea and restless leg syndrome interfere with REM sleep. A study of 102 peri- and postmenopausal women who reported sleep disturbance (with or without hot flashes) found that 53% had sleep apnea, restless legs, or both (Freedman & Roehrs, 2007). Therefore, it is important to evaluate women who complain of

> **CLINICAL PEARL**
>
> Patients who complain of poor sleep due to hot flashes should be evaluated for sleep apnea and restless leg syndrome. By correcting the underlying sleep disorder and restoring REM sleep, it is possible to reduce hot flashes at night.

nighttime hot flashes for possible sleep apnea or restless legs. Correcting the underlying sleep disorder should enable the patient to achieve more REM sleep. The increase in REM sleep may reduce nighttime hot flashes.

Exercise, dietary changes, and mind–body techniques can help to relieve menopausal symptoms while providing additional health benefits. Herbal treatments for hot flashes have shown mixed results. Menopause-related symptoms involving mood, cognition, memory, and energy may respond well to CAM. Some women prefer synthetic estrogen and progesterone, whereas others seek CAM treatments, especially as some research confirms their efficacy and potential to reduce cancer risks. In weighing the risks and benefits of treating menopausal symptoms, women need all the available information for informed consent in choosing CAM, hormone replacement therapy, or no treatment.

Herbs and Nutrients

Evidence suggests that certain herbs and nutrients can be physically, emotionally, and cognitively beneficial during menopause.

Soy and Isoflavones

In a review of 16 randomized trials of whole soy or soy isoflavone supplements, eight showed statistically significant improvements in one or more menopausal symptoms (Newton, Reed, LaCroix, Grothaus, Ehrlich et al., 2006). In animal studies, soy protected against breast cancer and other estrogen-sensitive cancers. The applicability of such animal studies to humans has been questioned. A meta-analysis of the effects of soy on breast cancer risk concluded that soy may be associated with a small decrease in breast cancer risk and that there is insufficient evidence to support high-dose isoflavone supplementation for prevention (Trock et al., 2006). Isoflavones have both estrogenic and antiestrogenic activity. Estrogen receptor binding effects need further study. Epidemiologic data and animal studies suggest that the health benefits of soy (lowering cholesterol and cancer prevention) are best obtained from whole soy (i.e., whole food) rather than from extracted components (for reviews of soy, see Albertazzi, 2006; Anderson, Anthony, Cline, Washburn, & Garner, 1999).

There is some data that soy may be a promising adjunct for increasing bone mass density and cognitive function in menopausal women. A DBRPC crossover study of 78 postmenopausal women comparing 60 mg/day isoflavones versus placebo for six months found that when subjects were taking isoflavones, their scores on cognitive performance and mood tests improved significantly (Casini, Marelli, Papaleo, Ferrari, D'Ambrosio et al., 2006).

Red clover (*Trifolium pratense*) contains mildly estrogenic isoflavones similar to those in soy. Daidzein, genistein, formononetin, biochanin A, coumestrol, and naringenin were estrogenic in AP assay (induced alkaline phosphatase in an endometrial carcinoma cell line), and all of these, except formononetin, bound to one or both recombinant human estrogen receptors (alpha and beta) (Booth, Overk, Yao, Burdette, Nikolic et al., 2006). A 12-week DBRPC study of 252 menopausal women (with at least 35 hot flashes per week) compared two commercial red clover extracts with placebo. The reductions in mean daily hot flash counts were similar for Promensil 82 mg isoflavones per day (5.4), Rimostil 57 mg isoflavones per day (5.1) and placebo (5.0) groups. Promensil somewhat accelerated the reduction in hot flashes (Tice, Ettinger, Ensrud, Wallace, Blackwell et al., 2003).

Hops (*Humulus lupulus*), traditionally used to brew beer, bind to estrogen receptors in vitro but do not stimulate uterine growth in ovariectomized rats (Beckham, 1995; Fackleman, 1998). Hops strobiles contain estrogenic prenylflavanone, 8-prenylnaringenin (8-PN), 6-prenylnaringenin (6-PN), isoxanthohumol (IX), and xanthohumol (XN). The effects of hops on P450 enzyme systems tend not to be clinically significant because the enzymes inhibited by hops are not relevant to most medications (Henderson, Miranda, Stevens, Deinzer, & Buhler, 2000).

Extracts of hops and red clover, genistein and 8-PN, activate the estrogen response element (ERE) in Ishikawa cells while extracts, biochanin A, genistein, and 8-PN induced ERE-luciferase expression in MCF-7 cells. Hops and red clover extracts as well as 8-PN upregulated progesterone receptor (PR) messenger RNA in the Ishikawa cell line. In the MCF-7 cell line, PR messenger RNA was significantly upregulated by the extracts biochanin A, genistein, 8-PN, and IX. Further research on hops and red clover may be of value for treatment of menopausal symptoms (Overk et al., 2005). Red clover and hops phytoestrogens also act as selective estrogen enzyme modulators, have antioxidant activity and interact with transcription factors such as NF-kappaB.

Animal studies suggest that red clover isoflavones decrease bone loss induced by ovariectomy, probably by reducing the rate of bone turnover via inhibition of bone resorption (Occhiuto, Pasquale, Guglielmo, Palumbo, Zangla et al., 2007). Isoflavones in soy foods and red clover may have a modest positive health effect on plasma lipid concentrations, bone mass density, and cognitive function. Assessment of the risks and benefits of these herbs in women with breast cancer and breast cancer survivors remains controversial. Including soy in the diet of postmenopausal women may be beneficial, but without definitive data the optimal dose range remains unknown.

Black cohosh (*Cimicifuga racemosa*), used extensively in Europe for over 60 years, reduces LH levels and hot flashes. Most studies show no estrogenic effect, no binding to estrogen receptors in vitro. In contrast to ERT, black cohosh has no significant side effects. No toxicity occurred in rats given 90 times the human dose for six months. In breast cancer cell cultures, black cohosh did not induce proliferation (Freudenstein & Bodinet, 1999), whereas it inhibited DNA synthesis and augmented the antiproliferative activity of tamoxifen in vitro (Fackleman, 1998; Foster, 1999; Lieberman, 1998). There is no evidence of mutagenicity or carcinogenicity. Although stimulation of some uterine growth in ovariectomized rats had been reported, a multinational study of 400 postmenopausal women given 40 mg/day *Cimicifuga racemosa* BNO 1055 black cohosh for 52 weeks found no cases of endometrial hyperplasia

(Raus, Brucker, Gorkow, & Wuttke, 2006). Overall the number and intensity of hot flashes was markedly reduced and the herb was well tolerated. Several controlled studies, including one DBPC study, showed efficacy equivalent to ERT (Foster, 1999; Lieberman, 1998).

Studies of black cohosh have yielded inconsistent results. For example, a DBRPC 12-week study assigned 95 menopausal women to: (1) *Actaea racemosa* (ethanol extract BNO 1055) equivalent to 40 mg/day black cohosh; (2) conjugated estrogens (CE 0.6 mg/day); or (3) placebo (Raus et al., 2006). Of the 62 completers, those taking BNO 1055 and CE showed similar reductions in all estrogen deficiency symptoms and improved sleep quality versus the placebo group. However, a one-year DBRPC study of 351 women (ages 45–55) found no difference between frequency or intensity of vasomotor symptoms in those given 160 mg/day black cohosh (Pure World, Inc., *Actaea racemosa* or *Cimicifuga racemosa*; 2.5% triterpine glycosides; 70% ethanol extract) versus placebo (Newton et al., 2006). This study, limited to women in late menopausal transition or postmenopausal, concluded that black cohosh is unlikely to have an important role in the treatment of vasomotor symptoms.

Differences in the outcomes of DBRPCs may be due to differences in herbal preparations, patient selection criteria, length of study, and symptom measurements. Levels of bioactive compounds can be significantly affected by extraction procedures. A major problem in assessing this research is that studies using proprietary products such as special ethanol extract *Actaea racemosa* BNO 1055 may not reveal the process that makes their product special. This leaves open the question of whether the difference in outcomes of studies using BNO 1055 versus other brands could be due to significant differences in the quality and efficacy of the products or to other factors. Given the high safety profile of black cohosh, it could be recommended for relief of menopausal symptoms in women who do not want HRT.

Licorice (*Glycyrrhiza glabra*), a common ingredient in herbal remedies, contains glycyrrhetic acid, the active component that structurally resembles adrenocortical steroids. It is reported to increase conversion of testosterone to estrogen and to block cancer-promoting estrogens. In vitro animal studies suggest strong estrogen receptor binding but no stimulation of uterine growth in ovariectomized rats. Side effects include headache, lethargy, sodium and water retention, potassium depletion, and, rarely, hypertension (at high doses) (Fackleman, 1998; Robbers & Tyler, 1999). A pilot study of nine women given 3.5 g of licorice (7.6% glycyrrhizic acid) daily found that licorice can increase serum parathyroid hormone and urinary calcium levels after only two months. The effect of licorice on calcium metabolism is probably influenced by several constituents, which have aldosterone-like, estrogen-like, and antiandrogen activity (Mattarello, Benedini, Fiore, Camozzi, Sartorato et al., 2006) In order to avoid these adverse effects, patients interested in trying licorice should be advised to use only the deglycyrrhizinated form. For women at high risk of breast cancer (e.g., strong family history) and those with breast cancer, licorice may be contraindicated.

Dong quai (*Angelica sinensis*), a component in Chinese tonics since 500 b.c., has estrogen-like activity and strong binding to estrogen receptors in vitro, stimulates uterine growth in ovariectomized rats, and induces progesterone secretion (Belford-Courtney, 1993; Fackleman, 1998). The water-soluble extract of dong quai regulates uterine contractions while the essential oil relaxes uterine muscles. One DBPC trial of dong quai alone for menopause had negative results (Hirata, Swiersz, Zell, Small, & Ettinger, 1997). However, dong quai is traditionally used in combination with other herbs. Considering that dong quai may have weak estrogen-agonistic activity, its use in herbal preparations for perimenopausal symptoms, especially in women with breast cancer, warrants caution. Controlled studies of dong quai are needed.

Vitex (*Vitex agnus-castus*), often combined with black cohosh, licorice, dong quai, and other herbs (see *Vitex agnus-castus* above), modulates prolactin secretion by binding to dopamine receptors. Vitex has not been studied in menopause. Nevertheless, anecdotal reports suggest that it alleviates affective symptoms, hot flashes, fluid retention, and weight gain. Vitex may protect against breast cancer by acting as an antagonist to excess circulating estrogen. No side effects have been reported. However, vitex slightly binds to estrogen receptors in vitro and modestly stimulates uterine growth in ovariectomized rats. It has been used to treat hyperprolactinemia and one of the authors (RB) has used it to counteract antipsychotic medication-induced prolactin elevations (Mayo, 1997; McCaleb, 1995; Wuttke et al., 2003).

Native Americans use blue cohosh (*Caulophyllum thalictroides*) as a uterine tonic and to prevent miscarriages. Blue cohosh has modest estrogen receptor binding and has been used for menopausal symptoms. There are no controlled trials of blue cohosh and it needs further study (Fackleman, 1998). Several reports have linked the use of blue cohosh with perinatal stroke and neonatal congestive heart failure.

Golden root, Arctic root, or roseroot (*Rhodiola rosea*), has been used traditionally in the Republic of Georgia and Siberia to enhance fertility. In an open study of 40 women with amenorrhea given *R. rosea* extract 100 mg b.i.d., normal menstrual cycles were restored in 25 subjects and 11 of these became pregnant. In 25 women, uterine length increased to normal size (Gerasimova, 1970). More recently, Patricia Eagon at the University of Pittsburgh found strong estrogen receptor binding in vitro. However, *R. rosea* (extract used in Rosavin by Amerden) did not elevate circulating estradiol levels, nor did it increase uterine size in ovariectomized rats (Eagon, Elm, Gerbarg, Brown, & Check, 2003). The discrepancy between the lack of estrogenicity in the Eagon study versus Gerasimova's observations may be due to differences in the source of the herb (wild grown vs. cultivated) and extraction procedures. Moreover, in rats given estradiol implants, *R. rosea* reduced the excessive increase in estradiol that normally occurs with these implants (Eagon, personal communication, 2003). Research on the use of *R. rosea* in treating hormonal disorders is warranted. Clinical experience with *R. rosea* in women with perimenopausal symptoms has been encouraging.

St. John's Wort (*Hypericum perforatum*) 900 mg/day given to 111 menopausal women in an open series for 12 weeks significantly improved self-esteem, feeling attractive, irritability, anxiety, and depression. Psychosomatic symptoms (insomnia, headache, and palpitations), vasomotor symptoms (sweating, flushing, and dizziness), and sexual desire also improved (Grube, Walper, & Wheatley, 1999). These findings warrant more rigorous study.

Flaxseed and wheat germ have been used to relieve hot flushes and night sweats. In a DBRPC trial comparing flaxseed to wheat germ for improvement of lipid profile, bone density, and physical symptoms in menopausal women, both supplements were equally effective in relieving the hot flushes, but neither improved bone mineral density or lipid profile (Dodin, Lemay, Jacques, Legare, & Forest, 2005).

Off-Label Use of Psychotropic Medication for Menopausal Hot Flushes

For women with severe hot flashes in whom CAM treatments are ineffective, the following psychotropic medications may provide relief: terazosin (Hytrin), clonidine (Catapres), gabapentin (Neurontin), or venlafaxine (Effexor). Both terazosin and clonidine are antihypertensive medications that also reduce sweating and hot flashes. In practice, the authors find that most patients tolerate terazosin (1 mg/day) better than clonidine.

Perimenopausal Disorders of Cognition, Memory, and Mood

Ginkgo, Dehydroepiandrosterone (DHEA,) and Rhodiola rosea
Many women complain of memory problems, cognitive slowing, difficulty multitasking, fatigue, and mental fogginess, often associated with depression, during the perimenopausal years. Trials of *Ginkgo biloba* have had mixed results. In a six-week DBRPC study of *G. biloba* in postmenopausal women, those in Stage +1 (mean age 55) performed better than those in Stage +2 (mean age 61) at baseline on tests of memory and cognitive function. After six weeks, the only clear benefits were in Stage +2 women, who showed greater mental flexibility (Elsabagh, Hartley, & File, 2005). In a 12-week DBRPC study of 57 postmenopausal women (aged 51–66), those given Gincosan (*G. biloba* 120 mg plus *Panax ginseng* 200 mg) showed no significant effects on mood, menopausal symptoms, attention, or memory compared to those on placebo (Hartley, Elsabagh, & File, 2004).

For patients whose DHEA or DHEA-sulfate levels are low normal or below normal for age (particularly menopausal women), the authors have found that treatment with 7-keto DHEA 25–75 mg/day may enhance mood, cognitive function, memory, and sexual function (see sections on DHEA in Chapters 2 and 4). A starting dose of 25 mg a.m. and a maintenance dose of 50 mg a.m. are usually sufficient. Side effects are usually minimal and include hirsutism, acne, anxiety, and agitation. Unlike DHEA, 7-keto DHEA does not convert to estrogen or testosterone and therefore does not cause hirsutism or acne. DHEA can cause manic symptoms in bipolar patients.

DHEA, DHEA-sulfate, and testosterone free and total levels should be checked before treatment. If testosterone is low, DHEA-

---

CLINICAL PEARL

In clinical practice, the authors observe that *Rhodiola rosea* is particularly helpful in improving memory, mental clarity, cognitive speed, energy, and mood in perimenopausal women.

---

sulfate may modestly increase levels enough to alleviate cognitive and sexual dysfunction, but not enough to correct androgen deficiency states. In comparison, treatment with testosterone leading to higher testosterone levels may increase long-term risk of breast cancer. Therefore, DHEA may provide a more modest but safer elevation of testosterone into the low normal range, enhancing DHEA-sulfate and sexual function. However, since there are no clear data on DHEA and long-term risk of breast cancer, this approach may be contraindicated in women with a personal or family history of breast cancer. 7-Keto DHEA, which does not convert to testosterone, estrogen, or progesterone, is preferable in such cases.

Although *R. rosea* has not been studied for cognitive enhancement in perimenopausal women, the authors find that it is particularly helpful in improving memory, mental clarity, cognitive speed, energy, and mood in perimenopausal women. Studies are needed to validate these clinical observations.

Case 3—Menopause and Depression

Sophie, a 49-year-old journalist, complained of gradually worsening depression since she began to experience menopausal changes. She felt tired from the moment she awakened and throughout the day. Success at work led to more challenging writing opportunities, but instead of feeling excited, she felt overwhelmed. Everything became a burdensome chore, as she felt like she was moving through sludge. It became harder to concentrate, to multitask, and to keep track of details. For the past five years, she had taken an SSRI, but it no longer seemed to be working. Sophie did not want to take additional medication because she was already experiencing loss of libido on her prescription antidepressant. She agreed to try *R. rosea* (Rosavin by Ameriden) starting with 100 mg 20 minutes before breakfast and increasing to a total of 200 mg 20 minutes before breakfast and 20 minutes before lunch. By the end of the first week she noticed more energy. Over the next three weeks she felt more alert. Her mind seemed sharper and she was able to keep track of details and make decisions more quickly. Her menstrual cycles, which had been irregular, returned to normal. After two months she reported the return of her long-lost libido.

Mind–Body Practices for Menopausal Symptoms

Although the relaxation and reduction in anxiety and tension derived from mind–body practices probably has multiple benefits for menopausal women, more specific physiological mechanisms may also be brought into play. While estrogen levels decline during menopause, this hormonal change is not a sufficient explanation for the symptomatology. Robert Freedman (2005, 2006) has proposed that elevated sympathetic noradrenergic activation contributes to hot flashes, possibly by narrowing the thermoneutral zone (the temperature zone within which hot flashes are not triggered) such that small elevations in core body temperature set off hot flashes. To explore the possibility that reducing sympathetic tone using a relaxation procedure might also reduce hot flashes, several studies were undertaken. In three controlled studies, using paced respiration (slow deep abdominal breathing at 6–8 breaths per minute) as a relaxation process (on the presumption that this would reduce sympathetic tone), hot flashes were significantly reduced (50%) by objective measures with no adverse effects. In the second study, 33 women with frequent menopausal hot flashes were randomly assigned to three groups: eight sessions of paced respiration training; muscle relaxation; or alpha-wave electroencephalographic biofeedback (control). Twenty-four-hour ambulatory monitoring of sternal skin conductance showed that only those trained in paced respiration had significant reductions in frequency of hot flashes compared with the other groups (Freedman & Woodward, 1992). The third study replicated the results. Although the slow-paced respiration significantly reduced hot flashes, there was no evidence of reduction in sympathetic activity based on measures of plasma catecholamines, 3-methoxy-4-hydroxyphenylglycol, and platelet alpha-receptors (Freedman, 2005).

We propose that the paced respiration reduced menopausal hot flashes by increasing parasympathetic tone (which was not measured) rather than by reducing sympathetic tone. (See Chapter 3 for detailed discussion of the effects of yoga breathing on the parasympathetic nervous system.) This interpretation suggests that slow yoga breathing should be studied as a treatment for vasomotor symptoms of menopause because it increases parasympathetic tone. Patients can obtain the CD *Respire 1* to pace their respirations at five breaths per minute. In most cases, this will enhance parasympathetic tone and relaxation (see Coherence and Resonant Breathing in Chapter 3).

The effects of Sudarshan Kriya Yoga (see Chapter 3) on oxidative stress were compared with the antioxidant effects of vitamin E and estradiol. In a 30-day controlled study of 190 menopausal women, 40 were given an 8 mg estradiol patch (HRT), 40 received 500 IU vitamin E per day, and 60 were given Sudarshan Kriya Yoga (SKY) only. Indicators of oxidative stress and antioxidant defense were measured. Malonic dialdehyde was used as a marker of membrane lipid peroxidation (damage to the lipid component of cell membranes by free radicals). Two important antioxidant enzymes were measured: glutathione peroxidase (the major antioxidant for neuroprotection) and erythrocyte superoxide dismutase. Significantly greater decreases in serum malonic dialdehyde occurred in the women given SKY than in those given either HRT or vitamin E. Moreover, antioxidant defenses showed significantly greater increases in glutathione peroxidase and erythrocyte superoxide dismutase (Geehta, Chitra, Kubera, & Pranathi, 2006). This study suggests that the beneficial effects of SKY practice on oxidative stress and antioxidant activity exceed those of vitamin E and estradiol in menopausal women.

Integrative Approach for Menopause-Related Disorders

1. Identify target symptoms: hot flashes, cognitive impairment, memory decline, low energy, sexual dysfunction.
2. Obtain patient and family history regarding menopause, cancer, and cancer risk factors that may be contraindications for hormones, phytoestrogen, or other herbal treatments.

3. Evaluate for sleep apnea and restless legs. If the history includes daytime fatigue, snoring, gaps in breathing, leg movements at night, or uncomfortable leg sensations relieved by walking, a sleep study with polysomnography is needed to diagnose sleep disorders.
4. Obtain lab work: hormone levels (follicle stimulating hormone, luteinizing hormone, estrogens, progesterone, DHEA, DHEA-sulfate, free testosterone, total testosterone, thyroid functions, and possibly prolactin.
5. For hot flashes, try Remifemin (black cohosh).
6. For hot flashes with problems in cognitive or memory function or low energy try *Rhodiola rosea* plus Remifemin.
7. For problems with cognition, memory, or low energy, try *R. rosea* first.
8. For more pervasive complaints (hot flashes, cognitive, memory, low energy, sexual dysfunction) in women with low DHEA-sulfate, a trial of DHEA or 7-keto DHEA is often helpful.
9. In women with low testosterone who complain of anorgasmia, testosterone supplementation may be beneficial.
10. A trial of a breathing program such as *Respire 1* with or without Ujjayi breathing (see Chapter 3) can be helpful in all women.

FEMALE SEXUAL ENHANCEMENT AND FERTILITY

People over age 40 and those taking medications that adversely affect sexual function are the predominant consumers of herbal and nutrient sexual enhancers. Although scientific evidence for sexual enhancement using herbs is limited, many cultures have a long history of use and products promising sexual enhancement are sold widely. Possible mechanisms of action include vasodilation, improved circulation, anti-inflammatory, antioxidant, hormonal, stimulant, and mood enhancement (Rowland & Tai, 2003). This discussion is limited to sexual enhancers for which there is some research evidence, frequent consumer use, or positive clinical experience in the authors' practices. Although most of the research has been for male sexual dysfunction, some CAM approaches also enhance female sexual function.

It is estimated that 10% of U.S. couples of childbearing age are infertile. Individuals and couples who are unable to conceive are often seen by mental health practitioners for anxiety, depression, and difficulty dealing with the effects of infertility on their self-image, relationships, and quality of life. Hormonal treatments, in vitro fertilization (IVF), and embryo transplant may add further to stress and emotional instability. Conversely, stress, depression, or alcohol use (twice a week or more) can adversely affect fertility. Depressed women have twice the infertility rate compared to nondepressed women (Lapane, Zierler, Lasater, Stein, Barbour et al., 1995; Ruiz-Luna, Salazar, Aspajo, Rubio, Gasco et al., 2005). Psychotherapy, treatment of anxiety and depression, lifestyle counseling, mind–body techniques for relaxation and stress reduction, and other CAM interventions can be helpful.

Muira puama or marapuama (*Ptychopetalum guyanna*), an herb from the rain forests of Brazil, is used as an aphrodisiac, nerve tonic, and antiarthritic (Mowrey, 1996). Muira puama combined with *Gingko biloba* (Herbal vX) was tested in an open series in 202 healthy women complaining of low sex drive. After one month, 65% reported improvements in libido, intercourse, sexual satisfaction, intensity of orgasm, and other measures (Waynberg & Brewer, 2000). There is no research regarding mechanisms of action. Controlled studies are needed to confirm these findings.

Maca (*Lepidium peruvianum myenii*/Chacon) is a Peruvian adaptogen used to improve energy, sexual function, fertility at high altitudes, stress tolerance, nutritional status, and menopausal symptoms (Quiros & Cardenas, 1997). Sterols, glucosinolates, and alkaloid components increase FSH, estrogen, and testosterone levels in female rats (Chacon, 1997; Quiros & Cardenas, 1997). An aqueous extract of yellow maca increased litter size in female mice and increased uterine weight in ovariectomized rodents (Ruiz-Luna, Salazar, Aspajo, Rubio, Gasco et al., 2005). Enlargement of the uterus indicates estrogenic effects. These findings cannot be extrapolated to humans until clinical trials are completed.

No toxicity or side effects have been reported in human or animal studies. However, the authors have found that maca may precipitate agitation or mania in bipolar patients. Therefore, it should be used cautiously and in lower doses in cases of bipolar disorder. Both aqueous and methanolic extracts of maca exhibited estrogenic activity in MCF-7 cells (Valentova, Buckiova, Kren, Peknicova, Ulrichova et al., 2006). Excess doses may cause overactivation or breast tenderness. Maca use may be contraindicated in patients with fibroids, estrogen receptor-related cancer risk, family history of breast cancer, or endometriosis. Information on maca is available at www.maca750.com and www.medicine-plants.com.

Arginine and ArginMax

Arginine, the precursor to nitric oxide (NO), has been used to enhance sexual function in women. NO is involved in the vasodilation of genitalia during sexual arousal. L-arginine may predispose to herpes infection. There are no long-term toxicity studies.

In a four-week DBRPC study of 77 women, 73.5% of the subjects taking ArginMax (a supplement containing L-arginine, *Panax ginseng*, *G. biloba*, damiana leaf, multiple B vitamins, folate, vitamins A, C, and E, calcium, iron, and zinc) reported improvements in their sex lives (improved desire, vaginal lubrication, frequency of intercourse and orgasm, and clitoral sensation) compared with 37.2% of those on placebo. ArginMax had no significant side effects (Ito, Trant, & Polan, 2001). An estrogen bioassay using human endometrial adenocarcinoma cell AP enzyme sensitive to estrogen stimulation found no estrogenic activity in ArginMax or in a sample of *P. ginseng* extract (Polan, Hochberg, Trant, & Wuh, 2004). In a study of 12 healthy subjects, *P. ginseng* or *G. biloba* had no significant effect on CYP activity (indicating that it would not interfere with the metabolism of medications metabolized by liver CYP enzymes; Gurley et al., 2002).

The effect of ArginMax for Women was studied in 108 women aged 22–73 years who reported lack of sexual desire in a four-week DBRPC trial. Premenopausal women on ArginMax reported significantly improved sexual desire and satisfaction with sex life (Female Sexual Function Index), frequency of desire, and intercourse compared with placebo group. Perimenopausal women primarily reported improvements in frequency of intercourse, satisfaction with sexual relationship, and vaginal dryness compared with placebo group. Postmenopausal women showed increased level of sexual desire (51%) compared with placebo (8%). ArginMax has not been found to have estrogenic activity (Ito, Polan, Whipple, & Trant, 2006). This study highlights two important issues. First, the effects of herbal treatments vary with hormonal status. Second, the more effective treatment approaches combine synergistic herbs and other nutrients.

DHEA for Sexual Arousal in Postmenopausal Women

In a double-blind randomized crossover study of 16 postmenopausal sexually functioning women, a single oral dose of 300 mg DHEA given 60 minutes before presentation of an erotic video segment significantly increased subjective ratings of physical ($p < 0.036$) and mental ($p < 0.016$) arousal compared to placebo (Hackbert & Heiman, 2002). The use of a single dose of 300 mg DHEA 60 minutes before sexual activity may enhance arousal and pleasure. The possible risks of intermittent use of relatively high-dose DHEA for sexual enhancement compared with the risks of testosterone or other commonly used products has not yet been evaluated.

Integrative Approach to Sexual Dysfunction in Women

1. History and physical examination.
2. Rule out medical conditions that could affect sexual function. Also, evaluate for iatrogenic factors such as medications that may impair libido, arousal, or orgasm: birth control pills or other hormonal products, antidepressants (particularly SSRIs, venlafaxine, and antipsychotics), blood pressure medications, and over-the-counter preparations.
3. Evaluate psychological, emotional, and relationship factors contributing to sexual dysfunction.
4. Obtain laboratory studies: DHEA, DHEA-sulfate, free testosterone, total testosterone, prolactin.
5. If stress or lack of sleep are significant causative factors, then advise lifestyle changes and mind–body practices such as yoga breathing, yoga postures, meditation, and exercise.
6. For lack of libido, try maca, *R. rosea*, Herbal-vX (muira puama + ginkgo), or DHEA.
7. For problems with arousal or orgasm, suggest ArginMax, maca, *R. rosea*, DHEA, or 7-keto DHEA. These treatments can be layered for combined effects.

Fertility in Women

Stress, anxiety, and depression may affect a woman's chance of becoming pregnant. A review of the scientific literature noted that unipolar and bipolar depression have been associated with lower fertility (Williams, Marsh, & Rasgon, 2007). Most studies find that women seeking fertility treatment have higher rates of depression and that these symptoms reduce the success of fertility interventions. The reviewers commented that most of the studies are small, have many confounding variables, and show methodological problems. However, the better quality studies also show a correlation between depression and fertility. Chronic anxiety and depression are associated with infertility in both animal and human studies (Berga & Loucks, 2006; Levy, Brizendine, & Nachtigall, 2006).

Herbs

In a small three-month DBRPC study on the effects of a blend of six herbs including *Vitex agnus-castus* (Mastodynon) in 96 women with fertility disorders, positive outcomes were defined as: pregnancy or spontaneous menstruation in amenorrheic subjects; pregnancy or increased levels of luteal hormones. The vitex group showed 57.6% positive outcomes versus 36% in the control group. Among those who were given vitex, 10 became pregnant versus 5 in the placebo group (Gerhard, Patek, Monga, Blank, & Gorkow, 1998).

In a DBRPC study, Fertilityblend (FB), containing chasteberry, green tea, L-arginine, vitamins (including folate), and minerals was compared to placebo in 93 women (24–42 years old) who had been unable to conceive for 6–36 months. After three months, 14 out of 53 women on FB (26%) became pregnant versus 4 out of 40 (10%) on placebo. In the FB group, the average number of days with luteal-phase basal temperatures above 98 degrees increased significantly (Westphal, Polan, & Trant, 2006). Larger and more long-term studies are needed to clarify the role of herbal blends as an alternative or adjunctive treatment for fertility disorders.

In the Republic of Georgia, among the people living at high altitudes in the Caucasus Mountains, it is customary at weddings to present the bride with a large bouquet of *Rhodiola rosea* roots to ensure the birth of healthy children. The authors have found that some women resume menstruating or become pregnant when given *R. rosea,* including several who had previously undergone standard fertility treatments without success. In an open study of 40 amenorrheic women (7 who had never menstruated and 33 who had missed three or more cycles after having had regular menses), *R. rosea* restored regular menstrual cycles in 25 subjects. Of these, 11 subsequently

CLINICAL PEARL

The authors have found that in some women being treated for fertility problems, *Rhodiola rosea* plus maca, adaptogens used to enhance fertility by people living at high altitudes, may result in pregnancy. Once pregnancy occurs, the herbs are to be discontinued.

became pregnant (Gerasimova, 1970; Saratikov & Krasnov, 1987b). Although this study used outdated methodology, it is consistent with traditional folk medicine and with the authors' clinical observations that *R. rosea* may restore regular menstrual cycles and may enhance fertility.

MALE SEXUAL ENHANCEMENT AND FERTILITY

Sexual function in men can be adversely affected by physical or psychological stress, poor nutrition, substance abuse, low hormone levels, environmental toxins, medical conditions (e.g., benign prostatic hypertrophy, hypertension, and vascular disease), and medications such as nonthiazide diuretics, benzodiazepines, and antidepressants (particularly SSRIs and venlafaxine). While standard treatments for sexual performance are effective in many cases, conventional treatments for loss of libido (sexual desire) are more limited.

Erectile Dysfunction
Although phosphodiesterase-5 inhibitors such as sildenafil (Viagra) improve erectile function in approximately 60–70% of men, many patients cannot tolerate side effects, including headache and nasal congestion. There are concerns about risks with this class of drugs, particularly interactions with nitrates, and pulmonary hypertension with long-acting drugs such as vardenafil (Levitra) and tadalafil (Cialis).

Yohimbine
Yohimbine (*Pausinystalia yohimbe*) is both a prescription drug and a dietary supplement used to treat erectile dysfunction. Proerectile

effects may be due to inhibition of adrenergic receptors innervating the genitals. Meta-analysis of seven well-done DBPC studies showed that 15–43 mg/day yohimbine was more effective than placebo for 40% of men with sexual dysfunction (Ernst & Pittler, 1998; Morales, Condra, Owen, Surridge, Fenemore et al., 1987). In one case series, yohimbine reversed sexual dysfunction from fluoxetine in eight out of nine men and women (Jacobsen, 1992). The prescription form comes in 5.4 mg pills and the usual dose is 18–42 mg/day. Yohimbine content in over-the-counter products is often negligible (Betz, White, & der Marderosian, 1995). The prescription form of yohimbine provides the best quality. Some patients, particularly the elderly, cannot tolerate the side effects: anxiety, nausea, dizziness, chills, sweating, headache, insomnia, and at higher doses, increased blood pressure. In patients with anxiety disorders, yohimbine can trigger anxiety or panic attacks.

Dehydroepiandrosterone (DHEA)
The Massachusetts Male Aging Study found an inverse correlation between the incidence of erectile dysfunction and serum DHEA levels. A DBRPC 24-week study of 40 men with serum DHEA-sulfate levels below 1.5 mol/L found that the men given DHEA 50 mg/day achieved higher scores on assessments of erectile function, orgasmic function, sexual desire, and intercourse satisfaction. Their scores constantly increased in all values during the 24 weeks. In contrast, the placebo group showed a trend toward improvement in their scores during the first 8 weeks (probably a placebo response), followed by a decline to below baseline in all scores except sexual desire (Reiter, Schatzl, Mark, Zeiner, Pycha et al., 2001).

Ginseng
Asian ginseng (*Panax ginseng*) is a common sexual stimulant in herbal preparations. There have been anecdotal reports of hypersexual behavior. Animal studies have shown increases in sperm count, testicular weight, testosterone level, and mating counts. Based on animal models, ginseng (like sildenafil) may increase nitric oxide synthesis (Kang et al., 1995). One three-month placebo-controlled study of 60 men found that those given *P. ginseng* 300 mg/day experienced better sexual performance than those given placebo (Choi, Seong, & Rha, 1995). Studies with more rigorous methodology are needed.

Ginkgo

Ginkgo (*Ginkgo biloba*) improves blood flow to the brain, retina, legs, genitalia, and penis. In an open, nonblinded study, 50 men with erectile dysfunction given ginkgo for six months were able to achieve erections (Sohn & Sikora, 1991). An open study of 63 patients with antidepressant-induced sexual dysfunction who improved on 240 mg/day ginkgo (Cohen & Bartlik, 1998) has been criticized for flawed methodology (Balon, 1999). Although ginkgo can be used to treat mild impotence in middle-aged men, as a monotherapy, it does not improve libido or orgasm.

Pycnogenol

Pycnogenol, a standardized extract of French maritime pine bark, *Pinus maritime*, inhibits the cyclooxygenase enzyme, reducing prostaglandin production and inflammatory reaction, and increases production of nitric oxide by nitric oxide synthase together with L-arginine as substrate for this enzyme. Penile erection requires the relaxation of the cavernous smooth muscle, which is triggered by nitric oxide. An uncontrolled self-report study comparing L-arginine with L-arginine plus Pycnogenol found that after three months on the combination treatment, 92.5% of the men reported normal erections (Stanislavov & Nikolova, 2003). This study is limited by lack of placebo control and lack of objective documentation of erectile function. Another uncontrolled nonrandomized study of 19 subfertile men given 200 mg Pycnogenol daily for 90 days found that the mean sperm morphology score (Ham's F-10 capacitation) increased by 38% and the mannose receptor binding assay scores improved by 19% (Roseff, 2002). While these findings are preliminary, they indicate a potential role for Pycnogenol in fertility enhancement.

Pycnogenol has no mutagenic activity, no observed adverse effects in dogs at 150 mg/kg, no teratogenicity or adverse effects on fertility. In 2,000 patients, a 1.5% incidence of minor side effects included gastrointestinal disturbance, dizziness, nausea, and headache (Rohdewald, 2002). Moreover, evidence suggests that Pycnogenol may have long-term health benefits: antioxidant, anti-inflammatory, antihypertensive, and cognitive enhancement.

Muira Puama or Marapuama *(Ptychopetalum guyanna)*

In an open study of 262 men complaining of lack of sexual desire and impotence treated with muira puama 1,500 mg/day for two weeks, 62% reported enhanced libido and 51% reported better erections (Waynberg, 1990). Controlled studies are needed to confirm these findings. In clinical practice, the authors find that approximately 30% of patients report significant improvement in sexual desire and satisfaction with muira puama, while the rest have no response at all. Based on these observations, muira puama is worth trying in men with low libido, as the following case illustrates.

Case 4—Muira Puama for Loss of Sexual Desire

George, a successful 62-year-old businessman, was married to a woman who was 25 years younger. While taking an SSRI for depression, his libido and erectile function declined. George's wife became dissatisfied with their sex life, which had been very active. During his first visit, he decided to try muira puama. One month later he returned to report that his libido was much improved, but he had developed some blood in his urine. When asked about his sexual activity, he said that he and his wife were having intercourse seven days a week. While this was a welcome change, the frequent inter-course was causing some urethral irritation and blood in the urine. The patient was advised to reduce his sexual activity to three or four times a week. On his follow-up visit a month later, George said that his urine was now clear, but his wife would like some additional firmness in his erections. Silde-nafil (Viagra) was added to his regimen. The following month George came for his visit carrying a bottle of champagne, a gift from his wife to his doctor.

Maca

Maca (*Lepidium peruvianum myenii*/Chacon), is used to enhance energy, sexual function, fertility at high altitudes, and stress toler-ance (Quiros & Cardenas, 1997). Sterols, glucosinolates, and alka-loid components increase testosterone levels in male rats (Chacon, 1997; Quiros & Cardenas, 1997). Black maca increased spermatogenesis, prevented high-altitude spermatogenic disruption, and improved sexual performance in normal rats and in rats with erectile dysfunction (Cicero, Bandieri, & Arletti, 2001; Gonzales, Nieto, Rubio, & Gasco, 2006; Zheng, He, Kim, Rogers, Shao et al., 2000). These findings cannot be extrapolated to humans until clinical trials are completed.

In a 12-week DBRPC trial of different maca doses (1,500 mg or 3,000 mg/day) compared with placebo, 57 men showed significant improvements in self-perception of sexual desire at Weeks 8 and 12 compared to placebo (Gonzales, Cordova, Vega, Chung, Villena et al., 2002). This effect was independent of anxiety, depression, serum testosterone, or estradiol levels. Although two men given placebo reported improvement in sexual desire at Week 4, none of the men on placebo reported improvement at Weeks 8 or 12. Among those given maca, the incidence of reported improvement was 40.0% at Week 8 and 42.2% at Week 12. The assessment of desire was based on one question using a scale of 0–5. It would be worthwhile to replicate these findings using additional validated assessments of sexual desire.

Seminal analysis performed on nine men given maca 1,500 mg or 3,000 mg/day for four months resulted in significantly increased seminal volume, sperm count, motile sperm count, and sperm motility with both doses ($p < 0.05$). In four subjects with low baseline serum follicle-stimulating hormone (FSH) levels, maca did not increase sperm counts. There was no increase in serum testosterone, luteinizing hormone, FSH, prolactin, or estradiol (Gonzales, Cordova, Gonzales, Chung, Vega et al., 2001).

No toxicity or side effects from maca have been reported in human or animal studies. Excess doses may cause overactivation. Maca use may be contraindicated in patients with prostate cancer.

Arginine and ArginMax

Arginine is an alpha-2-adrenoceptor antagonist, the precursor to nitric oxide. Sunflower seeds (which contain large amounts of arginine) have been used to treat impotence. The nitric oxide signaling pathway is relevant to the treatment of sexual dysfunction in men and women. L-arginine may predispose to herpes infection. There are no long-term toxicity studies.

A DBRPC study of 50 men with erectile dysfunction found 9 out of 29 responded to L-arginine versus 2 out of 17 on placebo. All nine responders had decreased nitric oxide excretion or production at baseline (Chen, Wollman, Chernichovsky, Iaina, Sofer et al., 1999). In a two-week DBRPC crossover study of 45 men with erectile dysfunction, a combination of L-arginine glutamate 6 mg/day and yohimbine 6 mg/day, yohimbine 6 mg/day alone, or placebo was taken one to two hours before sexual intercourse. Men with mild-to-moderate erectile dysfunction ($\geq$14 on Erectile Function Domain) had significantly better response to both interventions than men with lower scores (<14) compared to placebo (Lebret, Herve, Gorny, Worcel, & Botto, 2002).

Acetyl-L-Carnitine

Acetyl-L-carnitine plus propionyl-L-carnitine (ALC) significantly enhanced the efficacy of sildenafil (Viagra) in alleviating erectile dysfunction in a DBRPC study of 96 men after bilateral nerve-sparing retropubic prostatectomy. Compared to men given sildenafil alone or placebo, those given ALC plus sildenafil showed significantly greater improvements in erectile function, sexual intercourse satisfaction, orgasm, and general sexual well-being (Cavallini, Modenini, Vitali, & Koverech, 2005).

In a six-month DBRPC study, 120 men aged 60–74 were evaluated for sexual dysfunction, depressed mood, and fatigue associated with aging. Compared to placebo, testosterone undecanoate 160 mg/day and carnitines (propionyl-L-carnitine 2 g/day plus acetyl-L-carnitine 2 g/day) significantly improved erectile function score, Depression Melancholia Scale score, and fatigue. Carnitines were more effective than testosterone on erectile function score. While increasing testosterone levels with testosterone supplementation may enhance sexual function, this may also increase prostatic volume. Carnitines do not increase prostatic volume (Cavallini, Caracciolo, Vitali, Modenini, & Biagiotti, 2004).

Prostatic Enlargement and Sexual Dysfunction

Many men experience sexual dysfunction, in part due to prostatic enlargement in middle and late life when free testosterone declines and the prostate is stimulated by increasing levels of estradiol, pro-

CLINICAL PEARL

Carnitines (acetyl-L-carnitine and propionyl-L-carnitine) can enhance the response to sildenafil (Viagra) better than testosterone without causing an increase in prostatic volume.

lactin, sex hormone-binding globulin, and dihydrotestosterone (DHT) with elevation of the estrogen-testosterone ratio. Reducing the size of an enlarged prostate sometimes improves sexual functioning. Standard treatments for benign prostatic hypertrophy (BPH) include finasteride (Proscar), alpha-adrenergic blockers (terazosin, doxazosin, or tamsulosin), and surgery. Finasteride is expensive and tends to exacerbate sexual dysfunction (4% report total impotence; "Finasteride for Benign Prostatic Hypertrophy," 1992). Side effects of alpha-adrenergic blockers include tiredness, dizziness, depression, headache, abnormal ejaculation, and rhinitis ("Tamsulosin for Benign Prostatic Hyperplasia," 1997). The three most studied herbal treatments for BPH are saw palmetto (*Serenoa repens*), pygeum (*Pygeum africanum*), and stinging nettle (*Urtica dioica*).

Saw Palmetto

Sitosterols in saw palmetto (*Serenoa repens*) reduce DHT levels, DHT binding, and inflammation. Several studies, including a three-year trial comparing saw palmetto with finasteride, showed that saw palmetto significantly increased urinary flow rate and decreased residual urine volume by at least 50%. Eleven percent of the patients taking finasteride stopped because of side effects compared to 2% of those taking saw palmetto (headache and upset stomach; Bach, Schmitt, & Ebeling, 1997). However, a one-year DBRPC trial of 225 men with moderate to severe BPH symptoms found no significant difference between those given saw palmetto extract 160 mg b.i.d. and those given placebo on the American Urological Association Symptom Index (Bent, Kane, Shinohara, Neuhaus, Hudes, Goldberg et al., 2006). As with other herbals, the extraction procedures may affect the levels of active constituents. Supercritical fluid extraction may produce more effective formulations (Faloon, 1999). Saw pal-metto may be most effective for mild to moderate BPH. A combina-tion of saw palmetto, pygeum, and stinging nettle may yield even better results, but has not been tested.

Pygeum

Pygeum bark (*Pygeum africanum*) inhibits prostate cell growth and aromatase (reduces the estrogen-testosterone ratio), increases prostate secretions, and decreases inflammation, prolactin (reducing testosterone uptake in the prostate), and cholesterol (reduces DHT binding; Bassi, Artibani, De Luca, Zattoni, & Lembo, 1987). In a 60-day DBRPC study of 263 men, pygeum extract significantly reduced nocturia and micturition volume (Barlet, Albrecht, Aubert, Fischer, Grof et al., 1990) with no side effects. There is evidence of rapid improvement in nocturnal erections and sexual activity even in elderly men (Carani, Salvioli, Scuteri, Borelli, Baldini et al., 1991). The doses for pygeum range from 75 to 150 mg/day. The long-term har-vesting of bark from the fragile pygeum tree may not be sustainable (Simons, Dawson, & Duguma, 1998).

Stinging Nettle

Stinging nettle root extract (*Urtica dioica*) blocks prostate cell growth receptors, blocks 5-alpha-reductase, inhibits aromatase, inhibits sex-hormone-binding globulin binding, and is anti-inflammatory (Lichius & Muth, 1997). Although it was effective alone in a placebo-controlled trial (Krzeski, Kazon, Borkowski, Witeska, & Kuczera, 1993), the effect was more robust in combination with pygeum in a DBPC study (Sokeland & Albrecht, 1997). A six-month DBRPC partial crossover study of 620 men with BPH found that 81% of those given *Urtica dioica* reported improved lower urinary tract symptoms (LUTS) versus 16% on placebo. International Prostate Symptoms Scores (IPSS), Qmax, peak urinary flow rates, and postvoid residual volumes all improved significantly in the *Urtica dioica* group compared with placebo. The group treated with the herb were found to have a modest reduction in prostate size (3.8 cc; $p < 0.001$; Safarinejad, 2005). The usual dose is 300 mg/day.

PRO 160/120, a combination of 160 mg WS 1473 saw palmetto and 120 mg WS 1031 *Urtica dioica* stinging nettle root extract, was

CLINICAL PEARL

Although the efficacy of combinations of saw palmetto, pygeum, and stinging nettle have not been formally studied, in clinical practice, the authors find that using all three herbs together often produces better results than any one of them alone. Compared to prescription drugs, these natural compounds can be effective for BPH, cause fewer side effects, and they are relatively inexpensive.

tested in 257 men with moderate to severe LUTS due to BPH in a DBRPC 24-week trial. Those given PRO 160/120 showed significantly greater improvements on IPSS, flow measures, and sonographs compared to those on placebo (Lopatkin, Sivkov, Walther, Schlafke, Medvedev et al., 2005).

Another 60-week DBRPC study compared the efficacy and safety of PRO 160/120 (Prostal or Prostagutt Forte) with the alpha1-adrenoceptor antagonist tamsulosin (CAS 106463-17-6) in 140 elderly outpatients suffering from LUTS caused by BPH. IPSS total score was reduced by a median of 9 points in both groups: 32.4% of the patients in the PRO 160/120 group and 27.9% in the tamsulosin group were responders. Both drugs were well tolerated with only one adverse event in each group. The study supports noninferiority of PRO 160/120 compared to tamsulosin as a treatment for LUTS due to BPH (Engelmann, Walther, Bondarenko, Funk, & Schlafke, 2006).

Fertility in Men

Abnormalities in sperm cell count and morphology may be due to both genetic and environmental factors. Stress, poor nutrition, cigarette smoking, pesticide exposure, industrial exposure (heavy metals and toxic chemicals), free radical damage, oxidative stress, excess heat or cold, and even cell phone use have been implicated as causative factors (Aitken & Sawyer, 2003; Wdowiak, Wdowiak, & Wiktor, 2007). Although there are few studies of herbs or nutrients in subfertile men, there is a significant literature on improving and preserving sperm quality in animal livestock. We also know that in populations living at high altitudes, certain herbs, such as maca and *Rhodiola rosea* have been used for centuries to enhance fertility in both animals and humans. Maca was found to increase spermatogenesis in rats exposed to high altitudes (Gonzales, Gasco, Cordova, et al., 2004) Standard medical treatments for male fertility are limited. Improved nutrition, avoidance of excess heat, and removal of toxic exposures may be beneficial in some cases. Mind–body practices for stress reduction and antioxidants may be helpful.

Vitamins and Minerals

In a DBRPC trial 103 subfertile and 108 fertile men were given one of four regimens: folate 5 mg/day; zinc 66 mg/day; folate 5 mg/day plus zinc 66 mg/day; or placebo. Total normal sperm count increased after 26 weeks with folate plus zinc in both subfertile (77% increase) and fertile men (Wong, Merkus, Thomas, Menkveld, Zielhuis et al., 2002).

In a DBRPC study of 64 subfertile men, those with low selenium plasma levels who were given selenium (L-selenomethionine 100 mg/day) had increased sperm motility and pregnancy rates (11%) compared to no pregnancies in the placebo group (Scott, MacPherson, Yates, Hussain, & Dixon, 1998).

Nutrients

In a study of infertile men whose total sperm mobility was less than 50% of normal (n = 102), those who did not have azoospermia (n = 66) were given L-carnitine 1 g/day and acetyl-L-carnitine 500 mg b.i.d. for six months. After three months, in both groups a significant increase was observed in live sperm count, motility, membrane integrity, and linear movement compared to baseline and after six months, there was an increased capacity for cervical mucus penetration (De Rosa, Boggia, Amalfi, Zarrilli, Vita et al., 2005).

Integrative Approach to Sexual Dysfunction in Men

1. History and physical examination, including inquiring about symptoms of prostatic enlargement such as difficulty urinating or increased frequency of urination. In men who do not report urinary problems, high blood pressure may be the first indication of prostatic enlargement with urinary retention affecting renal function.

2. Evaluate psychological, emotional, relationship, nutritional, and environmental factors that may contribute to sexual dysfunction.

3. Rule out iatrogenic factors such as a history of prostatic surgery or medications that can interfere with sexual desire, erectile function, or orgasm: antidepressants (particularly SSRIs, venlafaxine, antipsychotics), blood pressure medication, over-the-counter medications.

4. Ameliorate contributory factors such as relational problems, emotional issues, stress, poor nutrition, substance abuse, cigarette smoking. If stress and fatigue are factors, advise lifestyle changes, exercise, and mind–body practices such as yoga breathing, yoga postures, and meditation.

5. Identify target symptoms: libido, erectile dysfunction, inability to climax, lower urinary tract symptoms.

6. Obtain hormone levels: DHEA, DHEA-sulfate, free testosterone, total testosterone, sex-hormone binding globulin.

7. Evaluate risk factors such as personal or family history of prostate cancer or benign prostatic hypertrophy (BPH).

8. Consider obtaining a prostate-specific antigen test or urological consultation.

9. If there are symptoms of BPH, try saw palmetto, pygeum, and stinging nettle.

10. For problems with libido, try *Panax ginseng*, DHEA, muira puama, maca, and *Rhodiola rosea*.

11. For erectile dysfunction, consider maca, *R. rosea*, ArginMax, muira puama, *P. ginseng*, ginkgo, DHEA, and carnitines. These treatments may be added as layers for combined effects.

12. For infertility consider folate, zinc, selenium, carnitine, maca, and *R. rosea*.

TABLE 6.1 Treatment Guidelines for Hormonal Conditions and Sexual Disorders

CAM	Clinical Uses	Daily Dose	Side Effects, Drug Interactions,* Contraindications
Arginine	erectile dysfunction	900 mg 1–4 times/day	May predispose to herpes
Asian ginseng (*Panax ginseng*)	erectile dysfunction	100 mg t.i.d.	Insomnia, GI, mania, may lower blood sugar, abuse potential. D/C pregnancy Caution: anticogulants, MAOIs, hypoglycemic meds
B vitamins	PMS		None in women
Black cohosh (*Cimifuga racemosa*)	menopausal symptoms, hot flashes, PMS, dysmenorrhea	8 mg/day standardized extract	High level of safety. Minimal side effects: GI, drop in BP, headache, dizziness. D/C: pregnancy Caution: antihypertensive medications Contraindication: estrogen-sensitive tumors
Calcium	PMS	600 mg b.i.d.	Mild GI. Take with meals to avoid kidney stone formation
Carbohydrate PMS Escape	PMS		No significant side effects Study needs replication
Chaste tree, chasteberry (*Vitex agnus-castus*)	PMS, menopause, female infertility, hyperpro-lactinemia	40 mg/day standardized extract	No significant side effects. Rare: allergic reaction, dry mouth, headache, nausea. D/C: pregnancy
Dehydroepian-drosterone (DHEA)	menopause, cognitive, memory, sexual function, osteoporosis	25–200 mg/day	Acne, hirsutism (DHEA) Caution: bipolars Contraindication: estrogen-sensitive cancer, prostate cancer

TABLE 6.1 *Continued*

CAM	Clinical Uses	Daily Dose	Side Effects, Drug Interactions,* Contraindications
7-Keto DHEA	menopause, cognitive, memory, sexual function	25–300 mg	Caution: bipolar Contraindication: estrogen-sensitive cancer, prostate cancer
Dong quai (*Angelica sinensis*)	menopausal symptoms	Use under supervision of trained herbalist	Rigorous studies needed. Used in combination with other herbs. Photosensitivity. Contraindication: anticoagulants, estrogen-sensitive cancer
Evening primrose oil (*Oenothera biennis*)	PMS— no evidence of efficacy		GI, headaches. Increased risk of seizures with phenothiazines
Gingko (*Ginkgo biloba*)	erectile dysfunction	120 mg b.i.d.	GI. D/C: pregnancy Contraindication: anticoagulants
Hops (*Humulus lupulus*)	estrogenic effects, insomnia		Inadequate evidence of efficacy. Allergic reactions, fatigue. Contraindication: estrogen-sensitive cancer D/C: pregnancy
Licorice (*Glycyrrhiza glabra*)	adrenocortical steroid-type effect		Headache, lethargy, sodium and water retention, potassium depletion, hypertension. Use deglycyrrhinated only. Contraindication: diuretics
L-tryptophan	PMDD, dysmenorrhea	2,000 mg t.i.d.	Pharmaceutical grade by prescription only is safe

Maca (*Lepidium myenii)*	improve erections, libido, fertility (possibly), menopause	6 pills/day	No toxicity. Contraindications: estrogen-sensitive tumors, prostate cancer, endometriosis
Magnesium	PMS	360 mg/day	Loose bowels
Muira puama (*Ptychopetalum guyanna)*	libido, erections, arousal, orgasm in men and women, fertility	1,000–1,500 mg	Promising. Needs further study. Works best with ginkgo and other sexual enhancers. Contraindications: estrogen-sensitive cancer
Omega-3 fatty acids EPA & DHA	depression bipolar	6–10 g/day	GI distress, belching, loose stools, may affect glucose metabolism in diabetics. Safe during pregnancy.
Pygeum (*Pygeum africanum)*	BPH	75–150 mg	None reported
Red clover (*Trifolium pratense)*	menopausal symptoms, estrogenic effects	500 mg (40 mg isoflavones)	May modulate effects of tamoxifen, HRT, and other estrogenic drugs. D/C: pregnancy Contraindications: bleeding disorders, anticoagulants, estrogen-sensitive tumors
Rhodiola rosea	menopause— related fatigue, mood, memory, amenorrhea, fertility, libido	200–600	Anxiety, insomnia, jitteriness, vivid dreams, headache Rare: palpitations, chest pain. Caution: bipolars
S-adenosyl-methionine (SAMe)	depression gall stones	400–800 mg b.i.d.	Nausea, loose bowels, activation, anxiety, headache, occasional palpitations, mania in bipolar

TABLE 6.1 *Continued*

CAM	Clinical Uses	Daily Dose	Side Effects, Drug Interactions,* Contraindications
Saw palmetto (*Serenoa repens*)	BPH	320 mg	Mild occasional GI, constipation, loose stools. May give false low PSA readings in patients with prostate cancer
Soy	hot flashes	20–60 g	Best results with whole soy or whole food
Stinging nettle (*Urtica dioica*)	BPH	300 mg	Mild GI, allergic reactions May increase effects of diuretic and antihypertensive medications
Yohimbine (*Pausinystalia yohimbe*)	erectile dysfunction	18–42 mg	Anxiety, dizziness, chills, headache, rise in BP, increased heart rate, insomnia, nausea, bronchospasm, vomiting Contraindications: hypertension, asthma, cardiovascular disease, impaired renal or liver function

■ Combination Products

ArginMax Arginine, ginkgo, ginseng	low libido, arousal disorders, erectile dysfunction	6 caps/day	Rare side effects of ginkgo or ginseng Contraindication: anticoagulants
Super Mira Forte maca, muira puama, chrysin, zinc, nettle root, ginger, bioperine, piperine	sexual enhancement		Could increase prostate cancer risk, monitor prostate-specific antigen Contraindication: prostate cancer

PMS = premenstrual syndrome; PMDD = premenstrual dysphoric disorder; BPH = benign prostatic hypertrophy; GI = gastrointestinal side effects; BP = blood pressure; D/C = discontinue.

*Common side effects are listed. There are additional rare side effects. Individuals with high blood pressure, diabetes, pregnancy (or during breast-feeding), cancer, or any chronic or serious medical condition should check with their physician before taking supplements. Patients taking anticoagulants should consult their physician before using supplements.

**May increase risk of cardiac stents in men with baseline homocysteine <15 µmol/liter.

CHAPTER 7 OUTLINE

1. **Herbs:** ginkgo, St. John's Wort

2. **Nootropics:** racetams

3. **Hormones:** melatonin, DHEA

4. **Vitamins and Nutrients:** Omega-3 fatty acids, *N*-acetylcysteine, and B vitamins

5. **Weight Gain:** herbs, medications

6. **Off-Label Use of Medication:** allopurinol, celecoxib

7. **Mind–Body Practices:** yoga postures, yoga breathing, meditation

Schizophrenia and Other
Psychotic Disorders

In patients with psychotic disorders, complementary and alternative medicine (CAM) treatments can be valuable adjuncts to
pharmacotherapy to improve residual symptoms, prevent or delay
side effects, and to ameliorate adverse effects of antipsychotic medications. This chapter discusses treatments that are of practical use
to enhance outcomes, medication compliance, and quality of life in
patients with schizophrenia and other psychotic disorders. While
controlled studies of the use of CAM in psychotic disorders are limited, given the devastating effects of psychotic disorders, the severity of short- and long-term medication side effects such as, weight
gain, sedation, fatigue, extrapyramidal symptoms (EPS), and tardive dyskinesia (see Sidebar 7.1), which adversely affect compliance and cause additional iatrogenic medical problems (e.g.,
obesity, diabetes, cardiovascular disease), and considering the low
side-effect risk with CAM, clinicians may consider using a lower
threshold of evidence in deciding to offer complementary treatments for these patients.

It is worthwhile to use CAM treatments with cognitive enhancing, neuroprotective, antioxidant, and anti-inflammatory effects in
schizophrenic patients. Reduced levels of antioxidant defense

SIDEBAR 7.1 **POSSIBLE SIDE EFFECTS OF ANTIPSY-CHOTIC MEDICATIONS**

Changes in neurotransmitters systems induced by antipsychotic medications, including dopaminergic nerves in the striatum, may be responsible for the following side effects.

1. Extrapyramidal symptoms (EPS) include dystonias (muscle spasms), oculogyric crises (spasm of muscles controlling eye movements), pseudoparkinsonism (muscle rigidity, tremor, bradykinesia), akinesia (difficulty initiating movement), and akathisia (motor restlessness).

2. Tardive dyskinesia (TD) consists of involuntary movements of the tongue, jaw, trunk, or extremities that can occur as choreiform (rapid, jerky, nonrepetitive), or athetoid (slow, sinuous, continual).

enzymes have been found in schizophrenic patients. Oxidative damage, toxins, and inflammatory processes may contribute to the development of schizophrenia (Sivrioglu, Kirli, Sipahioglu, Gursoy, & Sarandol, 2007). Neuroprotection is also needed to reduce the incidence and severity of side effects from antipsychotic medications. The study of substances with known neuroprotective effects in patients who require antipsychotic medications is an emerging area of CAM research (Bishnoi, Kumar, Chopra, et al., 2007).

HERBS

Ginkgo

Ginkgo has been shown to increase circulating and membrane levels of polyunsaturated fatty acids (PUFAs) (especially eicosopentanoic acid) and to protect against oxidative stress in rat studies (Drieu et al., 2000). Increasing PUFAs and reducing oxidative damage to neurons may be a means to reduce serious adverse effects of antipsychotic medications. Preliminary studies indicate that ginkgo may protect against the neural damage caused by antipsychotics that leads to the development of extrapyramidal symptoms (EPS).

In a 12-week double-blind, randomized placebo-controlled (DBRPC) trial, 56 patients with treatment resistant schizophrenia were given ginkgo 360 mg/day plus haloperidol 1/4 mg/kg/day and compared with 53 patients given placebo plus haloperidol 1/4 mg/kg/day. The ginkgo group showed greater improvement in positive and negative symptoms. Furthermore, 57% of the patients in the ginkgo group were rated as responders versus 38% of the placebo group. The rate of extrapyramidal symptoms (EPS) was less in the ginkgo group (Zhang, Zhou, Zhang, Wu, Su et al., 2001). Positive symptoms of schizophrenia include delusions, hallucinations, disorganized speech, grossly disorganized or catatonic behavior. Negative symptoms refer to flattening of affect, alogia (restriction in the fluency and productivity of thought and speech), and avolition (restriction in goal-directed behavior).

A double-blind, randomized controlled trial (DBRCT) evaluated the ability of ginkgo (EGb) to augment the effects of olanzapine. For eight weeks, 15 schizophrenics were given olanzapine with gingko and 14 were given olanzapine alone. Those given gingko augmentation had a significant reduction in positive symptoms on the Positive Syndrome Scale (PANSS). The group taking gingko also had significantly greater reductions in superoxide dismutase and catalase (indicating reduced oxidative stress) (Atmaca, Tezcan, Kuloglu, Ustundag, & Kirtas, 2005).

St. John's Wort

St. John's Wort might improve cognitive function in schizophrenia. In a double-blind, placebo-controlled (DBPC) crossover study with 16 normal subjects, Kira 1500 mg/day improved the ketamine-induced decrease in N100-P200 peak amplitude when compared to placebo. Ketamine impairs the NMDA system and produces schizophreniform symptoms (Murck, Spitznagel, Ploch, Seibel, & Schaffler, 2006). If St. John's Wort can reverse this cognitive impairment in normal subjects, it could potentially improve cognitive function in schizophrenics. Similar to prescription antidepressants, St. John's Wort can trigger mania in bipolar patients. Schizoaffective patients

---

CLINICAL PEARL

N-acetylcysteine, in appropriate doses, may serve as a complementary treatment to reduce some symptoms of schizophrenia. It may also prevent or reduce medication-induced damage to striatal tissues and side effects, particularly akathisia. In the United States, NAC is most readily available in 600 mg tablets. Two 600 mg tablets twice a day would approximate the doses used in clinical trials with schizophrenic patients.

---

or bipolar patients who may be misdiagnosed as schizophrenic could become manic or psychotic on St. John's Wort.

NOOTROPICS

Nootropics are cognitive enhancing and neuroprotective agents. See Chapter 4 for a discussion of nootropics and the mechanisms by which they may enhance and protect neuronal functioning.

An eight-week double-blind randomized, placebo-controlled (DBRPC) trial in 14 inpatients on haloperidol 30 mg/day compared augmentation with piracetam 3200 mg/day to placebo in 16 schizophrenic patients (Noorbala, Akhondzadeh, Davari-Ashtiani, & Amini-Nooshabadi, 1999). Positive symptoms and overall scores improved more on piracetam. Also, negative symptoms improved faster on piracetam. Racetams enhance cognition and help NMDA and AMPA glutamate receptors. Larger controlled studies of racetams, particularly aniracetam, would be valuable.

HORMONAL TREATMENTS: MELATONIN AND DHEA

Melatonin

Melatonin can alleviate symptoms of tardive dyskinesia (TD). In a six-week (with four-week washout) double-blind, placebo-controlled crossover study of 22 patients with schizophrenia for a mean length of 25 years, 17 out of 22 had reduced symptoms of TD on melatonin 10 mg sustained release compared to placebo. Seven patients on melatonin dropped 3 points on the Abnormal Involuntary Movement Scale (AIMS) versus one patient on placebo (Shamir, Barak, Shalman, Laudon, Zisapel et al., 2001).

Chronic schizophrenic patients have blunted nocturnal melatonin levels. In a DBRPC study of 40 schizophrenic outpatients on haloperidol 10 to 15 mg/day, subjects given melatonin 3 mg at bedtime did better on numerous measures of sleep and quality of life (Kumar, Andrade, Bhakta, & Singh, 2007).

In an eight-week study of rats randomized to olanzapine, olanzapine plus melatonin, melatonin alone, and untreated control, melatonin blocked weight gain from the olanzapine (Raskind, Burke, Crites, Tapp, & Rasmussen, 2007). This finding deserves study in humans considering the urgency of the epidemic of weight gain and increased risk of diabetes from atypical antipsychotics.

Dehydroepiandrosterone (DHEA)

Lower DHEA levels and DHEA/cortisol ratio correlated with higher psychopathology, worse memory, and worse EPS in 17 medicated schizophrenic inpatients (Harris, Wolkowitz, & Reus, 2001). Several studies of schizophrenia found low DHEA levels, lower DHEA-Sulphate in women, and abnormal DHEA rhythms (Strous, 2005; Strous, Maayan, Kotler, & Weizman, 2005). Whether DHEA supplementation could improve symptoms of schizophrenia is being studied. In a six-week DBRPC trial in 30 schizophrenic inpatients with SANS score ≥ 25, increasing DHEA doses to 100 mg/day for the last two weeks resulted in significant reductions in negative symptoms (more so in women) that correlated with increased levels of DHEA and DHEA-Sulphate (Strous, Maayan, Lapidus, Stryjer, Lustig et al., 2003).

A 12-week DBRPC study of 40 chronic schizophrenic patients found that DHEA (up to 150 mg/day) reduced negative symptoms, EPS, akathisia, and glucose levels better than placebo. There was no change in psychosis. A small subset showed a trend toward improved memory (Strous, Stryjer, Maayan, Gal, Viglin et al., 2007). The effects of DHEA in reducing negative symptoms and medication side effects may be due to several mechanisms.

DHEA potentiates N-methyl-D-aspartate (NMDA)-receptor activity, suppresses GABA inhibition, enhances frontal dopamine release, and enhances sigma-receptor activity.

NUTRIENTS AND VITAMINS

Neuronal injury from oxidative stress may contribute to the pathogenesis and progression of schizophrenia and tardive dyskinesia.

Omega-3 Fatty Acids: Eicosopentanoic Acid (EPA)

Alterations in membrane phospholipids may be involved in the development of schizophrenia (Horrobin, 1998) with possible effects on neurotransmitter systems (du Bois, Deng, & Huang 2005). Magnetic resonance spectroscopy (31P) is being used to investigate the neurochemical effects of omega-3 and omega-6 fatty acid supplementation in schizophrenic spectrum disorders (Sota, Allegri, Cortesi, Barale, Politi et al., 2007). Four out five double-blind controlled studies (total of 377 patients) found ethyl-eicosapentanoic acid (EPA) to be better than placebo in augmenting the action of antipsychotic medications. One of the four positive studies found the enhancing effect of EPA in clozapine (Clozaril) treated patients, but not in patients treated with other atypical antipsychotics (Emsley, Myburgh, Oosthuizen, & van Rensburg, 2002; Fenton, Dickerson, Boronow, Hibbeln, & Knable, 2001; Peet, Brind, Ramchand, Shah, & Vankar, 2001). Three open trials (total of 50 patients) showed positive effects using EPA plus DHA to augment antipsychotic medication (Arvindakshan, Ghate, Ranjekar, Evans, & Mahadik, 2003; Mellor, Laugharne, & Peet, 1995; Sivrioglu et al., 2007). One controlled trial of EPA as a monotherapy (no antipsychotics) versus placebo reported somewhat positive results (Peet et al., 2001).

A meta-analysis of four of the EPA augmentation studies found that omega-3 fatty acids did not significantly improve symptoms of schizophrenia (Freeman et al., 2006). Inconsistencies among studies may be due in part to differences in the age of participants, the length and severity of illness, the type of schizophrenia, the choice of antipsychotic medication, the kind and dosage of omega-3 fatty acid preparations, and the length of the augmentation treatment. Another review found evidence that purified ethyl-eicosapentanoic acid is modestly effective in reducing the doses of antipsychotic medication required to treat acutely ill schizophrenics (Berger, Smesny, & Amminger, 2006) Further studies are needed.

N-acetylcysteine (NAC)

Glutathione is the primary neuroprotective antioxidant in the brain. N-acetylcysteine increases intracellular glutathione levels (see discussion in Chapter 2) and has its own free radical scavenger properties. In a double-blind, randomized, placebo-controlled (DBRPC) study of 140 schizophrenics, NAC 1,000 mg b.i.d. was given for six months. Compared to placebo, patients given NAC showed significant gains in Clinical Global Impression (CGI) with a moderate effect size=0.40. In addition, NAC reduced symptoms of akathisia, a side effect of motor restlessness caused by antipsychotic medication (Berk, 2007).

Oxidative stress causing damage to striatal tissues has been implicated in the pathogenesis of psychotropic medication side effects, including tremor, stiffness, and akathisia (see Sidebar 2.1). A study of oxidative stress evaluated two groups of rats. One group of animals was treated with haloperidol (Haldol) 1.5 mg/kg/day for 21 days, while the other group was not. Haloperidol caused significant elevations of the levels of striatal superoxide (free radicals) and lipid peroxidation (free radical damage to membranes). N-acetylcysteine (NAC) was given to both groups of animals for 21 days in three doses, 50 mg/day, 500 mg/day, and 1,500 mg/day. In the animals not pretreated with haloperidol, 50 mg/day and 500 mg/day NAC reduced oxidative stress markers. However, in striatal tissues of animals not exposed to haloperidol, NAC 1500 mg/day increased levels of superoxide (free radical), decreased lipid peroxidation, and increased consumption of reduced glutathione. The increase in superoxide levels caused by haloperidol was blocked by all doses of NAC. The 1,500 mg/day dose of NAC prevented the haloperidol-induced rise in lipid peroxidation. It also improved the ratio of glutathione to reduced glutathione (Harvey, Joubert, du Preez, & Berk, 2007). The highest dose used in this study far exceeds, proportionately, doses used in human studies. In excessive doses, NAC may have some effects that promote oxidative processes. This suggests caution, for example, in using high dose intravenous NAC in humans.

CLINICAL PEARL

N-acetylcysteine (NAC) in appropriate doses may serve as a complementary treatment to reduce some symptoms of schizophrenia and to prevent or reduce medication-induced damage to striatal tissues and the ensuing side effects. A dose of 1200 mg twice a day would approximate the doses used in clinical trials.

These studies support the role of oxidative pathways in the pathophysiology of symptoms of schizophrenia and antipsychotic induced side effects.

B Vitamins

Vitamin B_6 may ameliorate side effects of antipsychotic medications. In a four-week DBRPC trial in 15 schizophrenic and schizoaffective patients with tardive dyskinesia (TD), B_6 400 mg/day markedly reduced TD symptoms (Lerner, Miodownik, Kaptsan, Cohen, Matar et al., 2001). A five-day DBRPC study of 20 schizophrenic and schizoaffective patients with neuroleptic-induced akathisia showed that patients given B_6 600 mg b.i.d. had greater improvement in subjective sense of restlessness, distress, global ratings compared to those given placebo (Lerner, Bergman, Statsenko, & Miodownik, 2004).

A combination of folate, B_{12}, and B_6 may be beneficial in schizophrenia. In a DBRCT, 42 schizophrenic inpatients with homocysteine levels greater than 15 (indicator of increased oxidative stress) were randomly assigned to receive either a daily vitamin combination (folate 2 mg, B_{12} 400 mcg, B_6 25 mg) or placebo. Compared to the placebo group, those on the vitamin regimen, showed significantly greater reduction in homocysteine levels and scores on Positive and Negative Symptom Scale (PANSS), as well as improved cognitive function (Levine, Stahl, Sela, Ruderman, Shumaico et al., 2006).

Weight Gain Secondary to Antipsychotic Medications

Weight gain is one of the most common side effects of psychotropic medications and one of the most challenging causes of medication discontinuation. The mechanisms responsible for this are not well understood, but may involved both glucose and lipid metabolism. Finding CAM treatments that do not cause weight gain is one solution. However, for patients who must stay on neuroleptics in order to feel well and to function, dealing with weight issues requires considerable effort on the part of both the doctor and the patient. Frustration over persistent weight gain may lead to the use of stimulants, unproven weight-loss products on the market, or in some cases, surgery. Controlling weight gain usually requires changes in eating and exercise habits. If the health care practitioner does not have the expertise or the time to advise and regularly support the patient's efforts to lose weight, then referral to a nutritionist, a healthy weight loss program (e.g., Weight Watchers), and a structured exercise program are indicated. Regular exercise (e.g., walking 20–30 minutes twice daily) should be encouraged.

Mind–body practices are a healthy means to assist in weight reduction. To the extent that Mind–body–spirit programs improve emotion regulation, reduce stress and tension, and improve mood and self-esteem, they may mitigate some of the factors that contribute to poor eating habits. In addition, they provide activity that can be practiced at any level, depending on the patient's physical condition.

Treatments for neuroleptic-induced weight gain and diabetes have been neither well-studied, nor widely used. Some conventional treatments which have shown promise include metformin, amantadine, topiramate, and zonisamide. In clinical practice, the authors find that Rimonabant, a cannabinoid-1 receptor antagonist approved in Europe but not yet FDA approved in the United States can be helpful in reducing weight gain.

Herbs, Nutrients, and Melatonin

There are few controlled studies of CAM treatments for psychotropic-induced weight gain. Chromium picolinate 500 mcg b.i.d. has been used in the treatment of diabetes and some patients find it modestly

---

SIDEBAR 7.2 **FUCOXANTHIN AND FAT METABOLISM**

As an antioxidant, fucoxanthin. It is active in low oxygen conditions and it is a proton donor (rather than an electron donor). Its primary action for weight loss is thought to be the upregulation of uncoupling protein-1 (UCP-1) (also called thermogenin) production. During the Krebs cycle (oxidation of carbohydrates, fats and proteins) protons (H^+) are captured (coupling process) in the formation of ATP (energy transport molecules). When the process is uncoupled, protons are lost and instead of capturing the energy in a usable form (ATP), the energy is lost and dissipated as heat. The upregulation of UCP-1 shifts the balance towards more uncoupling. Consequently, the cells must burn more carbohydrates and fats in order to produce the same amount of ATP. In other words, by reducing the efficiency of mitochondrial energy production, UCP-1 makes the system burn more supplies (fats and carbohydrates), increasing the metabolic rate (Leonid Ber, 2007, personal communication,).

---

helpful and affordable. Other glucose regulating herbs may be used, but in the absence of studies, it is difficult to recommend them.

In an eight-week study of female rats, olanzapine reduced nocturnal plasma melatonin levels by 55% and caused an 18% increase in body weight. In rats given olanzapine + melatonin, nocturnal melatonin levels returned to normal and there was only a 10% increase in weight. The normal age-associated weight increase in rats given neither experimental substance was 7%, but the increase in animals given melatonin alone was 5% (Raskind, Burke, Crites, Tapp, & Rasmussen, 2007). Whether the positive effects of melatonin in reducing weight gain in rats will be found in human studies remains to be seen.

Fucothin 200 mg capsules contain 5 mg fucoxanthin, a carotenoid derived from two seaweeds, wakame (*Undaria pinnatifida*) and kombu (*Laminaria japonica*), combined with a small amount of pomegranate seed oil extract (a source of conjugated linoleic acid) (see Sidebar 7.2).

Two clinical studies have shown that fucoxanthin can induce weight loss. In a 16-week DBRPC pilot study, different doses of the extract were given to 40 obese, nondiabetic women. In the groups who were given at least 15 mg/day fucoxanthin, the metabolic rate was 18.2% higher than in the placebo group. Significant differences in metabolic rate were evident by week 6 (Abidov & Roshen, in process). A larger DBRPC 16-week trial compared fucoxanthin to placebo in 110 obese non-diabetic women with BMI > 30 kg/m², body weight 203 to 212 pounds (92–96 kg). Participants were put on a 1,800 calories/day diet and made no changes in their usual physical activities. After 16 weeks the placebo group lost an average of 3 pounds (1.5% of initial body weight) versus the fucoxanthin group's average loss of 14.5 pounds (7% of initial body weight). The weight was preferentially lost from abdomenal fat tissues. Other benefits of fucoxanthin were reduction in C-reactive protein (associated with cardiovascular risk), decreased triglyceride levels, reduced blood pressure, and improvement in liver enzymes. The weight-loss product was well tolerated with no adverse side effects (Abidov, in press).

Fucothin has not been tested in patients with medication-induced weight gain. However, it shows promise as a potential, non-stimulant weight loss aid. As a seaweed derivative, fucoxanthine contains iodine that may be contraindicated in certain conditions, for example, thyroid disease and acne.

PRESCRIPTION MEDICATION AUGMENTATION STRATEGIES: OFF-LABEL USES

Allopurinol 300 mg/day was used to augment neuroleptics in 11 treatment resistant schizophrenics. Five out of 11 cases responded to allopurinol augmentation (Lara, Brunstein, Ghisolfi, Lobato, Belmonte-de-Abreu et al., 2001). Benefits may be due to the ability of allopurinol to boost adenosine which inhibits glutamate systems. In a 12-week DBRPC crossover trial of 35 poorly responsive schizophrenic/schizoaffective patients (22 completers), those given allopurinol 300 mg/d showed significant improvement in positive and negative symptoms compared to those given placebo. The better responders were those patients with refractory positive symptoms and a shorter illness duration (mean=15 years) (Brunstein, Ghisolfi, Ramos, & Lara, 2005). An eight-week DBRPC study of 46 schizophrenic inpatients compared haloperidol plus allopurinol to haloperidol plus placebo. The group with allopurinol augmentation showed significantly greater improvements in positive symptoms, general symptoms, Positive and Negative Symptom Scale (PANSS) and extrapyramidal symptoms (Akhondzadeh, Safarcherati, & Amini, 2005). The neuropsychiatric effects of allopurinol may be due to its inhibitory effect on purine degradation with enhancement of adenosinergic activity. Adenosine tends to exert effects (opposite of dopamine effects) which are antipsychotic, anxiolytic, sedative, and antiaggressive.

Schizophrenia may be associated with an abnormal immune response including increased release of proinflammatory cytokines. COX-2 inhibitors reduce such cytokines. In an eight-week DBRPC trial, 60 schizophrenics receiving risperidone 6 mg/day were assigned to augmentation with celecoxib 200 mg b.i.d. or placebo. Celecoxib augmentation produced more improvements in positive symptoms, general psychopathology, and PANSS total scores than placebo (Akhondzadeh, Tabatabaee, Amini, Ahmadi Abhari, Abbasi et al., 2007).

MIND–BODY PRACTICES: MEDITATION, YOGA BREATHING, YOGA POSTURES

Meditation is not generally recommended for schizophrenic patients because they tend to become increasingly upset with introspection, awareness, and focus on their internal delusional processes. However, gentle relaxing yoga postures and limited amounts of slow relaxing yoga breathing can have a calming, stabilizing effect (Raghuraj, Nagarathna, Saraswati, Nunn, & Telles, 1995; Scott, 1997).

A program of Ujjayi yoga breathing (a slow calming breath form, see Chapter 3) and reading spiritual literature was introduced to an outpatient chronic mental patient support group for schizophrenic women. The women expressed positive feelings about the program and found that it alleviated despair and enhanced their meaningful communication within the group (Brown, Gerbarg, & Muskin, 2003; Sageman, 2004) .

A randomized clinical trial (RCT) (rater blind) compared the effects of Yogasana (n=31) (yoga postures) versus exercise (n=30) as adjunctive treatments in the management of schizophrenia. Patients with an average CGI score ⎕⎕4 were given 15 days of training and 31/2 months of practice at home. Out of 61 subjects, 41 completed the study. After four months, the Yogasana group showed greater improvements in CGI (average=7.1), positive and negative symptoms, depression, and quality of life compared to the exercise group. The exercise group improved compared to their baseline (Duraiswamy, Thirthalli, Nagendra, & Gangadhar, 2007).

Yoga programs that are adapted to the needs of schizophrenic patients and provided under the supervision of a psychiatrist can be a beneficial adjunct to treatment.

TABLE 7.1 Treatment Guidelines for Schizophrenia

CAM	Clinical Uses	Daily Dose	Side Effects, Drug Interactions,* Contraindications
B vitamins **B complex** **B$_{12}$** **folate**	akathisia, tardive dyskinesia	1 tab/day 1,000 mcg 800 mcg	Caution: cardiac stents**
Vitamin B$_6$	tardive dyskinesia, akathisia, tremor	100 mg/day	Occasional toxicity reported in doses > 200 mg/day. Neuropathy at > 1,000 mg/day. Contraindications: renal impairment, protein deficiency
Bio-Strath	tardive dyskinesia, akathisia, tremor	1 Tbsp/b.i.d. or 3 tabs b.i.d.	Caution: cardiac stents**
DHEA	negative symptoms	25–100 mg/day	Acne, hirsutism, increased prostate-specific antigen Contraindications: estrogen-sensitive cancers. Caution: bipolar or schizoaffective
Ginkgo (***Ginkgo biloba***)	augment antipsychotics	120 mg b.i.d.	Minimal: headache Rare: agitation. D/C: prior to surgery Contraindication: anticoagulants
Melatonin	tardive dyskinesia, sleep	sleep: 9–12 mg at bedtime tardive dyskinesia: 10–20 mg hs	Occasional agitation, abdominal cramps, fatigue, headache, dizziness, vivid dreams D/C: pregnancy

Metanx® **Methylfolate, B₆** **pyridoxyl-5'** **phosphate** **methylcobal-** **amin**	decreases homocysteine if it is high, akathisia, tardive dyskinesia		Caution: cardiac stents**
N-acetylcysteine	akathisia	1,000–1,200 mg b.i.d.	Minimal at appropriate doses
Racetams	augment antipsychotics	aniracetam 750 mg b.i.d.	Minimal. Rare: anxiety, insomnia, agitation, irritability, headache
Rhodiola rosea	extrapyramidal symptoms, energy, mood, medication-induced fatigue	100–300 mg/d	Activation, agitation, insomnia, jitteriness Rare: increased blood pressure, chest pain, bruising. Caution: bipolar and schizoaffectives

D/C = discontinue; hs = at bedtime; b.i.d. = twice a day

*Common side effects are listed. There are additional rare side effects. Individuals with high blood pressure, diabetes, pregnancy (or during breast feeding), or any chronic or serious medical condition should check with their physician before taking supplements.

**May increase risk of restenosis in men only with baseline homocysteine <15 μmol/liter.

CHAPTER 8 OUTLINE

1. **Physical and Emotional Stress of Cancer and Cancer Treatments**
   a. cancer-related fatigue, chemotherapy, immune suppression
   b. adaptogens and antioxidants: *Rhodiola rosea*, ashwaganda, amrit Kalash, AdMax, Bio-Strath
   c. cancer-related pain: mind-body-spirit practices
   d. caregiver stress: mind-body-spirit practices

2. **Cardiovascular Disease**
   a. mind-body practices
   b. depression, anxiety, medical trauma, and cognitive function

3. **Chronic Fatigue Syndrome, Fibromyalgia Syndrome, Arthritis**
   a. S-adenosylmethionine, acupuncture, carnitines, St. John's Wort, *R. rosea*, mind–body practices

4. **Human Immunodeficiency Virus – HIV**
   a. S-adenosylmethionine, *R. Rosea*, carnitines, mind–body practices

5. **Irritable Bowel Syndrome**
   a. mind–body practices

Medical Illnesses

INTEGRATIVE APPROACHES FOR PATIENTS WITH CANCER

Mind–body–spirit practices can provide significant physical and psychological benefits for cancer patients and their caregivers. Unlike herbal supplements, mind–body practices raise no concerns about interference with chemotherapy drugs or increased cancer risks. For more detailed descriptions of the mind-body-spirit practices discussed below, see Chapter 3. Integrative treatments are being developed to offer a variety of choices tailored to the needs of patients (Chong, 2006). A majority of cancer patients use complementary and alernative medicine (CAM) along with their standard cancer treatments. Many believe that CAM contributes to their healing, immune defenses, energy, and sense of well-being. Some also report a feeling of greater control in their treatment (Helyer, Chin, Chui, Fitzgerald, Verma et al., 2006).

Psycho-Oncology: Physical and Emotional Stress of Cancer, Cancer Treatments, Cancer-Related Fatigue and Pain, Caregiver Stress

Concern about CAM interference with chemotherapy and radiation has focused on herbs that affect the induction of drug metabolizing enzymes and drug transporters. Altering the pharmacokinetics of chemotherapy drugs can lead to increased toxicities or inadequate drug levels for therapeutic effect. Bosch and colleagues (Bosch, Meijerman, Beijnen, & Schellens, 2006) reviewed interactions between herbs (and other supplements) and drugs used in oncology. Substantial evidence indicated that St. John's Wort, kava, echinacea, and grapeseed extract, can significantly affect metabolism of chemotherapy agents. The possibility of some interactions based on in vitro and animal studies was noted for some forms of vitamin E, quercetin, ginseng, garlic, B-carotene, mukul myrrh tree, hops, wu wei ai (*Schisandra chinensis*), gan cao, flavonoids (e.g., chrysin). Tests for activation of nuclear receptors or induction of metabolizing enzymes found no effect from the following herbs: curcumin, lycopene, resveritrol, and silymarin. Because of interspecies differences, findings in animal studies may not be applicable to humans. A review of phytoestrogens and cancer noted the presence of multiple antioxidants in herbs that may have anticarcinogenic activity (Piersen, 2003).

In an extensive review of the literature on the effects of antioxidants and other nutrients on chemotherapy and/or radiation treatment, Simone and colleagues (Simone, Simone, & Simone, 2007a; Simone, Simone, & Simone, 2007b) reported that 280 peer-reviewed studies, including 50 studies involving a total of 8,521 patients, consistently found no interference with cancer therapies. In fact, the antioxidants and nutrients enhanced anticarcinogenic effects, decreased treatment side effects, protected normal tissues, and increased patient survival. The authors point out that the widespread notion that antioxidants interfere with chemotherapy was based on a single study in which vitamin C became concentrated in cancer cells in mice. The study did not demonstrate interference with chemotherapy. The belief that folic acid interferes with methotrexate stems from a study of folinic acid (a prescription drug that has no relation to folic acid other than sounding similar). The review cited numerous studies showing that N-acetylcysteine, vitamins A, B_6, B_{12}, C, D, E, K, beta-carotene, other retinoids, selenium, and glutathione protected normal tissue and increased destruction of cancer cells.

The evidence that antioxidants do not interfere with chemotherapy and that they could increase its effectiveness may seem counterintuitive. However, two prescription antioxidants, amifostine and dexrazoxane, have been FDA approved and widely used during cancer chemotherapy and/or radiation. Cancer cells are different from normal cells and they are affected differently by antioxidants. Simone and colleagues (2007b) suggest that, "Cancer cells accumulate excessive amounts of antioxidants due to a loss of the homeostasis control mechanisms for the uptake of these nutrients" (p. 46). The presence of excess antioxidants can shut down the cellular oxidative reactions necessary for energy production. In addition, in cancer cells, antioxidants have been shown to affect gene expression, inhibit cell growth, and increase cell apoptosis.

Cancer patients often suffer from malnutrition, vitamin deficiencies, immunosupression, cardiac damage, and/or liver dysfunction due to the toxic effects of standard cancer treatments. Vitamins and nutrients can improve nutritional and immune status, protect vital organs, and reduce morbidity and mortality from cancer therapies.

The immune system helps to protect against cancer as well as infections. Cancer chemotherapy can compromise immune function. Mind–body practices can improve antioxidant and immune status (Tai Chi Gives Immune System a Boost, 2007; Das, Kochupillai, Singh, Aggarwal, & Bhardwaj, 2002; Kimura, Nagao, Tanaka, Sakai, & Ohnishi, 2005; Kochupillai, Kumar, Singh, Aggarwal, Bhardwaj et al. 2005; Lee, Huh, Jeong, Lee, Ryu et al., 2003).

Women who undergo treatment for ovarian or uterine cancer may experience the sudden unset of extreme menopausal symptoms. Alleviating the distress of the loss of sex hormones, without increasing their risk of cancer can be challenging. While the potential for chemoprotection of the reproductive/endocrine system by phytoestrogens remains unclear, evidence is mounting for other benefits including improved lipid profile and bone density; for example, with red clover, and soy. The lack of strong research data on phytoestrogens regarding efficacy in prevention, cancer survival, and symptom reduction makes it difficult to weigh the benefits against potential risks of interference with cancer treatments or possible stimulation of hormone-sensitive cancers (an area that has not been adequately studied). The risks associated with phytoestrogens may be less severe than those known to occur with prescription hormone replacement therapy (HRT). Black cohosh, for example, is a nonestrogenic herb that can be beneficial for menopausal symptoms. Some studies indicate that it may be almost as effective as HRT, and possibly safer. (For alternative treatments in menopause, see Chapter 6.)

Cancer-Related Fatigue, Chemotherapy, Immune Suppression

Fatigue is the most common and distressing complaint of cancer patients. A review of 21 studies of CAM treatments in which cancer-related fatigue was one of the outcomes measured, evaluated the available data as promising but limited (Sood, Barton, Bauer, & Loprinzi, 2007). A pilot study of acupuncture in 37 patients reported a mean improvement in postchemotherapy fatigue of 31% (Vickers, 2004). In a nonrandomized study of 14 cancer patients, four to five sessions of hypnosis significantly reduced hot flashes and improved fatigue and insomnia (Younus, Simpson, Collins, & Wang, 2003). In a retrospective study of 689 women with breast cancer who had been treated with surgery and chemotherapy, radiation or hormone therapy, 219 women receiving mistletoe in addition to standard therapy had less nausea, gastrointestinal symptoms, fatigue, and depression compared with 470 women on standard treatment alone (Schumacher, Schneider, Reich, Stiefel, Stoll et al., 2003). Oral levocarnitine 4 gm/day for seven days improved fatigue in 45 out of 50 patients with stage IV cancer receiving chemotherapy, who had low serum carnitine levels, in a Phase III open study (Graziano, Bisonni, Catalano, Silva, Rovidati et al., 2002). An eight-week multicenter, double-blind, randomized, placebo-controlled MCDBRPC study of the effects of oral levocarnitine (L-carnitine) twice daily on fatigue in 352 cancer patients is in process (Eastern Cooperative Oncology Group, 2007). Significant reduction in fatigue was found in a nonrandomized study of 63 cancer patients given an eight-week Mindfulness Based Stress Reduction (MBSR) program (Carlson & Garland, 2005).

Adaptogens Augment Chemotherapy While Protecting Liver and Bone Marrow

Adaptogens are herbs containing many bioactive compounds, including antioxidants and metabolic regulators. They have been shown to increase the capacity of organisms to resist damage from multiple stressors including toxins, radiation, free radicals, chemotherapy agents, infections, temperature extremes, and psychological stress. Extracts from adaptogenic plants have been found to improve immune parameters in ovarian cancer patients with immunosuppression from chemotherapy (Breckhman & Dardymov, 1969; Panossian & Wagner, 2005; Saratikov & Krasnov, 1987).

Rhodiola rosea

The authors have found that *Rhodiola rosea* is very beneficial for cancer-related fatigue. For a discussion of *R. rosea*, an adaptogenic medicinal herb, see Chapter 4. While *R. rosea* is used in oncology centers in the Russian Federation and Eastern Europe, studies of its effects on fatigue in cancer patients have not yet been published (Abidov, personal communication 2006).

The antifatigue properties of *R. rosea* have been studied in animals and humans (see Chapter 2) and may be due to the ability of *R. rosea* to increase and sustain cellular production of high energy molecules, ATP, and creatine phosphate (Abidov, Crendal, Grachev, Seifulla, & Ziegenfuss, 2003; Abidov, Grachev, Seifulla, & Ziegenfuss, 2004). Coincidentally, a nonblinded randomized placebo-controlled 28-week study of 58 patients with advanced non small cell lung cancer found that those who were given 10 intravenous 30-hour ATP infusions at two-to-four week intervals had statistically significant improvements in weight, serum albumin, muscle strength, energy, fatigue ($p < 0.0001$), and quality of life. Side effects included chest heaviness (Agteresch, Dagnelie, van der Gaast, Stijnen, & Wilson, 2000). While this treatment was effective, it has limited practicality because of the need for intravenous infusion. However, since *R. rosea* can be easily given by mouth, it would be worthwhile to study as a simpler way to increase ATP, particularly because it has already been found to improve muscle strength, energy, and fatigue in animal studies, normal subjects, and patients with other illnesses. Unlike stimulants such as amphetamines, *R. rosea* has shown no potential for abuse, and it does not deplete energy, induce dysphoric or abnormal mental states, or result in withdrawal symptoms.

Many chemotherapy drugs damage stem cells in the liver and bone marrow resulting in increased susceptibility to infections and other medical problems. If blood cell counts fall too low, it may be necessary to interrupt the chemotherapy. In studies of human cancers (Lewis lung carcinoma, Ehrlich's sarcoma, Pliss lymphosarcoma, NK/Ly tumor, and melanoma B16) transplanted into mice, *R. rosea* extracts demonstrated antitumor and antimetastatic activity. In addition, *R. rosea* protected liver and bone marrow cells from the chemotoxic effects of adriamycin and cyclophosphamide while at the same time it increased the effectiveness of the chemotherapy agents in destroying cancer cells and reducing metastases (Dement'eva & Iaremenko, 1987; Razina, Zueva, Amosova, & Krylova, 2000; Udintsev, Fomina, & Razina, 1992; Udintsev & Schakhov, 1989, 1990, 1991). *R. rosea* is an example of an adaptogen that could be used to alleviate fatigue and depression in cancer patients while providing two additional benefits: augmenting the effectiveness of chemotherapy drugs and reducing damage to the liver and bone marrow.

In 12 patients with superficial bladder carcinoma, *R. rosea* extract improved urothelial tissue, leukocyte integrines, and T-cell immunity with a trend toward reduction in frequency of relapse (Bocharova, Matveev, Baryshnikov, Figurin, & Serebriakova, 1995). A 95% ethanol extract of *R. rosea* stems showed cytotoxicity against prostate cancer cells (Ming, Hillhouse, Guns, Eberding, & Xie, 2005).

Much of the literature on *R. rosea* cancer research is published in non-English-language journals. The inability to access this literature, combined with reluctance to use herbal preparations in cancer patients and the lack of funding to test this adaptogen, have inhibited many Western oncologists from exploring the potential benefits of *R. rosea* and other adaptogenic herbs. Consumer interest and private sector funding may be needed to bring attention to this neglected area of research.

Adaptogen Combination Treatments

In a study of 28 women with stage III to IV ovarian cancer treated with cisplatin and cyclophosphamide, those who took AdMax 270 mg/day (combination of extracts from roots of *Leuzea carthamoides, R. rosea, E. senticosus* and fruits of *S. chinensis*) for four weeks following chemotherapy showed increases in T cell subclasses (CD3, CD4, CD5, and CD8), IgG and IgM compared with those who did not (Kormosh, Laktionov, & Antoshechkina, 2006).

Ayurvedic Medicine

Ayurvedic medicine is the ancient healing system of India, perhaps the oldest in the world. *Ayurveda* means "knowledge of life." Ayurvedic practitioners train for many years to learn the theory and practices, including the use of hundreds of herbal preparations. Clinicians trained in Western science often find it difficult to grasp theories based on such different principles. Nevertheless, those interested in integrating Eastern wisdom into their work, will find scientific evidence to support the use of some of the most popular treatments. The authors have found that for patients with extremely difficult, treatment resistant symptoms, referral to an Ayurvedic specialist may result in significant improvements and functional recovery. Sudha Prathikanti (2007) has written an excellent review of the history, theory, and modern uses of Ayurveda.

The theory of Ayurveda is based on balancing the individual's three constitutional doshas (vata, pitta, and kappa) which arise from the five elements of ancient philosophy (fire, air, water, earth, and space). Precise recommendations for lifestyle changes, diet, massage, yoga postures, herbal preparations, and other treatments, follow from the patient's history and pulse diagnosis. The authors have found that many patients in Western societies are so far out of balance in their lifestyles that Ayurvedic herbs alone are too mild to be effective. However, ashwaganda, Amrit Kalash, and Mentat (see Chapter 4) are often helpful. People who are deeply interested in mind–body–spirit practices or a more traditional lifestyle attuned to nature, may benefit most readily from the gentle, subtle Ayurvedic approach. Such individuals often find it more tolerable and effective than synthetic pharmaceuticals. To locate a trained Ayurvedic practitioner in your area, contact the National Ayurvedic Medical Association.

Ashwagandha (*Withania somnifera*)

Ashwagandha (*Withania somnifera*) is an adaptogenic herb that has been used in Indian medicine for its antistress, anti-inflammatory, antioxidant, analgesic, antidepressant, and immunomodulatory effects. An in vitro and in vivo study of selective tumor inhibition by an ashwagandha leaf extract found that one of the constituents, withanone, activated p53, a gene responsible for tumor cell apoptosis. The herbal extract selectively killed various human tumor cells, but not normal human cells (Widodo, Kaur, Shrestha, Takagi, & Ishii, 2007).

Amrit Kalash

Amrit Kalash, a proprietary Ayurvedic formula containing many herbs, including ashwagandha, enhanced immune function, and protected against free radical damage and toxic effects of chemotherapy in animal and cell culture studies. Amrit Nectar tablets (MA-7; containing 38 herbs) showed antioxidant activity and protected against toxicity from adriamycin and cisplatin (Dwivedi, Natarajan, & Matthees, 2005). It is reported to improve energy, well-being, sleep, and appetite, and to lessen vomiting and diarrhea. Amrit Kalash has also been found to increase tolerance of cancer treatment without interfering with the action of chemotherapy agents. Additional RCTs are needed to confirm safety and efficacy for cancer patients.

In clinical practice, the authors find that patients who take Amrit Kalash during a course of chemotherapy report improved energy, digestion, and sense of well being, as well as little or no hair loss.

Bio-Strath

Bio-Strath, a traditional Swiss herbal brewer's yeast preparation, contains a high concentration of B vitamins and antioxidants. When given to 177 cancer patients during radiation therapy in a DBRPC stratified trial, Bio-Strath improved energy, appetite, weight gain, and red blood cell counts compared with placebo. There was no effect on tumor growth or on the action of radiotherapy on the tumor (Schwarzenbach & Brunner, 1996).

CAM for Cancer-Related Pain

A review of CAM for relief of cancer-related pain concluded that hypnosis, imagery, support groups, acupuncture, and healing touch appear to be promising short-term interventions, but the lack of rigorous trials with adequate statistical power limits the ability to adequately assess their efficacy (Bardia, Barton, Prokop, Bauer, & Moynihan, 2006). Nevertheless, there is a sizable literature and a long history of clinical practice in the use of hypnosis and acupuncture for pain relief in many conditions. There is no reason to believe that the pain experienced by cancer patients would be less responsive to these approaches. Furthermore, in the authors' experience, hypnosis can be used to reduce chemotherapy related nausea and other side effects. Since it is known that anxiety is a major factor in the subjective experience of pain, mind–body techniques such as hypnosis, relaxation, yoga breathing, and meditation that alleviate anxiety should be beneficial for pain relief. In clinical practice, the authors have observed these effects. An additional mechanism by which yoga breathing can reduce or block pain perception is through stimulation of the vagus nerve which is involved in nocioception (discrimination of painful stimuli).

Mind–Body Practices

Mind-body-spirit practices can help reduce anxiety, depression, over-reactivity to cancer-related pain, insomnia, and fatigue. Many studies have shown that mind–body interventions derived from yoga (including breathing, meditation, relaxation, physical postures, centering, and visualization) ameliorate stress-related mental and physical disorders including asthma, high blood pressure, cardiac illness, elevated cholesterol, irritable bowel syndrome, cancer, insomnia, multiple sclerosis and fibromyalgia (Becker, 2000; Benson, 1996; Jacobs, 2001). The reduction of SNS overactivity, the increase of PNS tone, and the enhancement of autonomic balance and flexibility are integral to these therapeutic effects. The association between cardiac vagal (parasympathetic) tone and emotional regulation has been demonstrated in anxiety, stress, PTSD, depression, anger, aggression, and behavioral disorders in children and adults Beauchaine, 2001; Porges, 2001). In addition, the focus of Eastern philosophies on spiritual values and acceptance can help cancer patients adjust better to their situation with a greater sense of peace. For example, many people become distraught over their sense of losing control of their bodies. Learning to let go of the need for control and focusing on the present moment instead of worrying about what comes next, helps cultivate a greater sense of calmness.

Mindfulness-Based Stress Reduction (MBSR)

A randomized, wait-list controlled trial of mindfulness-based stress reduction (MBSR) in 90 heterogeneous cancer patients showed a 65% decrease in overall mood disturbance and 31% decrease in symptoms of stress (Speca, Carlson, Goodey, & Angen, 2000). An eight-week open study of MBSR based on the program of Kabat-Zinn (1990) in 49 patients with early stage breast cancer and 10 with early stage prostate cancer showed significant improvements in quality of life, symptoms of stress, and sleep quality. The immune profile shifted in a pattern consistent with improvement in depressive symptoms, including no changes in the number of lymphocytes, but a decrease in IL-10 production by natural killer (NK) cells, increase of IL-4 from T cells, and decrease in IFN-gamma from T cells (Carlson, Speca, Patel, & Goodey, 2003).

Tibetan Yoga

Lorenzo Cohen, director of the Integrative Medicine Program at M.D. Anderson Cancer Center in Houston, found that seven weeks of Tibetan yoga classes helped lymphoma patients fall asleep faster and sleep better with fewer sleep medications than patients not given yoga (Cohen, Warneke, Fouladi, Rodriguez, & Chaoul-Reich, 2004).

A 12-month study of women with recent cancer diagnoses compared the effects of a 12-week training in emotion regulation skills (n=54) (relaxation techniques, guided imagery, meditation, emotional expression, and adaptive reappraisals of cancer experiences) with an intervention decliner group (n=56) and a standard care control group (n=44). Compared to the other groups, at four months, the intervention group reported greater increases in perceived control, emotional well-being, coping efficacy, as well as greater decreases in perceived risk of recurrence, cancer worry, and anxiety (Cameron, Booth, Schlatter, Ziginskas, & Harman, 2007).

Iyengar Yoga

A seven-week randomized pilot study of heterogeneous cancer patients found that those participating in an Iyengar Yoga program (yoga postures) (n=20) gained significant improvements in quality of life, emotional function, and symptoms of diarrhea, but other measures of mood, tension, and depression did not reach statistical significance, possibly due to the small size of the study (Culos-Reed, Shields, & Brawley, 2005).

Kundalini Yoga

David Shannahoff-Khalsa describes Kundalini Yoga (KY) techniques for cancer patients (Shannahoff-Khalsa, 2006a, 2006b). He suggests starting with techniques for tuning in to induce a meditative state, spine flexing and shoulder shrugs for energy and fatigue. Techniques for reducing anxiety, depression, self-destructive behavior, mental fatigue, anger, fear, and negative thoughts involve various combinations of physical postures, yoga breath techniques, chanting, and specific thought repetitions. Techniques are also described to stimulate the immune system, fight cancer, and balance red and white blood cells. Although there are some studies showing that KY can ameliorate anxiety and obsessive–compulsive disorder (see Chapter 3), evidence for the other benefits is limited (immune stimulation) or anecdotal. The breath techniques of KY, including slow respiration against airway resistance with breath holds and the vibrational stimulations of chanting, have the potential to affect the stress response systems, parasympathetic activity, and immune parameters (see Chapter 3). However, each KY technique is time consuming. Although convincing patients to spend several hours a day performing the recommended combination of techniques may be challenging, it can be a rewarding experience for patients motivated to practice regularly.

Sudarshan Kriya Yoga

Sudarshan Kriya Yoga combines gentle yoga stretches, yoga breathing, meditation and yoga knowledge, spirituality, and community mindedness in a supportive group setting. Although no scientific studies have proven that yoga practices significantly alter the course of cancer, many individuals claim to have experienced such benefits. Research studies have shown that yoga practices can improve the physical condition, measures of immune function, symptoms of psychological distress, sleep, socialization, happiness, and overall quality of life for individuals with cancer and other chronic illnesses (Banerjee, Vadiraj, Ram, Rao, Jayapal et al., 2007; Culos-Reed et al., 2005; Moadel, Shah, Wylie-Rosett, Harris, Patel, Hall et al., 2007). A review of research on the use of yoga in cancer patients concluded that there is preliminary support for the feasibility and efficacy of yoga interventions for cancer patients, although controlled trials are lacking (Bower, Woolery, Sternlieb, & Garet, 2005).

In 26 women diagnosed with stage 0, I, II, and III breast cancer (BC) within the previous five years, mean age 54.2 (35–78), a study consisting of pre- and posttest within subject quantitative assessments with a two-week wait list control and postintervention in-depth qualitative assessments demonstrated significant (p<0.0001) improvements in quality of life, spiritual well-being, positive states of mind, and perceived stress following an eight-day Art of Living Sudarshan Kriya Yoga (SKY) Course. Benefits were sustained at five-week follow-up. Subjects reported mind–body–spirit experiences: positive emotions (100%) of love, joy, peace, centeredness, and mental clarity. They described the following benefits directly relating to breast cancer: letting go of "BC survivor" identity (33%), less fear of recurrence and fear of death (33%), healing of body image (33%). Transformation was expressed as increased sense of peace (100%), increased self-esteem and empowerment (83%), improved relationships (75%), breakthrough, letting go, or deepening (83%), spiritual transformation or strengthening (100%) (Warner, 2006).

Case 1—Breast Cancer Integrative Treatment

Beth sought therapy at the age of 50 while undergoing radiation for breast cancer because she was feeling overwhelmed, anxious, and depressed. Worry about her prognosis and treatment-related fatigue contributed to a constant state of stress. Beth had always been an active, physically attractive woman who looked young for her age. The loss of her hair was devastating to her self image causing her to feel self-conscious and insecure about her appearance, even in a wig.

Psychotherapy began with Beth sharing her feelings and building trust in the support and understanding of her therapist. She worked hard in therapy, keeping notes and conscientiously trying to apply what she learned to her daily life.

She discovered that as a child her role had been to try to make everything perfect to prevent family arguments, including negotiating and making peace between her mother and her aunts. The role of peacemaker was a recurring source of stress in her adult life as she tried unsuccessfully to mediate conflicts between the various adult children and their divorced parents. Her method of dealing with the uncertainties of life by anticipating every possible problem and taking preventive actions failed when she developed cancer. Without this defense, Beth felt helpless and terrified. Although there was substantial progress in therapy, the constant traumatic effects of the cancer diagnosis and radiation kept fueling her anxieties. Her therapist suggested that she take the Sudarshan Kriya Yoga Course to help reduce stress reactivity and anxiety.

Beth entered the course with skepticism, wondering what it was about, how it would help, and if it was some sort of weird cult, but she decided to suspend judgment and to see what impact it might have. Because she was on extended medical leave from work, Beth had time to do the daily 20 minutes of breathing and 10 minutes of relaxation afterward. She cried intensely after each session in the beginning, comparing it to an exorcism. Angry feelings about being ill had been pent up, because she had been trying to be the good, smiling, stoic patient. She released these feelings in the safety of her private breath practice. She also resolved painful emotions regarding a cousin who had died from cancer some months before and her mother whose life was claimed by the same disease in 1995. She came to terms with a landslide of negative feelings related to her illness, her family, and her life in general.

After completing the full complement of cancer treatment protocols—surgery, chemotherapy, and radiation—Beth felt healthy. Her blood tests and MRI were completely normal; her mammograms clear. However, as with many cancer survivors, there were scares. One CA27–29 blood test (which looks for markers of breast cancer) came back high. That threw her into turmoil, until her PET scan and bone

scan came back normal. Yoga breathing helped keep the anxiety down to a manageable level.

Beth returned to work full-time and resumed her very
busy life. She continued the SKY practice, but not every day.
When she took an advanced Sudarshan Kriya course in 2004,
she realized that things she had dismissed as inevitable
events in life were really stressors. She finished the course
with a greater respect for her body and mind. Beth described
how her feelings toward herself and others changed, "At the
end of my daily breathing practice I feel ready to start my day
with peace and compassion for other people. Yoga breathing
has opened my heart to love more freely and to enjoy life
more. I am more connected to other people by living from the
heart instead of the head."

Case 2—Yoga Breathing Reduces Prostate-Specific Antigen (PSA)

As men age, their prostates tend to enlarge and many worry
about developing prostate cancer. Stress and inflammation
may be contributory factors to prostatic hypertrophy. Every
year men anxiously await the results of their prostate-specific
antigen (PSA) testing to see if this cancer marker is stable.
Frank was a busy 57-year-old CEO of a large investment
firm. After years of chemotherapy had failed to eradicate his
prostate cancer, his PSA numbers were elevated to more than
three times normal levels. To counteract the high level of
stress he was experiencing, Frank was advised to take a yoga
breathing course. Two weeks after he completed the six-day
Sudarshan Yoga Breath Course and engaged in daily yoga
breath practice (20 minutes/day), his PSA was retested and
found to be normal. Nevertheless, seeing himself as "too
busy" to practice yoga every day, he stopped. Twelve weeks
later, when his PSA was elevated again, Frank resumed daily
yoga breathing. Although Frank won't take time to practice
yoga every day, he gets his PSA checked every three months
and whenever it starts to increase, he resumes his yoga
breath practices just long enough to bring the test numbers
back down to normal. Frank discovered that daily SKY

breathing was an effective way for him to lower his PSA to a normal level.

Professional and Family Caregiver Stress in Oncology

Caring for cancer patients is a highly stressful occupation. In addition to the daily stress of treating extremely ill and dying patients, oncology staff and faculty at academic hospitals and research facilities are under constant stress to obtain grants and produce research. Faculty wellness programs are attempting to reduce the physical and emotional toll and prevent adverse effects such as professional burnout and suicide.

Sudarshan Kriya Yoga

The Faculty Wellness Program at MD Anderson Cancer Center in Houston, Texas offered the five-day Sudarshan Kriya Yoga Basic Course three times to a total of 48 faculty and staff members. An online survey of the participants drew responses from 24 subjects (50% response rate) who reported the following items to be better/much better as a result of taking the course: anxiety/tension 38%/33%; ability to stay calm 42%/29%; mood 50%/25%; ability to focus 46%/4%; relationships outside of work 29%/12%; feelings of stress 38%/38%; sleep 33%/17%; anger/frustration 42%/17%; closeness with coworkers 21%/8%; optimism 29%/25% (Apted, 2006).

CARDIOVASCULAR DISEASE

The leading cause of death and disability in the United States and many other countries is cardiovascular disease (CVD). The potential role of CAM in prevention and treatment of CVD, as well as in recovery after acute episodes or surgery, is of growing interest. A review by Kim Innes and colleagues (2005) of the possible protective effects of yoga in reducing risk indices identified 70 studies, including one observational, 26 uncontrolled, 21 nonrandomized controlled, and two RCTs. Although many had methodological limitations, the reviewers concluded that, " . . . collectively, they suggest that yoga may reduce many IRS-related [insulin resistance syndrome] risk factors for CVD, may improve clinical outcomes, and may aid in the management of CVD and other IRS-related conditions." The reported benefits included improved glucose tolerance and insulin sensitivity, lipid profile, blood pressure, oxidative stress, coagulation profiles, sympathetic activation, and cardiovagal function (Innes, Bourguignon, & Taylor, 2005).

The positive effects of yoga on cardiovascular risk factors probably occur through downregulation of the sympathoadrenal system and the hypothalamic-pituitary-adrenal axis (HPA) and via stimulation of the vagus nerve leading to increased parasympathetic activity (see Chapter 3). Some of the physical consequences of these changes include decreased heart rate and blood pressure as well as increased heart rate variability (HRV) and baroreflex sensitivity (Brown & Gerbarg, 2005a). Psychological effects include reduction in stress reactivity, perceived stress, anxiety, sleep, and depression. Both the physical and psychological shifts would potentially have positive impact on glucose tolerance, insulin sensitivity, lipid profile, visceral adipose tissue, oxidative stress, coagulation factors, and endothelial function. The net result of any combination of these physiological mechanisms would be reduced risk for cardiovascular disease (Innes et al., 2005).

Mind–body practices, particularly those that include slow yoga breath techniques and relaxation training are an effective, low cost, low risk means to reduce morbidity and mortality from CVD. Health care providers can best serve their patients by explaining the potential benefits of mind–body practices, by referring patients to courses that match their emotional needs and their physical capacities, and by persistently monitoring and encouraging them to continue the practices. Patients with recent acute cardiac events, chest surgery, or poorly controlled hypertension, should avoid rapid intense yoga breathing or strenuous or head-down postures.

Patients with CVD are at increased risk from psychotropic medication side effects. CAM treatments for anxiety, PTSD, depression, and cognitive dysfunction can reduce these risks (see Chapters 2, 3, and 4). In a prospective study of 309 patients, one year after coronary artery bypass graft, 27.0% of the depressed patients had experienced a cardiac event compared with 10.2% of the nondepressed patients (Oz, 2004). Patients who have experienced myocardial infarction, cardiac arrest, or surgery may be left with symptoms of posttraumatic stress disorder or cognitive dysfunction secondary to cerebral ischemia. Appropriate CAM treatments can facilitate fuller recovery (see Chapters 3 and 4). In using vitamins, herbs, and nutrients, it is important to check for possible interactions with anticoagulants and other medications. B vitamins, including folate should be avoided in men with cardiac stents because they may accelerate occlusion in those whose homocysteine level is <15 μmol/liter.

CHRONIC FATIGUE SYNDROME, FIBROMYALGIA, AND ARTHRITIS

Complementary and alternative treatments (CAM) have shown some benefits for people with fibromyalgia syndrome (FMS) and chronic fatigue syndrome (CFS). These include SAMe (S-adenosylmethionine), St. John's Wort, *Rhodiola rosea* (Brown & Gerbarg, 2004), dehydroepiandrosterone (DHEA), cognitive-behavior therapy (CBT), acupuncture, meditation, and Qigong.

S-adenosylmethionine (SAMe)

Fibromyalgia syndrome (FMS) is a painful inflammatory condition that often leads to depression. Four double-blind placebo controlled studies (Jacobsen, Danneskiold-Samsoe, & Anderson, 1991; Tavoni, Vitali, Bombardieri, & Pasero, 1991; Tavoni, Jeracitano, & Cirigliano, 1998; Tavoni, Vitali, Bombardieri, & Pasero, 1987; Volkmann, Norregaard, Jacobsen, Danneskiold-Samsoe, Knoke et al., 1997) and three case series reported that SAMe improved both depression and pain in patients with fibromyalgia at doses equivalent to 800 mg/day. There were no side effects. Twelve studies have shown that SAMe has analgesic and anti-inflammatory effects in osteoarthritis (Di Padova, 1987). In seven controlled comparison studies, SAMe was equally as effective as nonsteroidal anti-inflammatory agents in reducing pain and inflammation but unlike other medications, SAMe did not cause gastric erosion or GI bleeding.

In a 16-week double-blind crossover trial, SAMe reduced pain and inflammation of knee osteoarthritis as effectively as a COX-2 inhibitor, celecoxib (Najm, Reinsch, Hoehler, Tobis, & Harvey, 2004). A two-year Phase IV study of over 20,000 people found that

SAMe significantly relieved arthritis symptoms with minimal side effects (Berger & Nowak, 1987). Mild arthritis may respond to SAMe 600 mg/day by week four. Moderate arthritis usually requires 1,200 mg/day SAMe for three to four weeks. Up to four months may be needed for severe arthritis (Bradley, Flusser, Katz, Schumacher, Brandt et al., 1994). After three months of SAMe in doses of 400 to 1,200 mg/day MRI studies showed accelerated cartilage regeneration (Konig, Stahl, Sieper, & Wolf, 1995). Because of its dual benefits and low side effect profile, SAMe is the preferred antidepressant for treatment of depression in the context of osteoarthritis, rheumatoid arthritis, or fibromyalgia.

Other Modalities: Acupuncture, Magnesium, Carnitines, St. John's Wort

A review of CAM treatments for CFS and FMS (Ernst, 2004) considered two out of nine acupuncture studies to be of good quality. These studies indicate that acupuncture can be a useful adjunctive treatment and that rigorous trials are needed. Two small RCTs provide modest evidence that magnesium may be helpful in a subgroup of CFS/FMS patients (Holdcraft, Assefi, & Buchwald, 2003). In an open comparison trial, 30 CFS patients were randomized to one of three groups: acetyl-l-carnitine alone; propionyl-carnitine alone; and acetyl-l-carnitine + propionyl carnitine. Those given acetyl-l-carnitine showed improvements in mental fatigue, those on propionyl-carnitine had improved general fatigue, and those receiving both carnitines improved in mental and general fatigue. Attention improved in all groups (Vermeulen & Scholte, 2004). St. John's Wort (brand Kira) 900 mg/day reduced fatigue, depression and anxiety in a six-week open series study of 19 CFS patients (Stevinson & Ernst, 1999). A six-week DBRPC study of 184 patients with somatoform disorders (somatization disorder) but not depression found that those given St. John's Wort Kira 600 mg/day did better than placebo, particularly those with autonomic dysfunction (Muller et al., 2004).

Rhodiola rosea

Extensive studies of cosmonauts in Swedish/Russian space research found that *Rhodiola rosea* strengthened the sympathetic nervous system (SNS) and parasympathetic nervous system (PNS) function

---

CLINICAL PEARL

In clinical practice, the authors find that *R. rosea* in doses ranging from 50 to 600 mg/day significantly enhances physical and mental energy and endurance in patients with CFS and FMS. While most patients require 200 to 600 mg/day, it is best to start with 50 mg/day in patients who tend to be sensitive, anxious, ill, or elderly and then increase by 50 to 100 mg every three to seven days as tolerated to avoid overstimulation.

---

while improving mental and physical endurance (Baranov, 1994; Brown & Gerbarg, 2004; Brown, Gerbarg, & Ramazanov, 2002; Polyakov, 1966). Several modern studies have shown that *R. rosea* reduces mental and physical fatigue while increasing alertness, accuracy, and mental focus, particularly under stress, in healthy subjects (Darbinyan, Aslanyan, Embroyan, Gabrielyan, Malmstrom et al., 2007; Shevtsov et al., 2003; Spasov, Mandrikov, & Mironova, 2000; Spasov, Wikman, Mandrikov, Mironova, & Neumoin, 2000). (For a more detailed discussion of *R. rosea* see Chapter 4). Based on this evidence the authors have given *R. rosea* in doses ranging from 50 to 600 mg/day to patients with CFS and FMS.

The authors believe that exhaustion of the stress response system with erratic activity of the SNS and reduced activity of the PNS constitutes the underlying pathology in CFS/FMS (Brown & Gerbarg, 2004; Stein & Hunter, 2004). Low respiratory sinus arrhythmia (RSA) and low heart rate variability (HRV) have been associated with FMS and CFS (Martinez-Lavin, Hermosillo, Rosas, & Soto, 1998). In a study of orthostatic and mental stress, 28 FMS patients showed hyporeactive SNS response when compared with 15 controls (Friederich, Schellberg, Mueller, Bieber, Zipfel et al., 2005). Compared with 19 age-matched healthy men, 19 men with FMS showed SNS hyperreactivity and low PNS activity with abnormal autonomic responses during postural changes (Cohen, Neumann, Alhosshle, Kotler, Abu-Shakra, & Buskila, 2001). Depression frequently precedes exhaustion of the stress response system. Fifty percent of people with FMS had major depression during the previous year or at the time of diagnosis of FMS.

Mind–body practices for FMS/CFS, including relaxation, hypnotherapy, and biofeedback provide some limited benefit while Qigong and Mindfulness Meditation are supported by uncontrolled studies (Ernst, 2004; Kaplan, Goldenberg, & Galvin-Nadeau, 1993; von Weiss, 2002). Yoga breathing can help normalize the activity of the SNS and PNS, reducing stress reactivity and improving mood, sleep, anxiety, cognitive function, and immune parameters (see Chapter 3). In a two-year prospective study of CAM use, 155 subjects with CFS of unclear etiology, average age 67 years, and mean symptom duration of 6.7 years, were assessed for fatigue and other symptoms at baseline, six months, and two years. Subjects reported that they derived the greatest subjective benefits from CoQ10 (69% of 13 subjects), dehydroepiandrosterone (DHEA) (65% of 17 subjects), and ginseng (56% of 18 subjects). Treatments at six months that predicted subsequent fatigue improvement were vitamins (p=.08), vigorous exercise (p=.09), and yoga (p=.002). Yoga appeared to be most effective for people who did not have unclear thinking associated with their fatigue. Magnesium and support groups were associated with worsening fatigue (Bentler, Hartz, & Kuhn, 2005).

Paul Lehrer and colleagues developed a method to use heart rate variability feedback to teach resonant breathing at the optimal rate for respiratory-cardiovascular function (usually 5 to 6 breaths per minute; see Chapter 3). Twelve women with fibromyalgia completed 10 weekly sessions of HRV biofeedback to learn to breathe at their resonant frequency (RF). By week 10, depression improved significantly. They were instructed to continue practicing resonant breathing 20 minutes twice a day. At the three-month follow-up the women showed significant improvements in depression, pain, and functioning (Hassett, Radvanski, Vaschillo, Vaschillo, Sigal et al., 2007).

External Qigong Therapy

A pilot study of 10 FMS patients were given five to seven external Qigong therapy (EQT) sessions of about 40 minutes each over a three-week period with testing at baseline, three weeks, and three months. The mean Tender Point Count (TPC) was reduced from

136.6 to 59.5, the mean McGill Pain Questionnaire (MPQ) from 27 to 7.2, the mean Fibromyalgia Impact Questionnaire (FIQ) from 70.1 to 37.3, and mean Beck Depression Inventory (BDI) from 24.3 to 8.3 (all p<0.01). At three-month follow up, some symptoms increased, but continued to be much better than at baseline. Two subjects reported complete remission (Chen, Hassett, Hou, Staller, & Lichtbroun, 2006). Although this was a small study, the large effect size supports the significance. Larger RCTs with follow-up sessions to maintain benefits are indicated for this promising treatment.

Sudarshan Kriya Yoga

Preliminary data suggest prolongevity effects of SKY breath practices (Brown & Gerberg, in press): improved lipid profile; enhanced immune system function increased antioxidant defense enzymes, glutathione (GSH) and superoxide dismutase (SOD); and reduced serum lactate (stress indicator) (Geehta et al., 2006; Sharma, Aggarwal, Sen, Singh, Kochupillai et al., 2002). Further studies are needed to confirm the positive effects of breath practices on lipid profile, antioxidant systems, and indicators of stress.

Integrative Approach to Treatment of CFS/FMS

1. Complete medical workup to rule out treatable organic illnesses.
2. Psychiatric evaluation to identify comorbid and contributory conditions such as anxiety, depression, OCD, PTSD, substance abuse, personality disorders, and relationship problems.
3. If anxiety, depression, or fatigue is prominent, trials of an SSRI, venlafaxine (Effexor), tricyclic antidepressants (TCAs) alone or with SSRIs, duloxetine (Cymbalta), pregabalin (Lyrica), or milnacipran (Ixel) are indicated. Milnacipran, is a strong norepinephrine reuptake inhibitor with some serotonin reuptake inhibitory effects.
4. For symptoms of fibromyalgia, SAMe (800–1600 mg/day) is the first CAM treatment of choice. It often works best in combination with a serotonin reuptake inhibitor (SSRI), tricyclic antidepressant (TCA), or serotonin norepinephrine reuptake inhibitor (SNRI).

5. For fatigue (mental and/or physical) *Rhodiola rosea* 50–600 mg/day is the first CAM treatment of choice. Start with 50 to 200 mg/day depending on the patients' physical condition, age, and sensitivity to stimulation. Capsules containing dried root extract may be opened to allow for dose adjustments. If there are no signs of overstimulation (anxiety, agitation, insomnia) then the dose may be increased by 50 to 200 mg/day every three to seven days up to a maximum of 600 mg/day. In elderly or medically fragile patients, start with lower doses and do increases more slowly.

6. Propionyl-L-carnitine (1,000–2,000 mg/day) can be beneficial for physical fatigue, while acetyl-L-carnitine (1,000–2,000 mg/day) tends to be better for mental fatigue. Patient response is variable, so it is worthwhile to try each alone and in combination to determine what works best for the individual.

7. The addition of acupuncture can be beneficial for pain, fatigue, and sleep.

8. A program of yoga breathing and gentle yoga postures can be quite helpful, for example, Qigong, Sudarshan Kriya, or gentle Kundalini. Patients need support and encouragement to locate an appropriate course, attend weekly sessions, and maintain their daily practices. The authors have found the Basic Course in Sudarshan Kriya taught by the Art of Living Foundation to be particularly helpful for the full range of physical and psychological symptoms in CFS/FMS, and the daily practice requires less than 30 minutes. For those unable to take the course, the HRV training in Resonance Breathing or Coherence Breathing using the Respire I CD (www.coherence.com) can be used (see Chapter 3).

HUMAN IMMUNE DEFICIENCY VIRUS (HIV), PERSONS LIVING WITH AIDS, AND HEPATITIS

About 30 to 50% of HIV+ patients experience depressive disorders associated with low immune response, disease progression, decreased expectations of survival, and lower quality of life.

> **CLINICAL PEARL**
>
> SAMe deficiency in HIV+ patients may contribute to depression, demyelination, and myelopathy. SAMe 800 to 1,600 mg/day can alleviate depression and improve liver function.

S-adenosylmethionine

Because HIV patients are often treated with medications that place a burden on liver metabolism and cause other side effects, an antidepressant such as SAMe that supports liver functions and is low in side effects should be considered. SAMe deficiency has been found in HIV-infected patients and this may contribute to the depression, demyelination, and myelopathy that sometimes occur. An open-label eight-week pilot study of 20 patients with HIV and major depression given SAMe 400 mg twice a day with folic acid (800 mcg/day) and B_{12} (1,000 mcg/day) found significant improvement in depression by week 4 with a drop in the mean HAMD scores from 27 to 9. Many patients with HIV are former drug abusers with abnormal liver functions due to hepatitis B and C. In this study, liver functions improved with the administration of SAMe. None of the patients had adverse side effects (Shippy, 2004).

Rhodiola rosea

Although no studies have been done in AIDS patients, the authors find that *R. rosea* can help to relieve fatigue, depression, and anxiety

> **CLINICAL PEARL**
>
> In the authors' clinical experience, *R. rosea* in combination with SAMe can alleviate the fatigue and cognitive interference associated with Interferon treatment.

in persons living with AIDS with minimal side effects. AIDs patients with hepatitis C may be treated with Interferon. The debilitating fatigue and cognitive interference caused by Interferon often responds to *R. rosea* in combination with SAMe.

Acetyl-L-Carnitine

Fatigue and antiretroviral toxic neuropathy are common severe problems in HIV patients. Different forms of carnitine have been helpful in CFS (see CFS/FMS section above). Similarly, acetyl-L-carnitine can relieve fatigue in patients with AIDS. Two open trials and one DBRPC study of 90 patients found that acetyl-L-carnitine also significantly relieved pain from peripheral neuropathy in AIDs patients (Youle & Osio, 2007).

Mind-Body-Spirit Practices

In persons living with AIDS, anxiety has a profound impact on quality of life and it can interfere with adherence to antiretroviral therapies. Anxiety disorders are correlated with subjective pain and the rate of disease progression in HIV. All components of heart rate variability, a marker of cardiac autonomic tone, were significantly reduced in a study of 21 HIV+ adults when compared with 18 healthy volunteers (Mittal, Wig, Mishra, & Deepak, 2004). Interventions that improve autonomic balance and tone may be beneficial (see Chapter 3). A study of the effectiveness of strategies for self-management of anxiety in an international sample of 1,072 persons from Norway, Taiwan, and the United States with HIV/AIDS found that 502 (47%) reported HIV-related anxiety. The most commonly used strategies for managing anxiety included talking with family and friends, watching television, walking, and talking with a health care provider. On a scale of 1 to 10, the highest overall ratings of effec-

---

CLINICAL PEARL

R. rosea and acetyl-L-carnitine or propionyl-L-carnitine can reduce fatigue in persons living with AIDS with very few side effects.

tiveness were given for prayer (8.1 SD 2.3), meditation (7.4 SD 2.7), relaxation techniques (7.2 SD 2.5), and exercise (7.3 SD 2.5). Women were more likely to use prayer (76%) versus 25% of men. Men were more likely to use alcohol (40%) versus 25% of women (Kemppainen, Eller, Bunch, Hamilton, Dole et al., 2006).

Mantra Repetition

A randomized study of 93 HIV-infected adults compared mantra repetition (n=46) to the effects of nonsense syllable repetition in a control group (n=47). Increased mantra practice (measured by wrist counters) was associated with a decrease in non-HIV related intrusive thoughts and an increase in quality of life, existential spiritual well-being, meaning/peace, and spiritual faith. Findings suggest that a mantra group intervention and individual practice may reduce emotional distress and improve spiritual well-being. After three months, the measures returned to baseline. The loss of efficacy over time was attributed to lack of practice, refresher sessions, and face-to-face follow-up (Bormann, Gifford, Shively, Smith, Redwine et al., 2006).

Mindfulness Meditation and Concentrative Meditation (Kundalini)

In a randomized crossover study of 78 men with HIV Centers for Disease Control (CDC) Stage II or III, who had previously practiced meditation for at least one year and were not taking psychotropic medications, 36 subjects were assigned to receive 20 minutes of mindfulness meditation first and 36 to engage in 20 minutes of concentrative meditation first. Both practices significantly improved scores on Social Efficacy and Health Behavior Self-Efficacy, but not on General Self-Efficacy (Khalsa, 2007). The concentrative meditation practice used in this study, Pauri Kriya, is a Kundalini technique similar to one used by Shannahoff-Khalsa. It includes controlled inhalation while mentally repeating syllables combined with finger movements followed by controlled exhalation while reciting syllables aloud (creates airway resistance) and coordinating finger movements.

Art of Living Foundation: Sudarshan Kriya Yoga

An RCT of 62 people (47 completers) living with HIV/AIDS found positive changes in well-being on the Mental Health Index (MHI) and the MOS-HIV Health Survey immediately following a course in yoga breathing, meditation, and yoga postures by the Art of Living Foundation. These improvements were lost over time on follow-up tests. The Daily Stress Inventory indicated an increase in the impact of stress over time after the program. Qualitative interviews revealed that participants in the yoga breathing course showed positive changes in how they were living their daily lives (Brazier, Mulkins, & Verhoef, 2006). This loss of positive effects over time is probably due to nonadherence to daily yoga practice and nonattendance at weekly follow-up sessions. This study illustrates the difficulties of maintaining yoga practices over time in HIV patients whose lives may be disrupted by physical problems and the multiple stressors they face.

Mind–body–spirit practices can enhance physical and mental well-being in HIV patients without adding to the burden of medications. Biopsychosocial approaches can address social interactions, health behaviors, and self-efficacy. Many Yoga programs report benefits for persons living with AIDS anecdotally (Stukin, 2001). However, controlled clinical studies are needed to develop the complementary role of mind–body–spirit practices in treatment. For long-term benefits, programs designed for HIV+ patients should include long-term follow-up with frequent refresher sessions, regular group meetings, monitoring, and support for continuation of regular practice. Linking yoga courses with other medical services in health care facilities would probably improve adherence.

IRRITABLE BOWEL SYNDROME (IBS)

Stress exacerbates gastrointestinal distress through release of neuropeptides and neurotransmitters triggering GI responses. The enteric nervous system produces the same neuropeptides and neurotransmitters as the CNS. A biopsychosocial model of functional GI disorders has led to increased interest in self-regulation or mind-body therapies including hypnosis, biofeedback, guided imagery, meditation, and relaxation techniques. These may work by reducing the perception of pain and stress leading to decreased SNS drive, blood pressure, heart rate, serum lactic acid, and tonic muscle tension. Autonomic dysfunction has been implicated in IBS.

Yoga Postures and Right Nostril Breathing

In a two-month RCT of 22 men aged 20 to 25 years with diarrhea-predominant IBS, conventional symptomatic treatment with loperamide 2 to 6 mg/day (n=11) was compared with a yoga intervention (n=9). The yoga intervention included 12 yoga postures and right nostril breathing twice a day. Both groups showed significant reductions in bowel symptoms and state anxiety. In the conventional treatment group, electrophysiologically recorded gastric activity increased, whereas, in the yoga group PNS response was enhanced (measured as heart rate parameters) (Taneja, Deepak, Poojary, Acharya, Pandey et al., 2004).

Relaxation and Guided Imagery

Chronic recurrent abdominal pain (RAP) affects 10 to 30% of school aged children. There are no conventional medications proven to be effective for functional abdominal pain in children. A randomized controlled study of 22 children, aged 5 to 18 years found that those trained in guided imagery and progressive muscle relaxation (n=14) had significantly greater decreases in the number of days with pain after one month (67% vs. 21% p=0.05) and after two months (82% vs. 45% p<0.01), as well as greater decreases in the number of days of missed activities than a comparison group given breathing exercises (n=8): abdominal breathing, "bubble breathing" (prolonged expiration to blow bubbles), and "breathing in fives" (full deep inhalation for count of 5, breath hold for 5, full exhalation for 5, and hold for 5) (Weydert, Shapiro, Acra, Monheim, Chambers et al., 2006). While this study is small, it does support the benefits of guided imagery and progressive relaxation for children with functional bowel disorders. In designing the program of guided imagery, the authors consulted numerous experts to devise the most effective approach. The choice of breath techniques may not have been ideal because children of different ages have different capacities and respond differently to breath practices. Also, it would be preferable to focus on breath techniques that increase PNS activity in order to reduce anxiety and quiet gastrointestinal activity.

In a four-week RCT, 25 adolescents aged 11 to 18 years with IBS were assigned to either a yoga intervention or a wait-list control. Following the yoga intervention, adolescents reported reduction in functional disability, emotion-focused avoidance, and anxiety (Kuttner et al., 2006).

Integrative Approach to Treatment of Irritable Bowel Syndrome

1. Medical workup to rule out organic causes.
2. Elimination of exacerbating dietary and substance abuse factors.
3. Assessment of psychological factors and comorbid conditions: anxiety, depression, PTSD, OCD.
4. Assessment of contributory environmental factors.
5. If GI symptoms are clearly exacerbated by stress and anxiety, a trial of mirtazepine (Remeron) at bedtime can be helpful because it is more calming to the GI tract than other antidepressants. It provides sedative and anxiolytic effects without risk of habituation as can occur with benzodiazepines, particularly in anxious individuals. However, Remeron can cause weight gain and daytime sedation (particularly in the first two weeks of treatment). Most patients will tolerate the initial sedation if they understand that it usually clears with time. However, for patients who cannot tolerate the daytime drowsiness or weight gain, tricyclic antidepressants (TCAs) such as amitriptyline, doxepin, and imipramine can reduce excess bowel activity in diarrhea-predominant IBS. However, TCAs can exacerbate constipation in constipation-predominant IBS and cause other side effects (dry mouth, arrhythmia, or hypotension).
6. Mind–body practices including self-hypnosis, guided imagery, progressive relaxation, slow yoga breathing against airway resistance (Ujjayi or alternate nostril breathing) to activate the PNS, and later meditation.
7. Most people benefit from resonant breathing or coherent breathing. (www.coherence.com). See also Chapter 3 on Anxiety Disorders.

TABLE 8.1 Treatment Guidelines for Psychological Aspects of Medical Illness

CAM	Clinical Uses	Daily Dose	Side Effects, Drug Interactions,* Contraindications
Ashwaganda (*Withania somnifera*)	stress, depression, augment chemotherapy	100–400 mg b.i.d.	Minimal
B vitamins			Caution: cardiac stent**
B$_1$ thiamine	anemia, fatigue	50 mg/day	
B$_2$ riboflavin	migraine	200 mg b.i.d.	
B$_{12}$ cobalamin	anemia, fatigue, peripheral neuropathy, Bell's palsy, depression	1,000 mcg/day	
Carnitines Alcar Acetyl-L-carnitine	chronic fatigue syndrome, mental fatigue	1,500 mg b.i.d.	Mild gastric upset, take with food
Propionyl-L-carnitine	fatigue	1,000–2,000 mg/day	
Folate	Anemia, fatigue	800 mcg/day	Caution: cardiac stents**
Fucoxanthin Brown seaweed	obesity, metabolic syndrome	1 pill t.i.d.	Minimal, more studies needed Caution: thyroid disease
Ginkgo (*Ginkgo biloba*)	cerebrovascular disease	120–240 mg/day	Minimal: headache, decreased platelet aggregation. D/C 2 weeks prior to surgery Contraindication: anticoagulants

TABLE 8.1 *Continued*

CAM	Clinical Uses	Daily Dose	Side Effects, Drug Interactions,* Contraindications
Ginseng *Panax Ginseng*	fatigue	400–800 mg/day	Activation GI, anxiety, insomnia, headache, tachycardia, decreased platelet aggregation. Caution: anticoagulants
Rhodiola rosea	chronic fatigue syndrome, fatigue, anxiety, depression, cognitive enhancement, memory	150–600 mg/day	Agitation, insomnia, jitteriness, headache. Rare: increased blood pressure, bruising, chest pain Caution: bipolars.
S-adenosyl-methionine (SAMe)	chronic fatigue, fibromyalgia, migraine, depression, liver disease, HIV/AIDS, Parkinson's	800–1,600 mg 400–2,000 mg 400–2,000 mg 400–2,200 mg 1,200–1,600 mg 800–2,400 mg 800–4,400 mg	Occasional GI, agitation, anxiety, insomnia. Rare: palpitations Caution: bipolar II Contraindication: bipolar I

■ **Combination Products**

CAM	Clinical Uses	Daily Dose	Side Effects, Drug Interactions,* Contraindications
Amrit Kalash (contains many Ayurvedic herbs)	fatigue, nausea, hair loss due to chemotherapy	1 tsp b.i.d.	Minimal
Bio-Strath B vitamins, antioxidants	Energy, appetite, weight, anemia, radiation	1–2 Tbsp b.i.d. 3 tabs b.i.d.	Caution: cardiac stent**

| Metanx 2.8 mg L-methylfolate, 25 mg pyridoxal 5'-phosphate, 2 mg methyl-cobalamin | cardiovascular risks, elevated homocysteine | 1–2 tabs/day | Minimal Caution: cardiac stent** |

D/C = discontinue; GI = gastrointestinal symptoms; hs = at bedtime; b.i.d. = twice a day; g = grams; mg = milligram; mcg = microgram; tsp = teaspoon; Tbsp = tablespoon

*Common side effects are listed. There are additional rare side effects. Individuals with high blood pressure, diabetes, pregnancy (or during breast-feeding), or any chronic or serious medical condition should check with their physician before taking supplements.

**May increase risk of restenosis of cardiac stents in men only whose baseline homocysteine is <15 μmol/liter.

CHAPTER 9 OUTLINE

1. **Mind–Body Practices**
2. **Herbs and Nutrients**: thiamine, magnesium, *N*-acetylcysteine, omega-3 fatty acids, S-adenosylmethionine, passionflower, ginseng, Kudzu
3. **Technology-Based Interventions**
4. **Fetal Alcohol Syndrome**
   a. prenatal prevention
   b. donepezil
   c. cholinergic enhancers

Substance Abuse

A survey of intravenous drug users recruited from a needle-exchange program and a methadone maintenance program found that 45% used at least one complementary and alternative medicine (CAM) treatment. Mind–body practices such as religious healing, relaxation techniques, and meditation were the most frequently used. The level of self-perceived effectiveness for CAM was high. For most participants, the use of CAM was related to their addiction (Manheimer, Anderson, & Stein, 2003). This study indicates that CAM is likely to be acceptable and considered effective by a substantial percentage of intravenous substance abusers. There is also growing evidence to support the use of mind–body practices, herbs, and nutrients as complementary interventions in the treatment of individuals with substance abuse disorders (Dean, 2003).

Difficulty in regulating affects such as anxiety, fear, and anger contribute to the abuse of substances. Interventions that improve affect tolerance and affect regulation help patients learn to deal with difficult emotions without using substances of abuse. Many people who suffer from addictions have poor nutritional status along with comorbid physical and emotional problems such as depression, anxiety disorders, posttraumatic stress disorder, traumatic brain injury, neurological deterioration, lung disease, liver disease, hepatitis, and HIV. Herbs, nutrients, antioxidants, and nootropics that ameliorate these conditions, as described in the other chapters in this book, can be valuable in such cases.

MIND-BODY PRACTICES

An excellent review of mindfulness-based cognitive interventions in the treatment of cooccurring addictive and mood disorders proposes that chronic use of addictive substances compromises areas of the brain responsible for affect regulation, attention, inhibitory control, and the ability to observe and moderate responses to intense emotions (Hoppes, 2006). Deficits in affect regulation increase vulnerability to relapse, particularly in early stages of recovery. By improving affect tolerance and affect regulation, mind–body approaches can enhance treatment outcome during the withdrawal, early recovery, and maintenance phases. Randomized clinical trials in this area are limited; however, several aspects of mind–body practices may contribute to their beneficial effects. Breath practices, yoga postures, relaxation, and meditation reduce states of arousal, tension, anxiety, insomnia, anger, depression, and PTSD (see Chapters 2 and 3). Patients report that during recovery, mind–body practices help them by putting a distance between the impulse to take substances of abuse and the compulsion to act on the impulse. Mind–body programs often incorporate aspects of Eastern psychology and Buddhist theory of mind regarding the nature of thoughts and emotions. This can change the relationship to mental contents, modify the appraisal of thoughts and feeling states, teach people to let go of their attachment to negative thoughts/emotions, redirect attention away from negative thoughts, and balance techniques for change with a philosophy of nonjudgmental acceptance. Mindfulness techniques and affect tolerance have been incorporated into Dialectical Behavioural Therapy (DBT) in the treatment of substance abuse (Linehan, Dimeff, Reynolds, Comtois, Welch et al., 2002).

Qigong

Qigong incorporates meditation, relaxation, guided imagery, concentration, and breathing exercises. The Chinese word *qi* translates as breath of life or vital energy, similar to the Sanskrit word, *prana*. *Gong* means "the skill to work with." By developing awareness of *qi* sensations in the body, practitioners learn to guide the flow of *qi*. Qigong masters are believed to possess the ability to emit energy (external *qi*), sending it to heal the recipient.

In a comparison control study of Qigong versus medication and placebo during opiate withdrawal, 86 male heroin addicts (DSM-III-R) admitted for mandatory treatment to the Changzhou Drug Treatment Center in the People's Republic of China were assigned to one of three treatment groups according to the order of their admission. One group practiced a simple form of Qigong (PanGu) together 2 to 2.5 hours/day and received emitted *qi* for 10 to 15 minutes/day from a Qigong master. The second group was treated with detoxification medication in tapering doses (lofexidine), physical exercise, and group counseling. The nontreatment group was only given emergency care for acute pain, diarrhea, or insomnia (diazepam or methaqualone). The Qigong group had significantly lower mean scores on the Chinese Standard Evaluation Scale of Withdrawal Symptoms starting from the first day of treatment ($p<0.05$). Mean Hamilton Anxiety scores (Ham-A) were comparable at baseline among the groups (33.5–37.4). However, by day 5 of detoxification, mean Ham-A dropped from 37.4 ± 7.5 to 8.2 ± 4.9 in the Qigong group versus from 33.5 ± 8.5 to 13.6 ± 6.4 in the medication group, and from 35.0 ± 4.7 to 21.3 ± 11.4 in the nontreatment group. On day 10, the Ham-A scores were 0.7 ± 1.0, 5.3 ± 3.1, and 7.3 ± 18.2 respectively (Li, Chen, & Mo, 2002). Although there are methodological problems in this study, such as the inability to separate effects of group Qigong practice from interventions by the Qigong master, it provides evidence that Qigong practices may accelerate detoxification and reduce withdrawal symptoms. The physiological mechanisms by which these effects occur may be similar among mind-body practices that use breath, posture, relaxation, imagery, concentration and meditation.

Once withdrawal is achieved, maintenance of abstinence becomes the focus of treatment. Recently detoxed patients are often anxious, depressed, and under severe psychosocial and financial stress—conditions that promote relapse. Sedatives, anxiolytics, and some sedating antidepressants must be used with caution due to the high risks of abuse and dependence. Mind–body practices can be valuable complementary treatments with standard rehabilitation services, counseling, and self-help groups such as Alcoholics Anonymous and Narcotics Anonymous.

Sudarshan Kriya Yoga

After one week of detoxification, 60 hospitalized, alcohol dependent patients were randomly assigned to receive two weeks of either Sudarshan Kriya Yoga (SKY) breathing or continued standard treatment with counseling and benzodiazepines for sleep. The SKY intervention was limited to the breath practices given 45 minutes every other day without the other group interventions used in the general courses. There were greater mean reductions in scores on BDI and levels of cortisol in the SKY group than in the control (Vedamurthachar, Janakiramaiah, Hegde, Shetty, Subbakrishna et al., 2006). While this study suggests a beneficial effect of SKY in reducing anxiety and cortisol levels in recently detoxed alcoholic patients, the statistical reporting needs some clarification and the study needs replication.

In a two-week study, community clinic patients with opioid dependence (DSM-IV) on agonist maintenance were randomly assigned to standard treatment (n=14) or to standard treatment plus a 5-day course called Nav-Chetna Shivir (n=15) which included two to three hours per day of yoga breathing (Sudarshan Kriya Yoga), meditation, singing, and discussing healthy living. At the end of two weeks, there was no significant difference between groups on the Addiction Severity Index. The WHO Quality of Life Brief scale showed significant change in the yoga augmented group in the physical (p<0.001), psychological (p<0.01), and social relationship (p<0.01) domains compared to no significant change in the control group. The Stages of Change Questionnaire showed significantly increased motivation in the yoga group compared to the control (Yadav, Dhawan, Sethi, & Chopra, 2006).

Hatha Yoga

In a six-month study, 61 patients treated for opioid addiction in a methadone maintenance program were randomized to receive either conventional weekly group psychotherapy or a weekly Hatha Yoga group. After six months, there were no significant differences between the two groups on psychological, sociological, and biological measures. The study concluded that the alternative Hatha Yoga treatment was not more effective than conventional group therapy treatment (Shaffer, LaSalvia, & Stein, 1997). The study highlights issues that can arise when researchers set up studies and interpret Eastern practices. The benefits of most mind–body techniques accrue from regular daily practice. The finding that once-a-week Hatha Yoga was as effective as once-a-week group psychotherapy is very promising. Framing the outcome as a negative may discourage further exploration of the documented positive effects. The findings of this study indicate that it would be worthwhile to evaluate the complementary effects of combining Hatha Yoga with standard treatment for methadone maintenance.

Many patients with substance abuse have comorbid psychiatric conditions that complicate their treatment. The following complex case illustrates some of the risks, benefits, and adaptations involved in treating such challenging patients.

Case 1—Alcoholism, Marijuana Addiction, Bipolar Disorder, and Severe PTSD

Throughout her childhood, Lenore had been horribly tortured and sexually abused by several males in her family. As an adult her memories of trauma were easily triggered. For example, anytime she felt slighted, criticized, or rejected by anyone she would start binge drinking and engage in dangerous behaviors. She had no control over these reactions. During one binge she fell out of a third-story window and had to be hospitalized. She was too erratic to take medications. Although she was intelligent and appealing, she could not keep a job or form any friendships.

Her psychiatrist recommended the Sudarshan Kriya Yoga breathing course. The first time Lenore took the course, she opened up quickly in the safe and welcoming atmosphere. After confiding some details of her life to the group, she became terrified because she had allowed herself to trust other participants. She fled from the course, started drinking, and became despondent. Lenore and her psychiatrist realized that she needed to go more slowly. She responded well to talking with her psychiatrist and the yoga teacher about ways to proceed more slowly. First she was taught basic Ujjayi breathing. The calming effect enabled Lenore to begin to feel better. After several months of practicing Ujjayi for 10 minutes twice a day, Lenore felt ready to try the SKY course again. Her yoga teacher and her psychiatrist worked out a plan to help Lenore keep herself from opening up too quickly. With better preparation, Lenore responded well. She described the breathing as both gently energizing and soothing, "The breathing gives me a kind of uplift—a high, but I also feel more balance, calmer, and more in control so take better care of myself. After the breathing I have some hope and I am able to trust people and myself more."

Today, Lenore is attending school, holding down a job, taking medications (an atypical antipsychotic and an antidepressant) as prescribed, continuing cognitive behavioral therapy, and making friends. She is no longer tormented by traumatic memories or flashbacks. Although Lenore participated in Alcoholics Anonymous, she had never achieved a year of abstinence before. After completing the yoga course she was able to exceed a year of sobriety.

Some patients with severe emotional trauma may initially feel overwhelmed in the group experience or during yoga breathing. However, as in this case, collaboration between the psychiatrist and the yoga teacher was the key to supporting the patient with more preparation, encouragement and some technical modifications. Both the patient and her psychiatrist attribute the marked improvements in her emotional, cognitive, and interpersonal functioning to the addition of the SKY course and daily breath practices to her treatment regimen of medications and cognitive behavioral therapy.

Religious and spiritual programs have been widely used in the treatment of substance abuse. Yoga programs have been used in substance abuse treatment in India for many years (Nespor, 2000). Much of this work is published in Indian language publications or in documents from Indian religious institutions. These studies may not meet modern methodological and reporting standards. Western readers may consider such studies to be biased. While we can continue to wonder to what extent the benefits of such programs are due to their spiritual, emotional, philosophical, or physical practices, the controlled clinical studies beginning to appear and the neurophysiological studies of yoga practices may lead us to better understand the synergistic interplay of these important components.

HERBS AND NUTRIENTS

A small number of studies have documented benefits of herbs and nutrients in the treatment of substance abuse disorders. Individuals who abuse substances often have poor nutritional status and comorbid anxiety, depression, bipolar disorder, PTSD, cognitive impairments, ADD, and traumatic brain injury. Herbs and nutrients are particularly appropriate in substance abusers because they circumvent the tendency for abuse and dependence associated with prescription medications, they tend to be lower in side effects, and they put less burden on liver metabolism (compared to many prescription medications), particularly in patients who may have reduced liver reserves due to abuse-related liver diseases (alcoholic cirrhosis, hepatitis, HIV). Vitamins and cognitive enhancers can help to improve brain function that may be compromised by years of substance abuse, poor nutrition, and traumatic brain injuries (see Chapter 4 for a discussion of cognitive enhancers).

Vitamin B1 (thiamine)

Vitamin B_1 (thiamine) deficiency is known to be associated with chronic alcohol consumption. Severe deficiencies of thiamine contribute to Wernecke's encephalopathy, Korsakoff psychosis, polyneuropathy, and myopathy. Numerous studies have shown that thiamine supplementation can ameliorate some of the neurological sequelae of chronic alcoholism. In addition, animal studies indicate that thiamine deficiency may increase alcohol consumption (Zimatkin & Zimatkina, 1996). Thiamine supplementation is a well-established complementary treatment for alcoholism.

Magnesium

Acute alcohol administration can cause sudden severe vasoconstriction and decreased cerebral blood flow. Alcohol use, particularly "binge drinking" is associated with headaches, strokes, sudden death, and worse outcomes in patients with brain injury. Low levels of intracellular and extracellular magnesium modulate a cascade of events involved in cerebrovascular constriction. In rat studies, infusion of magnesium was found to attenuate alcohol-induced vasoconstriction. In humans, intravenous magnesium sulfate relieved alcohol-associated headaches (Altura, & Altura, 1999; Barbour, Gebrewold, Altura, & Altura, 2002). Although animal studies suggest that magnesium may improve alcohol-associated brain injury, clinical studies in nonalcohol related brain injury have not shown benefits (Schouten, 2007; Temkin, Anderson, Winn, Ellenbogen, Britz, Schuster et al., 2007; Winn, Temkin, Anderson, & Dikmen, 2007).

Taurine and Acamprosate

Taurine, an amino acid and antioxidant, prevented toxic damage to the liver during alcohol withdrawal in rats by reducing acetaldehyde levels (Watanabe, Hobara, & Nagashima, 1985). Supplementation with taurine (1–4) gm/day reduced alcohol withdrawal symptoms better than placebo in a RCT study of 60 patients (Ikeda, 1977). Taurine has also been used to reduce alcohol craving. Acamprosate, a medication derived from taurine, is more effective than taurine for reducing alcohol craving in clinical practice. For this reason, and because medical insurance will cover the cost of acamprosate, few patients will require taurine.

Acetyl-L-Carnitine (Alcar)

Alcohol abuse is associated with low serum carnitine levels. Abstinent alcoholics treated with acetyl-L-carnitine (Alcar) 2,000 mg/day for three months showed better performance on neuropsychological testing than control subjects (Tempesta, Troncon, Janiri, Colusso, Riscica et al., 1990). Several rat studies have shown that Alcar protects against alcohol induced metabolic abnormalities, including glutathione (major antioxidant) depletion (Calabrese, Scapagnini, Catalano, Dinotta, Bates et al., 2001; Calabrese, Scapagnini, Latteri, Colombrita, Ravagna et al., 2002). Acetyl-L-carnitine may have a role in the prevention and treatment of cognitive deficits associated with alcohol abuse. One rodent study found that Alcar protected against tremor during alcohol withdrawal and reduced alcohol consumption (Mangano, Clementi, Costantino, Calvani, & Matera, 2000).

N-acetylcysteine

Animal studies have indicated that N-acetylcysteine (NAC) inhibits cocaine-seeking behavior. In a DBRPC crossover trial, 15 hospitalized nontreatment-seeking patients with cocaine dependence were given four doses of either NAC (600 mg) or placebo. In rating their responses to watching slides depicting cocaine and cocaine use, subjects reported less interest and less desire to use cocaine while they were taking NAC. This study suggests that NAC may reduce cocaine cue reactivity (LaRowe, Myrick, Hedden, Mardikian, Saladin et al., 2007).

A four-week open pilot study in 23 treatment-seeking cocaine-dependent patients tested NAC in doses of 1200 mg/day, 2,400 mg/day or 3,600 mg/day. The two higher doses of NAC were associated with better retention rates. A majority of the 16 subjects who completed the study either terminated cocaine use completely or significantly reduced their cocaine use during NAC treatment. All three doses were well-tolerated. These findings support the value of further trials of NAC as an adjunct for treating individuals with cocaine dependence (Mardikian, LaRowe, Hedden, Kalivas, & Malcolm, 2007).

Omega-3 Fatty Acids from Fish Oils

In a DBRPC three-month study, 13 substance abusers given 3,000 mg/day of fish oils versus 11 patients given placebo, showed a progressive decrease in anxiety in those given the fish oils (Buydens-Branchey & Branchey, 2006). This effect may be related to the fact that ethanol (alcohol) reduces n-3 PUFAs (polyunsaturated fatty acids) in nerve cell membrane. The use of omega-3 fatty acids in patients with alcohol abuse warrants further study.

S-adenosylmethionine

S-adenosylmethionine (SAMe) has significant potential as a valuable treatment for all stages of alcoholism. Many alcoholics suffer from depression and use alcohol as a self-medication. While SAMe is an effective antidepressant with few side effects (see Chapter 2 for a discussion of SAMe), unlike prescription antidepressants, it does not put a burden on liver metabolic systems and does not cause elevations of liver enzymes (a common side effect of SSRI's). In fact, SAMe has been shown to improve liver function (Hote, Sahoo, Jani, Ghare, Chen et al., 2007) and to reduce alcohol-induced liver toxicity through several mechanisms. First, SAMe reduces serum alcohol levels, but does not increase serum acetaldehyde levels. Second, SAMe protects liver mitochondria from damage by alcohol (Lieber, 2002). Third, SAMe maintains glutathione (the main antioxidant) supplies.

In a 30-day DBRPC study of 64 alcoholics (DSM III) with at least a six-year history of alcohol abuse, SAMe 200 mg IM/day significantly improved anxiety, depression, fatigue, anorexia, insomnia, and nausea/vomiting while enhancing treatment compliance and abstinence compared to placebo. Patients given SAMe had lower gamma-GT levels (indicator of liver function) and lower serum alcohol levels compared to no change in those given placebo. In the SAMe group, 14/28 patients had documented abstinence, compared to 5/27 in the placebo group (p<0.01) (Cibin, Gentile, & Ferri, 1988). This study showed efficacy at a relatively low dose of SAMe, 200 mg IM , equivalent to 400 mg p.o. The evidence for SAMe antidepressant and hepatoprotective effects is compelling. Although further studies of oral SAMe in the treatment of alcoholism are needed, the authors believe that the evidence base is sufficient to justify the use of SAMe in the treatment of depression, anxiety, and hepatic dysfunction in alcoholics.

Studies of hepatic stellate cells found that the antifibrinogenic properties of SAMe combined with dilinoleoylphosphatidylcholine (DLPC) may be explained by the inhibition of collagen producing mRNA and the prevention of the leptin-stimulated tissue inhibitor of metalloproteinase TIMP-1 production. In addition, SAMe blocked the generation of H_2O_2 (a tissue damaging free radical) and restored the reduced glutathione (GSH) (major tissue protecting antioxidant) levels (Cao, Mak, & Lieber, 2006).

Ethanol (alcohol) decreases SAMe synthesis and reduces intracellular SAMe levels. Ethanol also reduces the enzymatic activity of methionine adenosyltransferase (MAT) II (see Chapter 2, Figure 2.1). MAT II catalyzes the synthesis of SAMe, which is vital for the activation and proliferation of T helper CD4(+) lymphocytes. Ethanol impairs immune function by decreasing MAT II and SAMe (Akhondzadeh, Kashani, Mobaseri, Hosseini, Nikzad, & Khani, 2001). The reduction in SAMe and MAT II may have additional

---

CLINICAL PEARL

Supplementation with SAMe may improve mood as well as cognitive, hepatic, and immune function in individuals who abuse alcohol.

---

adverse effects on mood and cognitive function. Supplementation with oral SAMe can reverse these deficits.

The decline in dopamine and SAMe levels induced by methamphetamine in rat studies may underlie the damage to brain functions (Cooney, Wise, Poirier, & Ali, 1998). Although the use of SAMe in the treatment of methamphetamine addiction is not yet supported by clinical studies, based on this preclinical data and considering the low level of risks and the numerous known health benefits, Dr. Richard Brown has used SAMe in methamphetamine addicts (who do not have bipolar disorder) to accelerate recovery as part of a holistic approach. This is a good example of accepting a lower level of evidence for a specific treatment based upon an understanding of the mechanisms of action and weighing the minimal risks in a situation where there are limited standard treatment options.

Passionflower (*Passiflora incarnata*)

A study of mice found that an extract of *Passiflora incarnata* reversed tolerance of and dependence on morphine, nicotine, ethanol, diazepam, and delta-tetrahydrocannabinol (Dhawan, Dhawan, & Chhabra, 2003). In a 14-day DBRPC study, 65 patients with opioid dependence (DSM-IV) were randomly assigned to treatment with clonidine plus *Passiflora* extract or clonidine plus placebo extract. There was no difference in the effectiveness of both treatments in reducing physical symptoms of withdrawal based on the Short Opiate Withdrawal scale (SOWS). However, the addition of *Passiflora* to clonidine accelerated the onset of action and significantly diminished the psychological symptoms of withdrawal (Frezza, Surrenti, Manzillo, Fiaccadori, Bortolini et al., 1990). This study is a good example of the appropriate use of an herb to complement the effects of a standard treatment. The use of *Passiflora* as a complementary treatment in opioid withdrawal warrants further study using additional psychological measures. Potential side effects include dizziness, confusion, ataxia, sedation, and prolonged QT intervals.

Other Herbs that Reduce Alcohol Intake in Animal Studies

Numerous plant extracts have been found to reduce alcohol intake without suppressing appetite in rat strains inbred to prefer alcohol. These include St. John's Wort, *Tabernanthe iboga* (ibogane), *Panax ginseng*, and *Salvia miltorrhiza* (Danshen; Overstreet, Rezvani, Cowen, Chen, & Lawrence, 2006).

Panax ginseng

Panax ginseng may reduce dependence and tolerance for cocaine, amphetamines, and morphine, based on animal studies (Huong, Matsumoto, & Yamasaki, 1997; Kim, Kang, & Seong, 1995; Oh, Kim, & Wagner, 1997). These effects may be due to increasing central nervous system dopamine levels.

Pueria labota or Kudzu

Pueria labota or Kudzu root (containing diadzin, diadzein, puerparin) was shown to decrease alcohol intake in rodent studies. In addition, in a small pilot DBRPC study, veterans diagnosed with alcoholism were randomly assigned to receive either Kudzu root extract 1.2 mg b.i.d. (n=12) or placebo (n=17). After one month, no statistically significant differences were noted in craving or sobriety scores (Shebek & Rindone, 2000). A DBRPC study of "heavy" alcohol drinkers studied kudzu extract versus placebo for seven days. Subjects on kudzu showed significant reduction in the number of beers (their favorite brand) consumed and the volume of each sip with a parallel increase in the number of sips and the time to consume each beer (Lukas, Penetar, Berko, Vicens, Palmer et al., 2005).

Mentat

Mentat, a traditional Ayurvedic herbal formula, contains ashwaganda (*Withania somnifera*), bacopa (*Bacopa monniera*), morning glory (*Evolvulus alsinoides*), gotu kola (*Centella asiatica*), musk root (*Nar-*

dostachys jatamansi), Indian valerian (*Valeriana jatamansi*), triphala, guduchi (*Tinospora cordifolia*), and mucuna (*Mucuna pruriens*). Mentat showed promise in reducing relapse in abstinent alcoholics in one small open series (Trivedi, 1999). Ashwaganda (one constituent in Mentat) has been reported to decrease opiate withdrawal symptoms in animal studies. These approaches need further clinical trials (Kulkarni & Ninan, 1997; Ramarao, Rao, Srivastava, & Ghosal, 1995).

Donepezil (Aricept)

Donepezil (Aricept) has been shown to reduce methamphetamine craving in rats (Hiranita, Nawata, Sakimura, Anggadiredja et al., 2006). This would suggest that Huperzine-A, and other cholinesterase inhibitors (sage, passionflower, galanthus, Ba Wei De Huang Wan), might prove helpful in reducing craving. Research to explore these possibilities is needed.

COMPLEMENTARY TECHNOLOGY-BASED INTERVENTIONS

James Lake provides an in-depth discussion of the following technology-based interventions (Lake, 2007).

Virtual reality gradual exposure has been used to excite alcohol, nicotine, marijuana, and cocaine craving followed by cognitive therapy to prevent response and induce desensitization to cues for abuse. This technology is in early development and requires further study.

Cranioelectrotherapy stimulation (CES) uses a weak electrical current (e.g., 100 Hz) given to the ears or scalp. CES is reported to reduce anxiety in substance abusers during withdrawal from drugs, but most clinicians are likely to have difficulty referring to therapists experienced in this technique and treatments are not reimbursable by insurance. Biofeedback can also ameliorate anxiety during the withdrawal phase.

Data on *acupuncture* for drug detoxification from alcohol, nicotine, and opiates is mixed. Studying the effect of acupuncture is complicated by the observations that merely inserting needles anywhere in the body (not in specific meridians) can release endogenous opiates in the brain which have beneficial effects for many stress-related conditions.

INTEGRATIVE APPROACHES

1. Correct nutritional imbalances with thiamine, folate, multi-B vitamins, and an A–Z multivitamin. Brewer's yeast, taken as two rounded tablespoons twice a day (Lewis Labs), is an inexpensive source of B vitamins and trace minerals.
2. For additional neuroprotection, administer 3,000 to 6,000 mg/day fish oils (omega-3 fatty acids); 600 to 800 mg/day magnesium; and 1,000 to 3,000 mg/day acetyl-L-carnitine.
3. Refer to self-help support groups such as Alcoholics Anonymous and Adult Children of Alcoholics. Refer family members to Alanon.
4. Prescription medications that may be helpful include the following:
   a. Naltrexone, acamprosate, or both for alcohol dependence.
   b. Topiramate 200 to 400 mg/day or isradipine may reduce craving for alcohol, cocaine, and other drugs.
   c. Rimonabant is being used for marijuana dependence. It must be ordered from Canada or Europe while awaiting approval by the U.S. FDA. Informed consent includes possible depression as a side effect.
   d. Valproate is useful for bipolar patients with alcoholism.
4. Evaluate the patient for possible ADD/ADHD. In such cases, stimulants may reduce drug dependence.
5. Refer the patient to easily accessible mind–body–spirit practices such as yoga, Qigong, vipassana meditation, dialectical behavior therapy with mindfulness, or others.
6. SAMe may be used to improve mood, liver function, immune function, for neuroprotection, and to help reduce alcohol intake. The risk of SAMe induced mania in bipolar patients must be considered.

In formulating the treatment plan, the following factors should be considered:

1. Discuss with the patient the treatment options and prioritize the target symptoms
2. Determine the feasibility of doing the intervention, taking into account the cost and likelihood of compliance.

CLINICAL PEARL

Mind–body–spirit programs can improve emotion regulation, reduce physical symptoms of withdrawal, and enhance motivation and compliance. Many patients in recovery report that these programs help them reconcile feelings about their past, including guilt, shame, anger, and remorse. They may also discover a new purpose and meaning in life. Patients with substance abuse problems should be encouraged to participate in mind–body–spirit practices.

3. The time frame and phase of treatment may determine the immediate goals
   a. The first two weeks may be focused on detoxification, physical stabilization, and engagement in treatment.
   b. The first three months require reduction in dysphoria and craving as well as keeping the patient in treatment.
   c. During the first year of abstinence significant brain recovery can occur.

FETAL ALCOHOL SYNDROME

Fetal alcohol spectrum disorders (FASD) are due to brain damage from prenatal alcohol exposure. The patients may have mental retardation, hyperactivity, behavioral and sexual disorders, and abnormal craniofacial development. Multiple mechanisms probably contribute to the neuronal damage including oxidative damage, mitochondrial damage, activation of caspase enzymes (leading to apoptosis, cell death), and depletion of PUFAs (polyunsaturated fatty acids) (Das, 2006). Damage is most marked in the hippocampus and cerebellum. Cholinergic neurons in the brain are particularly subject to injury and apoptosis. Despite public health efforts at prevention, 15 to 20% of women in the United States admit to drinking alcohol during pregnancy.

Animal studies have shown that neuroprotective compounds (choline, piracetam, Mentat, antioxidants, silymarin bioflavonoid, and the flowers of *Pueraria thunbergiana*) administered during pregnancy or in the postnatal period, if the mother is breat-feeding, can protect neonates from some of the neurological sequelae of maternal alcohol consumption (Bhattacharya, 1994; Neese, La Grange, Trujillo, & Romero, 2004; Thomas, Garcia, Dominguez, & Riley, 2004). Mentat contains 24 Indian medicinal herbs including brahmi (Bacopa) and ashwaganda. In one study, *Puerariae flos*, the flower of *Pueraria thunbergiana* (another name for Kudzu), significantly protected human neuroblastoma cells (SK-NMC) from ethanol-induced apoptosis and prevented increased capsase-3 mRNA expression (Jang, Shin, Kim, Chung, Yim et al., 2001).

Human studies are needed to translate these findings into clinical practice. FASD is a devastating lifelong condition for which there is no specific cure. Although CAM studies have not yet been reported in individuals with FASD, it is possible to apply treatments that have been beneficial in brain damage, ADHD, and learning disabilities to patients with FASD. Theoretically, any of the substances described for cognitive enhancement in this chapter and in Chapter 4 could be of help.

Based on similarities between FASD and other types of brain injuries, Dr. Richard Brown has treated adolescent and adult FASD patients in a county indigent rural mental health clinic to ameliorate cognitive and behavioral symptoms of the disorder. If cholinergic function in the hippocampus (part of the limbic system involved in sensory processing and memory) is disrupted due to traumatic brain injury, impairments in auditory sensory gating, inattention, and memory may develop (Arciniegas, 2001). Noting that donepezil (Aricept) improves cholinergic function and hippocampal gating in military veterans with traumatic brain injury (Silver, McAllistar, & Yudofsky, 2005), and considering that damage to the hippocampus and cholinergic function are prominent features of FASD, Dr. Brown administered donepezil to patients with FASD to improve cognitive function. He found that improvement could take at least three months and was manifested as a reduction in hyperactivity, better attention and impulse control, and greater capacity to engage in vocational rehabilitation. Donepezil may not be tolerated by preadolescent children who could become overstimulated. However, research on the use of milder cholinergic enhancers such as centrophenoxine, huperzine-A, and CDP-choline for children with FASD would be worthwhile (see Chapter 4).

TABLE 9.1 Treatment Guidelines for Substance Abuse

CAM	Clinical Uses	Daily Dose	Side Effects, Drug Interactions,* Contraindications
Acetyl-l-carnitine	alcohol withdrawal, craving	1,500 mg b.i.d.	Mild gastric upset, take with food
B vitamins			Caution: cardiac stents**
B₁ thiamine	brain damage	50 mcg	
B₁₂ cobalamin	due to alcohol	1,000 mcg	
folate	and poor	800 mcg	
B complex B50 or B100	nutrition	1 tab/day	
Bio-Strath		1 Tbsp b.i.d. 3 tabs b.i.d.	
Magnesium	loose bowels, vaso-constriction	600–800 mg	Minimal
N-actylcysteine	cocaine craving	2,400–3,600 mg	Minimal
Omega-3 Fatty Acids	nerve cell membrane function	6,000 mg	Gastrointestinal upset
Passionflower (*Passaflora incarnata*)	anxiety, opiate withdrawal	60 drops/day	Dizziness, confusion, ataxia, vasculitis, QT prolongation, sedative effects
Kudzu (*Pueria labota*)	craving	500 mg t.i.d.	Works infrequently
S-adenosyl-methionine (SAMe)	depression, liver cirrhosis, hepatitis	400–2,200 mg 1,100–1,600 mg mg/day	Occasional: nausea, diarrhea, agitation, anxiety, insomnia. Rare: palpitations Caution: bipolar II Contraindication: bipolar I

b.i.d. = twice a day; t.i.d. = three times a day; mcg = microgram.

*Common side effects are listed. There are additional rare side effects. Individuals with high blood pressure, diabetes, pregnancy (or during breast-feeding), or any chronic or serious medical condition should check with their physician before taking supplements.

**May increase risk of restinosis of cardiac stents in men only with baseline homocysteine ,<15 μmol/L.

CHAPTER 10 OUTLINE

1. **Body as a Whole**
   a. asthenia, fatigue, somnolence: *R. rosea, E. senticosus, P. ginseng*, ADAPT, maca
   b. hyperhydrosis (sweating): terazosin, gabapentin
   c. weight gain: amantadine, metformin, zonisamide, *R. caucasicum, R. rosea*

2. **Gastrointestinal**
   a. dry mouth: pilocarpine, huperzine, donepezil
   b. nausea: ginger, acupressure, Amrit Kalash
   c. hepatic dysfunction: S-adenosylmethionine, Chinese herbs, milk thistle
   d. constipation and hemorrhoids: triphala, magnesium, butcher's broom, horse chestnut

3. **Nervous System**
   a. akathisia: melatonin, B_6, N-acetylcysteine
   b. restless leg syndrome: lemon balm, passionflower, valerian
   c. tardive dyskinesia: melatonin, B_6
   d. cognition and memory: *R. rosea*, ADAPT, aniracetam, huperzine, donepezil, galantamine, artichoke
   e. insomnia: melatonin, coherence breathing, yoga breathing, exercise

4. **Sexual Dysfunction and Hormonal Changes:** *R. rosea, muira puama*, ArginMax, maca, 7-keto DHEA, vitex

5. **Cardiovascular System,**
   a. pedal edema: butcher's broom, horse chestnut

6. **Musculoskeletal System:** CoQ10

7. **Respiratory System:** sambucol, astragalus, reishi, Bio-stim, yoga breathing

8. **Hematological Disorders:** *R. rosea, E. senticosus*, shark liver oil, astragalus, lithium

9. **Hair Loss:** Amrit Kalash, B vitamins, zinc, selenium, dercos, nizoril 2%

CAM to Counteract Medication Side Effects

Intolerance of medication side effects is a major cause of nonadherence to treatment. Dose reduction or switching to a different medication is usually the first approach. However, for many patients, switching or reducing doses results in a return of symptoms. In such cases, complementary and alternative medicine (CAM) may alleviate or eliminate troublesome side effects. Approaches to alleviating side effects include herbs, nutrients, hormones, mind–body practices, and off-label uses of prescription medications. Many of these have not been formally studied as antidotes to side effects. Nevertheless, in clinical practice, we find these treatments can provide substantial relief. Patients are extremely appreciative when the doctor takes their side effects seriously, makes an effort to resolve the problem, and enables them to stay on their medications by reducing the burden of unpleasant side effects. In this chapter, we focus on ways to counteract medication side effects that are commonly encountered in practice.

For some supplements dosage guidelines are included. For others no dosages are offered because there is so much variation among different brands that the practitioner must examine the concentration of the active ingredient as well as the milligrams per tablet on the product label in order to determine an appropriate starting dose. To simplify this, we have listed some brand names of products with known concentrations. See the Quality Product List, Appendix A for more information. Where there is no specific dose recommended, the practitioner should start by following the instructions on the product label and increase gradually while monitoring for side effects. For off-label uses of prescription medications as antidotes for side effects, readers should consult the *Physicians Desk Reference* (PDR) for complete prescribing information, adverse effects, precautions, and drug interactions.

BODY AS A WHOLE

Complementary and alternative treatments can ameliorate medication-induced fatigue, somnolence, sweating, and weight gain.

Asthenia, Fatigue, Somnolence

Many drugs used in psychiatry and general medical practice cause fatigue or somnolence that can be mistaken for a symptom of depression. A careful review of all of the patient's medications may reveal the culprit to be: a psychotropic; an older antihypertensive such as terazosin (Hytrin), catapres (Clonidine), or methyldopa (Aldomet); an antihistamine; an opiate pain reliever; a beta blocker such as atenolol, metoprolol, or propranolol; a drug to alleviate symptoms of benign prostatic hypertrophy e.g., terazosin (Hytrin) or tamsulosin (Flomax); or a chemotherapy agent. The doctor primarily responsible for the medical treatment can be asked to find a therapy that is less likely to cause fatigue. If that is not possible, the following CAM treatments may increase daytime energy (mental and physical) without causing addiction. *R. rosea*, *E. senticosus*, and *P. ginseng* can be combined. If this combination is not sufficient, maca may be added. ADAPT-232 contains *R. rosea*, *E. senticosus*, and *S. chinensis*.

1. *Rhodiola rosea* 450–750 mg/d
2. *Eleutherococcus senticosus* 500 mg b.i.d.
3. *Panax* (Korean) *ginseng* 300 mg or more/day
4. ADAPT-232 two to four tablets/day
5. Lepidium meyenii (Maca-750) three to four tablets twice a day

Hyperhydrosis (Excess Sweating)

Daytime excessive sweating (hyperhydrosis) and night sweats are side effects of venlafaxine (Effexor) and occasionally other antidepressants. Excess sweating can be controlled with terazosin (Hytrin), an antihypertensive agent. The antisweating (antihyperhydrotic) effect can usually be attained with a small dose of 1 to 5 mg/day terazosin. Patients who are already taking antihypertensive medication may need dose adjustments and those prone to hypotension may need monitoring (see PDR for side effects and prescribing information).

Sometimes 300 to 900 mg/day gabapentin (Neurontin) reduces sweating. This is an off-label use of gabapentin. Slow, deep breathing can also be helpful (see Chapter 3).

Weight Gain

Many drugs, including SSRI antidepressants, mood stabilizers (lithium and valproate), and antipsychotics cause insulin resistance leading to serious weight gain and increased risks for diabetes, hyperlipidemia, and cardiovascular disease. Patients often despair when they gain weight despite a careful diet and regular exercise. It is best to substitute a drug that is less likely to cause weight gain; for example, switching from valproate (Depakote) to oxcarbazepine (Trileptal), lamotrigine (Lamictal), aripiprazole (Abilify), or ziprasidone (Geodon) when clinically indicated. If no substitute can be found, then a frank discussion with the patient is needed to formulate a weight management plan with the following components:

1. Monitoring weight, blood sugar, and lipid profile.
2. Increased aerobic exercise with at least 20 minutes a day of brisk walking, biking, swimming, heavy gardening, or the equivalent. For some patients, 20 to 50 minutes/day will be needed.
3. Carefully review the patient's diet and refer to a dietician to make further adjustments.
4. A structured weight loss program such as Weight Watchers.
5. Trials of medications and supplements that may help with weight control.

Medications that may be used to help patients overcome weight gain secondary to medication include:

1. Amantadine (Symmetrel) is a dopamine agonist, usually starting at 100 mg/day. Doses are slowly increased as tolerated up to 100 to 200 mg b.i.d. Side effects, particularly nausea, may limit the amount the patient can tolerate.
2. Metformin (Glucophage) is an oral hypoglycemic agent that is generally safe and unlikely to cause hypoglycemia in nondiabetic patients.
3. Zonisamide (Zonegram) and topiramate (Topomax) are both anti-convulsants that may induce weight loss.

There are innumerable supplements advertised to reduce weight. Many of them contain stimulants and lack any scientific support. Alternatively, several products are being developed that shift metabolism such that the body utilizes fat rather than carbohydrate as fuel for energy production. These effects occur through a variety of mechanisms including increasing lipolysis (the break down of triglycerides into fatty acids for utilization in mitochondrial energy production) and reduction of perilipins (proteins that cover the surface of lipid droplets and interfere with lipolysis). (see Chapter 7 for a review of the research on Fucoxanthin for weight loss).

Rhododendron caucasicum plus Rhodiola rosea

A combination of *Rhododendron caucasicum* plus *Rhodiola rosea* has been shown to enhance weight loss. When taken at the beginning of a meal, *R. caucasicum* blocks the absorption of about 20% of fat in the food. In addition, this herb contains antioxidants (polyphenols, propanolanoids, and proanthocyanidins) that support cellular repair and energy production. *R. rosea* accelerates fat burning two ways: by stimulating lipolysis and by reducing perilipins (Adamchuk, 1969; Adamchuk & Salnik, 1971).

In a double-blind placebo-controlled study of 273 obese men and women with body mass index of 29 to 34 kg/m^2, half the subjects were given one tablet of Rhodalean-400 (200 mg *R. rosea* + 200 mg *R. caucasicum*) three times a day for 20 weeks, while the other subjects were given placebo. Both groups were required to walk 20 minutes after lunch and dinner and to limit daily caloric intake to 1,800 calories/day. Of the 246 subjects who completed the study, those given Rodalean-400 had a mean weight loss of 9.3±1.4 kg (20.5±3.1

pounds) compared to 1.2±1.6 kg (2.6±3.5 pounds) in the placebo group. Postprandial cortisol levels were 17% lower in the Rhodalean-400 group than in those taking placebo. In addition, those given Rhodalean-400 had lower levels of perilipins. There were no side effects (Abidoff & Nelubov, 1997).

A different formulation of Rhodalean-200 (100 mg *R. rosea*+100 mg *R. caucasicum*) t.i.d. accelerated weight loss in a double-blind placebo-controlled study of 45 women who had given birth within the previous year and who had stopped lactating. On average, the women were 42 pounds above their ideal weight. They were required to maintain a calorie intake of 1,750 to 1,850 cal/day by reducing consumption of carbohydrates and fat. Those given Rhodalean lost 5 to 6% of their body weight (8–10 pounds) after six weeks compared to the placebo group who lost 0.4 to 0.7% (0.7–1.1 pounds). Among those on Rhodalean, 11.5% of the weight loss occurred from the waist area versus only 1.7 to 2.2% for those on placebo. There were no adverse effects (Abidoff, 1997).

While there have been no studies of *R. rosea* and *R. caucasicum* to counteract weight gain secondary to prescription medications, in clinical practice the authors have found some benefit, particularly by increasing the *R. rosea* up to 600 mg/day. The weight loss usually takes six to eight weeks to take effect in patients on psychotropics and requires at least 20 minutes of walking once or twice every day. It is important to inform the patient at the beginning not to expect the metabolic shift to become evident for six to eight weeks. Although these herbs are low in side effects, *R. rosea* can cause anxiety (in patients sensitive to stimulants) or manic symptoms in bipolar patients.

GASTROINTESTINAL

Dry Mouth
Mild dry mouth caused by antidepressants, mood stabilizers, or antipsychotics can be alleviate with lemon flavored sugar free lozenges such as Cepacol. Patients should be warned not to use hard candies containing sugar and to give careful attention to dental hygiene because reduction in saliva is associated with an increase in dental caries.

Dry mouth is usually an anticholinergic side effect. Other anticholinergic symptoms include blurred vision, constipation, and memory loss. These effects can be ameliorated with cholinergic agents (see Chapter 4).

1. For severe dry mouth, pilocarpine (Salagen) can be prescribed (see PDR for dosing and side effects).
2. Huperzine-A 200 to 400 mcg/d.
3. Donepezil (Aricept) starting with 2.5 mg/d. Some insurance companies only pay for Aricept for patients diagnosed with Alzheimer's disease. If the patient's insurance plan will not cover Aricept, then Huperzine-A is a less expensive alternative.

Nausea and Vomiting

Nausea and vomiting can sometimes be relieved by taking ginger tea or ginger capsules 40 minutes prior to ingestion of medications. Candied ginger is also useful, and can be carried in a plastic bag should nausea occur while driving, on public transportation, or at work. Acupressure bands (Sea Bands) applied to acupressure points at the wrist can relieve nausea. For severe nausea secondary to chemotherapy, Amrit Kalash (an Ayurvedic herbal compound) can be helpful.

Hepatic Dysfunction

Many medications used in psychiatry and general medical practice can cause hepatitis as indicated by elevations in liver enzymes. For a detailed discussion of the benefits of S-adenosylmethionine (SAMe) for liver function, see Chapters 2 and 9. Numerous studies have shown that SAMe can prevent or reverse abnormal liver function cause by other medications (e.g., anticonvulsants and mood stabilizers). In clinical practice, the authors find that SAMe is also effective in counteracting hepatic dysfunction caused by antidepressants, particularly SSRIs. The effectiveness of SAMe for improving liver function is enhanced further by polyenylphosphatidylcholine (Liverpro from Life Extension Foundation).

For bipolar patients, who should not be given SAMe, two Chinese herbal compounds containing bupleurum have shown efficacy in improving liver function tests (LFTs) in practice: Ease Two or Ease Plus (www.HealthConcerns.com or www.CraneHerb.com). A physician or licensed herbalist must order these herbs for patients. Follow dosing recommendations on the labels.

For very mild elevations in liver function tests, milk thistle (*Silybum marianum*) can be tried.

Constipation and Hemorrhoids

Constipation caused by medications, such as antipsychotics and tricyclic antidepressants, often responds to Triphala (an Ayurvedic herb) two to four capsules/day or magnesium 600 to 800 mg/day.

The pressure of straining during bowel movements can exacerbate hemorrhoids. Herbs that strengthen the walls of blood vessels, helping to heal and prevent hemorrhoids, include Butchers Broom (CircuCaps) and Horse Chestnut Extract.

NERVOUS SYSTEM

For a detailed discussion of the research on CAM treatments for extrapyramidal symptoms (EPS), see Chapter 7.

Akathisia

Akathisia, motor restlessness can be a side effect of antipsychotic or antidepressant medication. Preliminary studies in animals and humans have shown reduction in akathisia with:

1. Melatonin 9 to 10 mg hs
2. Vitamin B_6 600 mg b.i.d.
3. N-acetylcysteine 1,000 to 1,200 mg b.i.d.

Restless Leg Syndrome

Restless leg syndrome (RLS) is characterized by abnormal, uncomfortable sensations or movements of the legs, usually worse at night or at rest, often relieved by walking around. Antipsychotics, and antidepressants, particularly SSRIs can cause RLS with secondary loss of sleep. A combination of the following herbs can be helpful: lemon balm, passion flower, and valerian (see Chapter 3).

Tardive Dyskinesia

Tardive Dyskinesia (TD) is a disturbing side effect of antipsychotic medications that includes repetitive abnormal athetoid movements of the face, mouth, tongue, arms, hands, and sometimes the neck, trunk, and legs. CAM treatments found to reduce TD may be used alone or in combination:

1. Melatonin sustained release 9 to 10 mg at bedtime
2. Pyridoxine (B6) 400 mg/day

Impairment of Cognition and Memory or Word Finding Problems

Many patients report cognitive impairment, decreased memory, or word finding problems while using antidepressants, anxiolytics, mood stabilizers, and antipsychotics. See Chapter 4 for details of useful CAM treatments:

1. R. rosea 450 to 750 mg/day
2. ADAPT-232: two to four tablets/day
3. Aniracetam 750 mg b.i.d.
4. Huperzine-A 200 to 400 mcg b.i.d.
5. Donepezil (aricept) 5 to 10 mg/d
6. Galantamine 4 to 32 mg/day. If the patient does not have insurance coverage for this prescription medication, the herb galanthus (4–32 mg/d) is less expensive and works as well.
7. Artichoke extract may be of benefit in cognitive impairment secondary to chronic use of benzodiazepines.

Insomnia

Insomnia due to overstimulation by antidepressants or other medications may respond to a change in the dosing schedule or the use of more sedating antidepressants at night. For more details on breath practices see Chapter 3. CAM treatments for insomnia include:

1. Melatonin 3 to 9 mg at bedtime. Regular melatonin helps reduce sleep onset latency and extended release melatonin helps sustain sleep. A combination may be needed depending on the patient's sleep pattern.
2. Coherence breathing using Respire I CD
3. Slow yoga breathing, particularly Ujjayi (victorious breath) or alternate nostril breathing.
4. Daytime exercise, ideally six hours before bedtime.

SEXUAL DYSFUNCTION AND HORMONAL CHANGES

Many of the CAM treatments used for sexual dysfunction in general can be applied to the same disorders when they are secondary to medication. For more details see Chapter 6.

Anorgasmia

Anorgasmia due to antidepressants may be relieved by maca, *R. rosea*, and *muira puama*.

Erectile Dysfunction

Erectile dysfunction may respond to ArginMax or maca.

Loss of Libido

Libido may be enhanced with *R. rosea*, maca, *muira puama*, or 7-keto DHEA.

Irregular Menses, Galactorrhea, Mastalgia

Atypical antipsychotic medications, some older neuroleptics, and rarely SSRIs can cause elevated prolactin levels. This may lead to irregular menses, irritability, galactorrhea (breast milk secretion), or mastalgia (breast pain). When it is not possible to discontinue the medication, these side effects may improve with *Agnes cactus-vitex* (Vitex), a phytoestrogen.

Valproate has been associated with increased risk of polycystic ovary disease. When this occurs, it may be necessary to switch medications. Keeping in mind that insulin resistance also predisposes to polycystic ovary disease, the use of metformin (oral hypoglycemic agent) can be beneficial.

CARDIOVASCULAR SYSTEM

Pedal Edema

Some patients develop pedal edema (swelling of the feet and ankles due to leakage of fluid from veins into tissues while taking antipsychotics, mood stabilizers, or SSRIs. By strengthening the veins, CAM treatments can reduce pedal edema:

344 HERBS, NUTRIENTS & YOGA IN MENTAL HEALTH

1. Butcher's broom (Sanhelios CircuCaps 900 mg/day).
2. Horse chestnut extract (Nature's Way Standardized Extract 1 tablet b.i.d.)

MUSCULOSKELETAL SYSTEM

Muscle pain and weakness are a common side effect of statin drugs used to treat abnormal lipid levels. Over time, statin drugs tend to deplete levels of coenzyme Q10 (CoQ10). CoQ10 is essential for the healthy functioning of muscle tissue, including the heart. Patients on maintenance statin drugs should have their CoQ10 levels checked. If the levels are low, or if they develop symptoms of muscle pain or weakness, then supplemental CoQ10 is indicated. Ubiquinone or ubiquinol, forms of CoQ10, are probably more effective.

RESPIRATORY SYSTEM

Modafinil (Provigil), a medication used to increase alertness in patients with narcolepsy or brain injury (poststroke or traumatic brain injury) has been found to increase the incidence of upper respiratory infections. Respiratory infections can be reduced by CAM immune stimulators:

1. Sambucol (concentrated extract of elderberries) (Nature's Way 1 tsp b.i.d.)
2. Astragalus and reishi mushrooms
3. Bio-stim (anti-aging-systems.com)
4. Yoga breathing

HEMATOLOGICAL DISORDERS

Reduction in blood cell counts is a rare side effect of many medications, but it is not uncommon with valproate (Depakote). In general, if this occurs, the medication should be discontinued. The one exception is Depakote. Modestly reduced cell counts often occur with Depakote and frequently respond to the following natural CAM treatments enabling the patient to continue the mood stabilizer.

1. For decreased red blood cells, if the hematocrit is not lower than 32, try *R. rosea*, *E. senticosus*, or shark liver oil. Toxicity from contaminants and gastrointestinal disturbances with low quality shark oil has been reported. Therefore, the authors recommend only high quality shark oil products such as Immunofin two to six capsules/day (Lane Labs) or shark liver oil from Life Extension Foundation (see "Quality Herbal Products" chart in Appendix A).
2. For decreased white cell counts, if the total count is above 3,500 and the neutrophil count is above 1,500 try shark liver oil, two to six capsules/day Immunofin, *E. senticosus* (Eleuthero or Siberian ginseng) 500 mg b.i.d., astragalus, or lithium 600 mg/day or more.
2. For decreased platelets, if the platelet count is at least 80,000 and there is no bruising or bleeding, try shark liver oil (Immunofin), two to six capsules/day.

If any of the cell counts drop below the minimal levels mentioned above, then the Depakote should be discontinued and the CAM treatment continued until cell counts return to normal. A hematologist should be consulted if cell counts continue to decline or fail to improve.

HAIR LOSS

Hair loss secondary to mood stabilizers, antidepressants, or chemotherapy may improve with:

1. Amrit Kalash (Maharishi Ayurved)
2. B vitamins: B50 Complex, B100 Complex, Bio-Strath
3. Zinc 50 mg/d
4. Selenium 200 mcg/d. Some evidence suggests that chronic selenium deficiency may increase the risk for diabetes. This is being studied.
5. Dercos shampoo (antiaging-systems.com)
6. Nizoral 2% shampoo (by prescription only)

APPENDIX A

Guide to Quality Products

TABLE A.1 Guide to Quality Herbal Products

Herb	Manufacturer	Brand Name	Sources	Cost/day*
Ashwaganda *(Withania somnifera)*	Kare-n-herbs Ayurceutics	Tranquility-Kare Pegasus	*Karenherbs.com* *Ayurceutics.com*	$1.80–3.60
Brahmi *(Bacopa monniera)*	major brands Paradise Herbs	Bacopa	health food stores	$1.50–3.00
Black cohosh *(Cimifuga racemosa)*	Enzymatic Therapy Nature's Best	Remifemin Black Cohosh	*remifemin.com* *naturesbest-co.uk*	$0.60
Butcher's Broom	Bioforce Sanhelios	Higher Dose Circu Caps	800-641-7555	$0.26
Chamomile *(Matricaceia recuitita)*	major brands	Chamomile	health food stores	$0.25
Galantamine *(Galanthus navalis)*	Smart Nutrition Ameriden	Galantamine	smartnutrition.net ameriden.com	$2.00–4.00
Ginkgo *(Ginkgo biloba)*	Nature's Way Pharmaton Swanson	Gingold Ginkoba Time-Release Ginkgo	health food stores, pharmacies *swansonvitamins.com*	$0.35

Ginseng, Asian or Korean (*Panax ginseng*)	Hsu's Ginseng	Panax Ginseng	800-388-3818 *hsuginseng.com*	$0.20–0.40
	Action Labs	PowerMax-4x	800-932-2953	
Ginseng, American	Hsu's Ginseng	American Ginseng		
Ginseng, Siberian (*Eleutherococcus senticosus*)	Hsu's Ginseng	Eleuthero	800-388-3818 *hsuginseng.com*	$0.20–0.40
Hops (*Humulus lupulus*)	major brands	Hops	health food stores	$0.10
Horse Chestnut	major brands		health food stores	$0.25
Kava (*Piper methysticum*)	Nature's Way NaturesHerbs Natrol	Standard Extract Kava Power Kavatrol	health food stores	$0.40–1.20
Kudzu (*Pueria labota*)	Swanson Vitamins	Kudzu	*swansonvitamins.com*	$0.45/pill
Lemon Balm (*Melissa officianalis*)	major brands	Lemon Balm	health food stores	$0.25
Maca (*Lepidium meyenii*)	Medicine-Plants	Maca750™	*Medicine-Plants.com*	$1.80
Milk Thistle (*Silybum marianum*)	major Brands Nature's Best	Milk Thistle	health food stores *naturesbest.com.us*	$0.06
Muira Puama (*Ptychopetalium guyanna*)	Smart Nutrition	Muira Pauma	*smart-nutrition.net*	$0.20–0.30
Passionflower (*Passaflora incarnata*)	major brands	Passion flower	health food stores	$0.50–1.50

TABLE A.1 *Continued*

Herb	Manufacturer	Brand Name	Sources	Cost/day*
Pycnogenol Maritime Pine	Nature's Best	Pycnogenol	*naturesbest.co.uk*	$0.30
Pygeum (*Pygeum africanum*)	Nature'sWay	Pygeum	health food stores	$0.10
Red clover (*Trifolium pratense*)	see combination products	Red clover	health food stores	$0.66
Rhodiola rosea	Ameriden International	Rosavin™ 100 mg Rosavin Plus™ 150 mg	888-405-3336 *ameriden.com*	$0.60–4.00
	SwedishHerbal Institute—ProActive BioProducts	Arctic Root SHR-5	877-282-5366 x701 *proactivebio.com*	$0.65–3.00
	Kare-n-Herbs Medicine-Plants	Energy Kare Rosavin100™	*karenherbs.com* *Medicine-Plants.com*	
Sage (*Salvia officianalis*)	major brands Nature's Answer	Sage	health food stores willner.com	$0.29/ml
Salvia lavandulaefolia	major brands	Salvia	health food stores	$6.00/oz
Saw palmetto (*Serona repens*)	Nature's Way Life Extension	Saw Palmetto	health food stores *lef.com*	$0.40
Schizandra chinensis	Gaia Herbs Nature's Way	Schizandra	*Gaiaherbs.com* health food stores	$1.80 per gram
St. John's Wort (*Hypericum perforatum*)	Alokit, Lichtwar Healthcare Nature's Way	Kira (LI-160) Perika	*MyPharmacy.com*, *iherb.com* health food stores	$0.75–3.50
Stinging nettle (*Urtica dioica*)	major brands	Stinging nettle	health food stores	$0.09

Valerian officianalis	major brands	Valerian	health food stores	$0.04–0.08
Vinpocetine (***Vinca minor***)	Life Extension Smart Nutrition Intensive Nutrition	Vinpocetine	*lef.com* *smart-nutrition.net* *intensivenutrition.com*	$0.50
Vitex agnus cactus **Chaste tree, chasteberry**	major brands	Vitex	health food stores	$0.25
Yohimbine** *Pausinystalia Yohimbe*		Actibine Yocon Aphrodyne	physician prescription	$1.00–4.00

Cost /day* = cost per day. Costs of products may vary. This table lists approximate costs at the time of publication. Unless noted otherwise all prices are costs/day based upon recommended treatment dosages. Herbs that are available in health food stores are also available on the Internet.

**Recommend use only under supervision of a physician.

TABLE A.2 Guide to Quality Vitamins, Nutrients, Nootropics, Nutriceuticals, and Hormones

Nutrient	Manufacturers and Distributors	Brand Name	Sources	Cost/day*
Acetyl-l-carnitine	Life Extension Foundation (LEF) Smart Nutrition	Acetyl-L-Carnitine ALCAR	800-544-4440 *lef.org* *smart-nutrition.net*	$0.50–1.50
Alpha-lipoic acid	major brands	Alpha-lipoic Acid	health food stores, Internet	$0.07–0.14
Aniracetam	(IAS) International Antiaging Systems Smart Nutrition	Aniracetam	*antiaging-systems.com* *smart-nutrition.net*	$1.50
B vitamins B$_{12}$ sublingual	major brands Twin Labs GNC	B-12 DOTS Liquid B-12	health food stores General Nutrition Center	$0.06
Centro-phenoxine meclofenoxate	(IAS)	Lucidril	*antiaging-systems.com*	$0.50–2.50
CDP-choline	Smart Nutrition LEF	CDP-choline	800-479-2107 *smart-nutrition.net* 800-544-4440 *lef.org*	$2.00–4.00
Dehydroepian-drosterone	major brands	DHEA	health food stores	$0.15–0.55
7-Keto DHEA	LEF Living Fountain Smart Nutrition Swanson Vitamins	7-Keto DHEA	800-544-4440 *lef.org* *wwhoniline.com* *smart-nutrition.net* *swansonvitamins.com*	$0.20–1.60
GABA Y-aminubutyric acid	Pharma Foods Int.	Pharma-GABA	*pharmafoods.co.jp/ english/index.html*	not listed

Huperzine-A	Smart Nutrition General Nutrition Centers (GNC)	Huperzine	800-479-2107 *smart-nutrition.net*	$0.10–0.40
5-Hydroxy-tryptophan	major brands Smart Nutrition	5-HT	health food stores *smart-nutrition.net*	$6.00
Idebenone	Thorne Research Smart Nutrition	Idebenone	800-932-2953 *smart-nutrition.net*	$3.20–10.00
Inositol	IAS	Inositol	*antiaging-systems.com*	$1.50–3.00
Melatonin	LEF, IAS, Natrol Schiff, Solgar Living Fountain	Melatonin	health food stores *wwhonline.com*	$0.05–0.20
N-acetyly-cysteine	Puritan's Pride	NAC	*puritansale.com*	$0.16–0.24
Nicergoline	IAS	Nicergoline	*antiaging-systems .com*	$0.70–4.20
Omega-3 Fatty acids	Vital Nutrients IAS Nordic Naturals Twin Labs, Solgar	Ultra Pure Fish Oil	1-888-328-992 *vitalnutrients.net* antiaging-systems.com health food stores	$1.60–2.60
Phosphatidyl serine (not bovine)	Jarrow and others	Phosphatidyl-serine	health food stores	$0.50
Picamilon	IAS Smart Nutrition	Picamilon	*antiaging-systems.com* *smart-nutrition.net*	$0.40–1.20
Piracetam	IAS Smart Nutrition	Piracetam	*antiaging-systems.com* *smart-nutrition.net*	$1.80
S-adenosyl-L-methionine (SAMe) Ademetionine (only use tablets in blister packs)	Nature Made Jarrow, Geroformula Now Foods GNC, LEF IAS	SAMe other pharmacies Donamet®, Samyr®	800-276-2878 *naturemade.com* health food stores, CVS, *lef.org* antiaging-systems.com	$1.00–4.00

TABLE A.2 *Continued*

Nutrient	Manufacturers and Distributors	Brand Name	Sources	Cost/day*
Selegiline L-deprenyl	liquid or tablet IAS	L-Deprenyl, Emsam®, Jumex®	by prescription US pharmacies IAS	$0.50–14.00
Ubiquinone Ubiquinol (CoQ10)	LEF	Ubiquinol	*lef.org*	$2.00
Vinpocetine	LEF Smart Nutrition Intensive Nutrition	Vinpocetine	800-544-4440 *lef.org* *smart-nutrition.net* *intensivenutrition.com*	$0.50

Cost /day* = Cost per day. Costs of products may vary. This table lists approximate costs at the time of publication.

LEF = Life Extension Foundation; IAS = International Antiaging Systems; GNC = General Nutrition Centers.

TABLE A.3 Guide to Quality Combination Products

Complex	Contents	Manufacturers and Distributors	Contact	Cost/day*
ADAPT-232®	R. rosea, E. senticosus, S. chinensis	Swedish Herbal Institute ProActive Bio Products, Inc.	877-282-5366 x701 proactivebio.com	$1.00–1.50
Amrit Kalash®	many Ayurvedic herbs	Maharishi Ayur Ved	800-255-8332 mapi.com	$2.00
ArginMax®	Arginine, ginkgo, ginseng, vitamins, antioxidants	Daily Wellness	pharmacies	$0.15 per pill
B vitamin complex	varies with brand	major brands	health food stores	$0.06
Bio-Strath®	B vitamins + antioxidants	Nature's Answer	800-681-7099 health food stores	$1.00
Cerefolin®	2 mg methyl-cobalamin, 5.6 mg, L-methyl-folate, 600 mg N-acetyl-cysteine	PamLab	PamLab.com health food stores	$1.35
Clear Mind™	R. rosea, R. caucasicum, Rives nigrum	Ameriden	ameriden.com	$1.30–3.60
Cognitex®	Vinpocetine, ashwaganda, hops, ginger, rosemary, PtdSer-DHA, PtdCholine, α-glyceryl phos-phoryl choline, phosphatides	Life Extension Foundation	lef.com	$1.80

TABLE A.3 *Continued*

Complex	Contents	Manufacturers and Distributors	Contact	Cost/day*
Deplin®	7.5 mg L-methyl-folate	PamLab	*PamLab.com* health food stores	$1.33
Ease 2™	many Chinese herbs for liver support	CraneHerb HealthConcerns	*CraneHerb.com* *HealthConcerns.com*	$1.00
Ease Plus™	many Chinese herbs for liver support	CraneHerb HealthConcerns	*CraneHerb.com* *HealthConcerns.com*	$1.00
EZ- Energy™	*R. rosea* 70mg, *S. chinensis,* *E. senticosus,* *A. mandshurica,* *R. carthamoides*	Ameriden	*ameriden.com*	$0.65–1.30
FertilityBlend	chasteberry, green tea, L-arginine, vitamins, minerals	Daily Wellness	*fertilityblend.com*	$2.65
FucoTHIN™	brown seaweed pomegranate seed oil	Garden of Life	health food stores	$1.00
Horse Chestnut Complex	horse chestnut butchers broom rutin grapeseed oil	Nature's Best	*naturesbest.co.uk*	$0.30
Immune Stimulators				$0.60–1.20
RM10	10 mushrooms	Garden of Life	health food stores	
Noxylane4 Double strength	mushrooms	Lane Labs	*lanelabs.com*	
MycoDefense	mushrooms	Natures Way	*naturesway.com*	
Host Defense	mushrooms	New Chapter	*new-chapter.com*	

Kan Jang®	Andrographis *E. senticosus*	Swedish Herbal Institute ProActive Bio Products Inc.	877-282-5366 x70 *proactivebio.com*	$1.30
Kare-n-Liver®	*S. chinensis* 100mg *E. senticosus* 100mg	Kare-n-Herbs	*kare-n-herbs.com*	$0.40
Mentat (BR16-A)	includes: Bacopa, gotu kola, ashwaganda, triphala, morning glory, arjuna	Himalaya	*himalaya-proselect .com* 888-688-6600	$0.40–0.80
Metanx®	L-methylfolate 2.5 mg, pyridoxal 5'-phos-phate 25 mg, methylcobala-mine 2 mg	PamLab	*PamLab.com*	$0.85 per pill
Neurogen™	*R. rosea, Galanthus wornorii,* vitamin C	Ameriden	*ameriden.com*	$1.30–2.60
Student Rasayana MA-SR	Bacopa plus many Ayurvedic herbs	Maharishi Ayur Ved	800-255-8332 *mapi.com* health food stores	$0.16–0.32
Vigodana	*R. rosea*, Mg, B_6, B_{12} folate	Dr. Loges GmbH&Co	*claydoc.com*	$1.00
Vitex Promensil	*Agnus cactus-vitex* calcium, vitamin D	Novogen health food and other stores	*promensil.com*	$0.65

Cost /day* = Cost per day. Costs of products may vary. This table lists approximate costs at the time of publication. Unless noted otherwise all prices are costs/day based upon recommended treatment dosages.

Useful Resources for Integrative Mental Health Care

BOOKS

Bratman D. & Girman A.M. (2003). *Mosby's handbook of herbs and supplements and their therapeutic uses.* St. Louis, MO: Mosby.

Ernst, E. Pittler, M.H., & Wider, B. (Eds.). (2006). *The desktop guide to complementary and alternative medicine: An evidence-based approach* (2nd ed.). London: Mosby. Concise, well-organized as a quick reference resource.

Feuerstein, G. (1998). *Yoga traditions: Its history, literature, philosophy, and practice.* Prescott, AZ: Hohm Press. Scholarly classic with exceptionally clear presentations of this complex subject.

Harkness, R., & Bratman, S. (2003). *Mosby's handbook of drug–herb and drug–supplement interactions.* St. Louis, MO: Mosby.

Lake, J. (2007). *Textbook of integrative mental health care.* New York: Thieme. Structured presentation of CAM treatments based on assessment of the levels of evidence.

Lake, J., & Spiegel, D. (2007). *Complementary and alternative treatments in mental health care.* Washington. DC: American Psychiatric Publishing. Chapters are written by experts in different areas of CAM, for example, Chinese medicine, homeopathy, Ayurvedic treatments, mindfulness, yoga, and qigong.

Muskin, P. R. (Ed.) (2000). *Complementary and alternative medicine and psychiatry. American Psychiatric Press Review of Psychiatry, 19*(1).

Weintraub, A. (2004). *Yoga for depression: A compassionate guide to relieve suffering through yoga.* New York: Broadway Books.

JOURNALS

Alternative Medicine Review: A Journal of Clinical Therapeutics
BMC Complementary and Alternative Medicine
Complementary Therapies in Medicine
Evidence-Based Complementary and Alternative Medicine
Focus on Alternative and Complementary Therapies: An Evidence-Based Approach
Herbalgram: Journal of the American Botanical Council

Integrative Medicine
International Journal of Yoga Therapy
Journal of Complementary and Alternative Medicine
Yoga Journal

WEBSITES

American Psychiatric Association: *www.psych.org*

American Psychiatric Association Caucus on Complementary, Alternative, and Integrative Care: *http://APACAM.org*

ConsumerLab.com: *www.consumerlab.com.* Rates many brands of herbs and supplements on some measures of quality and labeling accuracy. Does not assess for shelf life.

Coherence: *www.coherence.com*

Dr. Richard Brown & Dr. Patricia Gerbarg: Integrative Psychiatry Updates: *www.haveahealthymind.com*

Drugs.com: *www.drugs.com.* Concise, updated presentation of CAM including risks and interactions.

Federation of State Medical Boards. *Model Guidelines for Physician Use of Complementary and Alternative Therapies in Medical Practice. www.fsmb.org/pdf/2002 _grpol_complementary_alternative_therapies.pdf*

HeartMath: *www.HeartMath.com*

Interactive Metronome: *www.interactivemetronome.com*

Journey to the Wild Divine: *www.wilddivine.com*

National Center for Complementary and Alternative Medicine, National Institutes of Health, Department of Health and Human Services: *www.nccam.nih.gov*

National Library of Health Complementary and Alternative Medicine Specialist Library (NeLCAM): *www.library.nhs.uk/cam*

National Library of Medicine: *www.nlm.nih.gov*

Natural Medicines Comprehensive Database: *www.naturaldatabase.com*

OchsLabs. Introduction to LENS. *www.ochslabs.com*

Open Focus: *www.openfocus.com*

The Research Council for Complementary Medicine: *www.rccm.org.uk/default.aspx? m=0*

Stone Mountain Center: *www.stonemountaincenter.com.* Information about LENS neurotherapy treatment and training.

Supplement Watch: *www.supplementwatch.com*

U.S. Food and Drug Administration: *www.fda.gov/medwatch*

US Pharmacopeia: *www.usp.org*

MIND–BODY PRACTICES

The Art of Living Foundation: *www.artoflivingus.org*

International Association for Human Values: *www.IAHV.org* (disaster relief programs)

Project Welcome Home Troops: *www.ProjectWelcomeHomeTroops.org*

Mind and Life Institute: *www.mindandlife.org* (information on training, practices, and research)

National Qigong Association: *www.nqa.org*

National Ayurvedic Medical Association: *www.Ayurveda-NAMA.org*

LifeForce Yoga: *www.yogafordepression.com*

Glossary of Medications

ANTIDEPRESSANTS

Monoamine Oxidase Inhibitors
Selegiline (Eldepryl, EMSAM)

Selective Serotonin Reuptake Inhibitors
Citalopram (Celexa)
S-Citalopram (Lexapro)
Fluoxetine (Prozac)
Fluvoxamine (Luvox)
Paroxetine (Paxil)
Sertraline (Zoloft)

Other Antidepressants
Bupropion (Wellbutrin)
Mirtazapine (Remeron)
Nefazodone (Serzone)
Trazodone (Desyrel)
Venlafaxine (Effexor)

ANTIPSYCHOTICS

Atypical Antipsychotics
Aripiprazole (Abilify)
Clozapine (Clozaril)
Olanzapine (Zyprexa)
Quetiapine (Seroquel)
Risperidone (Risperdal)
Ziprasidone (Geodon)

Typical Antipsychotics
Haloperidol (Haldol)

ANXIOLYTICS AND SEDATIVE HYPNOTICS

Benzodiazepines
Alprazolam (Xanax)
Clonazepam (Klonopin)
Diazepam (Valium)
Lorazepam (Ativan)
Oxazepam (Serax)

Nonbenzodiazepines
Buspirone (Buspar)
Zolpidem (Ambien)

MOOD STABILIZERS USED FOR BIPOLAR DISORDER

Carbamazepine (Carbatrol, Tegretol)
Gabapentin (Neurontin)
Lamotrigine (Lamictal)
Lithium
Oxcarbazepine (Trileptal)
Topiramate (Topomax)
Valproate (Depakote)

MEDICATIONS USED FOR ADD/ADHD

Psychostimulants
Amphetamine (Adderall)
Methylphenidate (Concerta, Ritalin)

Selective Norepinephrine Reuptake Inhibitor
Atomoxetine (Strattera)

Medications Used for Cognitive Decline
Donepezil (Aricept)
Memantine (Namenda)

References

Abdou, A. M., Higashiguchi, S., Horie, K., Kim, M., Hatta, H., & Yokogoshi, H. (2006). Relaxation and immunity enhancement effects of gamma-aminobutyric acid (GABA) administration in humans. *Biofactors, 26*(3), 201–208.

Abdul, H. M., & Butterfield, D. A. (2007). Involvement of PI3K/PKG/ERK1/2 signaling pathways in cortical neurons to trigger protection by cotreatment of acetyl-L-carnitine and alpha-lipoic acid against HNE-mediated oxidative stress and neurotoxicity: Implications for Alzheimer's disease. *Free Radical Biology and Medicine, 42*(3), 371–384.

Abidoff, M. T. (1997). (Report No. Grant 77-1997). Moscow, Russia.

Abidoff, M. T., & Nelubov, M. (1997). Russian anti-stress herbal supplement promotes weight loss, reduces plasma perilipins and cortisol levels in obese patients: Double-blind placebo controlled clinical study. *Stress and Weight Management at Russian Perestroika/Healthy Diet, 97.*

Abidov, M. (in press). The effect of Xanthigen, a phytomedicine containing fucoxanthin and pomegranate seed oil, on body weight and liver fat, serum triglycerides, C-reactive protein, and plasma aminotransferases in obese non-diabetic female volunteers: A double-blind, randomized, and placebo-controlled trial. *International Journal of Obesity.*

Abidov, M., Crendal, F., Grachev, S., Seifulla, R., & Ziegenfuss, T. (2003). Effect of extracts from *Rhodiola rosea* and *Rhodiola crenulata* (*Crassulaceae*) roots on ATP content in mitochondria of skeletal muscles. *Bulletin of Experimental Biology and Medicine, 136*(6), 585–587.

Abidov, M., Grachev, S., Seifulla, R. D., & Ziegenfuss, T. N. (2004). Extract of *Rhodiola rosea radix* reduces the level of C-reactive protein and creatinine kinase in the blood. *Bulletin of Experimental Biology and Medicine, 138*(1), 63–64.

Abidov, M., & Roshen, S. (in press). Effect of fucoxanthin and santhigen, a phytomedicine containing fucoxanthin and pomegranate seed oil, on energy expenditure rate in obese non-diabetic female volunteers with non-alcoholic fatty liver disease: A double-blind, randomized, and placebo-controlled trial. *Bulletin of Experimental Medicine.*

Ackerman, P. T., Dykman, R. A., Holloway, C., Paal, N. P., & Gocio, M. Y. (1991). A trial of piracetam in two subgroups of students with dyslexia enrolled in summer tutoring. *Journal of Learning Disabilities, 24*(9), 542–549.

Adamchuk, L. B. (1969). *Effects of* Rhodiola *on the process of energetic recovery of rat under intense muscular workload.* Unpublished doctoral dissertation, Tomsk State University and Medical Institute, Tomsk, Russia. (In Russian)

Adamchuk, V. , & Salnik, B. U. (1971). Effect of *Rhodiola rosea* extract and piridrol on metabolism of rats under high muscular load. *Institute of Cytology of Russian Academy of Science.* (In Russian)

Agakishiev, R. S. (1962). Longevity in Caucasian Republic of Dagestan. In V. V. Alpatov (Ed.), *Problems of gerontology* (pp. 34–72). Moscow: Moscow Publishing House of Academy of Sciences of the USSR. (In Russian)

Agteresch, H. J., Dagnelie, P. C., van der Gaast, A., Stijnen, T., & Wilson, J. H. (2000). Randomized clinical trial of adenosine 5'-triphosphate in patients with advanced non-small-cell lung cancer. *Journal of the National Cancer Institute, 92*(4), 321–328.

Aitken, R. J., & Sawyer, D. (2003). The human spermatozoon—Not waving but drowning. *Advances in Experimental Medicine and Biology, 518,* 85–98.

Akhondzadeh, S., & Abbasi, S. H. (2006). Herbal medicine in the treatment of Alzheimer's disease. *American Journal of Alzheimer's Disease and Other Dementias, 21*(2), 113–118.

Akhondzadeh, S., Kashani, L., Mobaseri, M., Hosseini, S. H., Nikzad, S., & Khani, M. (2001). Passionflower in the treatment of opiates withdrawal: A double-blind randomized controlled trial. *Journal of Clinical Pharmaceutical Therapy, 26*(5), 369–373.

Akhondzadeh, S., Mohammadi, M. R., & Khademi, M. (2004). Zinc sulfate as an adjunct to methylphenidate for the treatment of attention-deficit hyperactivity disorder in children: A double blind and randomized trial. *BMC Psychiatry, 4,* 9.

Akhondzadeh, S., Naghavi, H. R., Vazirian, M., Shayeganpour, A., Rashidi, H., & Khani, M. (2001). Passionflower in the treatment of generalized anxiety: A pilot double-blind randomized controlled trial with oxazepam. *Journal of Clinical Pharmacy and Therapeutics, 26*(5), 363–367.

Akhondzadeh, S., Noroozian, M., Mohammadi, M., Ohadinia, S., Jamshidi, A. H., & Khani, M. (2003). *Melissa officinalis* extract in the treatment of patients with mild to moderate Alzheimer's disease: A double blind, randomised, placebo controlled trial. *Journal of Neurological and Neurosurgical Psychiatry, 74*(7), 863–866.

Akhondzadeh, S., Safarcherati, A., & Amini, H. (2005). Beneficial antipsychotic effects of allopurinol as add-on therapy for schizophrenia: A double blind, randomized and placebo controlled trial. *Progress in Neuropsychopharmacology and Biological Psychiatry, 29*(2), 253–259.

Akhondzadeh, S., Tabatabaee, M., Amini, H., Ahmadi Abhari, S. A., Abbasi, S. H., & Behnam, B. (2007). Celecoxib as adjunctive therapy in schizophrenia: A double-blind, randomized and placebo-controlled trial. *Schizophrenia Research, 90*(1–3), 179–185.

Albertazzi, P. (2006). A review of non-hormonal options for the relief of menopausal symptoms. *Treatments in Endocrinology, 5*(2), 101–113.

Aleynik, S. I., & Lieber, C. S. (2003). Polyenylphosphatidylcholine corrects the alcohol-induced hepatic oxidative stress by restoring s-adenosylmethionine. *Alcohol and Alcoholism, 38*(3), 208–212.

Almeida, J. C., & Grimsley, E. W. (1996). Coma from the health food store: Interaction between kava and alprazolam. *Annals of Internal Medicine, 125*(11), 940–941.

Alpert, J. E., Papakostas, G., Mischoulon, D., Worthington, J. J. 3rd, Petersen, T., Mahal, Y et al.(2004). S-adenosyl-L-methionine (SAMe) as an adjunct for resistant major depressive disorder: An open trial following partial or nonresponse to selective serotonin reuptake inhibitors or venlafaxine. *Journal of Clinical Psychopharmacology, 24*(6), 661–664.

Altura, B. M., & Altura, B. T. (1999). Association of alcohol in brain injury, headaches, and stroke with brain-tissue and serum levels of ionized magnesium: A review of recent findings and mechanisms of action. *Alcoholism, 19*(2), 119–130.

Alvarez, X. A., Mouzo, R., Pichel, V., Perez, P., Laredo, M., Fernandez-Novoa, L. et al. (1999). Double-blind placebo-controlled study with citicoline in APOE genotyped Alzheimer's disease patients. Effects on cognitive performance, brain bioelectrical activity and cerebral perfusion. *Methods and Findings in Experimental Clinical Pharmacology, 21*(9), 633–644.

Amaducci, L. (1988). Phosphatidylserine in the treatment of Alzheimer's disease: Results of a multicenter study. *Psychopharmacology Bulletin, 24*(1), 130–134.

American Psychiatric Association. (1987). *Diagnostic and statistical manual of mental disorders* (3rd ed. rev.). Washington, DC:

American Psychiatric Association. (1994). *Diagnostic and statistical manual of mental disorders (4th ed.).* Washington, DC:

Anderson, J. J., Anthony, M. S., Cline, J. M., Washburn, S. A., & Garner, S. C. (1999). Health potential of soy isoflavones for menopausal women. *Public Health and Nutrition, 2*(4), 489–504.

Andreatini, R., Sartori, V. A., Seabra, M. L., & Leite, J. R. (2002). Effect of valepotriates (valerian extract) in generalized anxiety disorder: A randomized placebo-controlled pilot study. *Phytotherapy Research, 16*(7), 650–654.

Antalis, C. J., Stevens, L. J., Campbell, M., Pazdro, R., Ericson, K., & Burgess, J. R. (2006). Omega-3 fatty acid status in attention-deficit/hyperactivity disorder. *Prostaglandins Leukotrienes and Essential Fatty Acids, 75*(4–5), 299–308.

Apted, J. (2006, February). Faculty wellness and yoga breathing. In *Proceedings World Conference Expanding Paradigms: Science, Consciousness & Spirituality* (pp. 110–118). New Delhi: All India Institute of Medical Sciences.

Arciniegas, D. B. (2001). Traumatic brain injury and cognitive impairment: The cholinergic hypothesis. *Neuropsychiatry Reviews, 17*–20.

Arciniegas, D. B., Topkoff, J. L., Rojas, D. C., Sheeder, J., Teale, P., Young, D. A. et al. (2001). Reduced hippocampal volume in association with p50 nonsuppression following traumatic brain injury. *Journal of Neuropsychiatry and Clinical Neuroscience, 13*(2), 213–221.

Arendt, J. (1997–1998). Jet lag/night shift, blindness and melatonin. *Transactions of the Medical Society of London, 114*, 7–9.

Arias, A. J., Steinberg, K., Banga, A., & Trestman, R. L. (2006). Systematic review of the efficacy of meditation techniques as treatments for medical illness. *Journal of Alternative Complementary Medicine, 12*(8), 817–832.

Arnold, L. E. (2001). Alternative treatments for adults with attention-deficit hyperactivity disorder (ADHD). *Annals of the New York Academy of Sciences, 931*, 310–341.

Arnold, L. E., & DiSilvestro, R. A. (2005). Zinc in attention-deficit/hyperactivity disorder. *Journal of Child and Adolescent Psychopharmacology, 15*(4), 619–627.

Arnold, O., Saletu, B., Anderer, P., Assandri, A., di Padova, C., Corrado, M., et al. (2005). Double-blind, placebo-controlled pharmacodynamic studies with a nutraceutical and a pharmaceutical dose of ademetionine (SAMe) in elderly subjects, utilizing EEG mapping and psychometry. *European Neuropsychopharmacology, 15*(5), 533–543.

Arrigo, A., Casale, R., Buonocore, M., & Ciano, C. (1990). Effects of acetyl-L-carnitine on reaction times in patients with cerebrovascular insufficiency. *International Journal of Clinical Pharmacological Research, 10*(1–2), 133–137.

Arvindakshan, M., Ghate, M., Ranjekar, P. K., Evans, D. R., & Mahadik, S. P. (2003). Supplementation with a combination of omega-3 fatty acids and antioxidants (vitamins E and C) improves the outcome of schizophrenia. *Schizophrenia Research, 62*(3), 195–204.

Asayama, K., Yamadera, H., Ito, T., Suzuki, H., Kudo, Y., & Endo, S. (2003). Double blind study of melatonin effects on the sleep-wake rhythm, cognitive and noncognitive functions in Alzheimer type dementia. *Journal of the Nippon Medical School, 70*(4), 334–341.

Atmaca, M., Kumru, S., & Tezcan, E. (2003). Fluoxetine versus *Vitex agnus castus* extract in the treatment of premenstrual dysphoric disorder. *Human Psychopharmacology, 18*(3), 191–195.

Atmaca, M., Tezcan, E., Kuloglu, M., Ustundag, B., & Kirtas, O. (2005). The effect of extract of *ginkgo biloba* addition to olanzapine on therapeutic effect and antioxidant enzyme levels in patients with schizophrenia. *Psychiatry and Clinical Neuroscience, 59*(6), 652–656.

Ayers, M. E. (1987). Electroencephalographic neurofeedback and closed head injury of 250 individuals. In *National head injury syllabus* (pp. 380–392). Washington, DC: Washington National Head Injury Foundation.

Bacci Ballerini, F., Lopez Anguera, A., Alcaraz, P., & Hernandez Reyes, N. (1983).

Treatment of postconcussion syndrome with S-adenosylmethionine. *Medicina Clinica (Barcelona), 80*(4), 161–164. (In Spanish)

Bach, D., Schmitt, M., & Ebeling, L. (1997). Phytopharmaceutical and synthetic agents in the treatment of benign prostatic hyperplasia (BPH). *Phytomedicine, 4,* 309–313.

Bacopa monniera. (2004). Monograph. *Alternative Medicine Review, 9*(1), 79–85.

Baghai, T. C., Moller, H. J., & Rupprecht, R. (2006). Recent progress in pharmacological and non-pharmacological treatment options of major depression. *Current Pharmacological Design, 12*(4), 503–515.

Balon, R. (1999). Ginkgo biloba for antidepressant-induced sexual dysfunction? *Journal of Sex and Marital Therapy, 25*(1), 1–2.

Bambauer, K. Z., Adams, A. S., Zhang, F., Minkoff, N., Grande, A., Weisblatt, R., Soumerai, S. B., & Ross-Degnan, D. (2006). Physician alerts to increase antidepressant adherence: fax or fiction? *Archives of Internal Medicine, 166*(5), 498–504.

Bandelow, B., Wedekind, D., & Leon, T. (2007). Pregabalin for the treatment of generalized anxiety disorder: A Novel pharmacologic intervention. *Expert Review of Neurotherapy, 7*(7), 769–781.

Banerjee, B., Vadiraj, H. S., Ram, A., Rao, R., Jayapal, M., Gopinath, K. S. et al. (2007). Effects of an integrated yoga program in modulating psychological stress and radiation-induced genotoxic stress in breast cancer patients undergoing radiotherapy. *Integrative Cancer Therapy, 6*(3), 242–250.

Barak, A. J., Beckenhauer, H. C., & Tuma, D. J. (1996). Betaine, ethanol, and the liver: A review. *Alcoholism, 13*(4), 395–398.

Baranov, V. B. (1994). *Experimental trials of herbal adaptogen effect on the quality of operation activity, mental and professional work capacity. Contract 93-11-615 Stage 2 Phase I.* Moscow: Russian Federation Ministry of Health, Institute of Medical and Biological Problems (IMBP). (In Russian)

Barbour, R. L., Gebrewold, A., Altura, B. T., & Altura, B. M. (2002). Optical spectroscopy and prevention of deleterious cerebral vascular effects of ethanol by magnesium ions. *European Journal of Pharmacology, 447*(1), 79–86.

Bardia, A., Barton, D. L., Prokop, L. J., Bauer, B. A., & Moynihan, T. J. (2006). Efficacy of complementary and alternative medicine therapies in relieving cancer pain: A systematic review. *Journal of Clinical Oncology, 24*(34), 5457–5464.

Barlet, A., Albrecht, J., Aubert, A., Fischer, M., Grof, F., Grothuesmann, H. G., et al. (1990). Efficacy of *Pygeum africanum* extract in the medical therapy of urination disorders due to benign prostatic hyperplasia: Evaluation of objective and subjective parameters. A placebo-controlled double-blind multicenter study. *Wien Klinische Wochenschrift, 102*(22), 667–673. (In German)

Baskaya, M. K., Dogan, A., Rao, A. M., & Dempsey, R. J. (2000). Neuroprotective effects of citicoline on brain edema and blood-brain barrier breakdown after traumatic brain injury. *Journal of Neurosurgery, 92*(3), 448–452.

Bassi, P., Artibani, W., De Luca, V., Zattoni, F., & Lembo, A. (1987). Standardized extract of *Pygeum africanum* in the treatment of benign prostatic hypertrophy. Controlled clinical study versus placebo. *Minerva Urologica e Nefroogica (Turin)1*, 39(1), 45–50. (In Italian)

Bastani, F., Hidarnia, A., Kazemnejad, A., Vafaei, M., & Kashanian, M. (2005). A randomized controlled trial of the effects of applied relaxation training on reducing anxiety and perceived stress in pregnant women. *Journal of Midwifery and Women's Health, 50*(4), e36–40.

Bateman, B., Warner, J. O., Hutchinson, E., Dean, T., Rowlandson, P., Gant, C., Grundy, J., Fitzgerald, C., & Stevenson, J. (2004). The effects of a double blind, placebo controlled, artificial food colourings and benzoate preservative challenge on hyperactivity in a general population sample of preschool children. *Archives of Disease in Childhood, 89*(6), 506–511.

Beauchaine, T. (2001). Vagal tone, development, and Gray's motivational theory: Toward an integrated model of autonomic nervous system functioning in psychopathology. *Developmental Psychopathology, 13*(2), 183–214.

Beauchaine, T. P., Katkin, E. S., Strassberg, Z., & Snarr, J. (2001). Disinhibitory psychopathology in male adolescents: discriminating conduct disorder from attention-deficit/hyperactivity disorder through concurrent assessment of multiple autonomic states. *Journal of Abnormal Psychology, 110*(4), 610–624.

Beauregard, M., & Levesque, J. (2006). Functional magnetic resonance imaging investigation of the effects of neurofeedback training on the neural bases of selective attention and response inhibition in children with attention-deficit/hyperactivity disorder. *Applied Psychophysiology and Biofeedback, 31*(1), 3–20.

Becerra, J., Fernandez, T., Harmony, T., Caballero, M. I., Garcia, F., Fernandez-Bouzas, A. et al. (2006). Follow-up study of learning-disabled children treated with neurofeedback or placebo. *Clinical EEG Neuroscience, 37*(3), 198–203.

Becker, I. (2000). Uses of yoga in psychiatry and medicine. In P. R. Muskin (Ed.), *Complementary and alternative medicine in psychiatry* (Vol. 19, pp. 107–145). Washington, DC: American Psychiatric Press.

Beckham, N. (1995). Phyto-oestrogens and compounds that affect oestrogen metabolism, part II. *Australian Journal of Medical Herbalism, 7*(2), 27–33.

Belford-Courtney, R. (1993). Comparison of Chinese and Western users of *Angelica sinesis*. *Australian Journal of Medical Herbalism, 5*(4), 87–91.

Bell, I. R., Edman, J. S., Morrow, F. D., Marby, D. W., Perrone, G., Kayne, H. L. et al. (1992). Brief communication. Vitamin B1, B2, and B6 augmentation of tricyclic antidepressant treatment in geriatric depression with cognitive dysfunction. *Journal of the American College of Nutrition, 11*(2), 159–63.

Bell, I. R., & Pappas, P. A. (2007). Homeopathy. In J. Lake, & D. Spiegel (Eds.), *Complementary and alternative treatments in mental health care* (pp. 195–224). Washington, DC: American Psychiatric Publishing.

Bellon, A. (2006). Searching for new options for treating insomnia: Are melatonin and ramelteon beneficial? *Journal of Psychiatric Practice, 12*(4), 229–243.

Benjamin, J., Agam, G., Levine, J., Bersudsky, Y., Kofman, O., & Belmaker, R. H.

(1995). Inositol treatment in psychiatry. *Psychopharmacology Bulletin, 31*(1), 167–175.

Benson, H. (1996). Mind over maladies. Can yoga, prayer and meditation be adapted for managed care? Interview by Jim Montague. *Hospital Health Network, 70*(8), 26–27.

Bent, S., Kane, C., Shinohara, K., Neuhaus, J., Hudes, E. S., Goldberg, H. et al.(2006). Saw palmetto for benign prostatic hyperplasia. *New England Journal of Medicine, 354*(6), 557–566.

Bent, S., Padula, A., Moore, D., Patterson, M., & Mehling, W. (2006). Valerian for sleep: A systematic review and meta-analysis. *American Journal of Medicine, 119*(12), 1005–1012.

Bentler, S. E., Hartz, A. J., & Kuhn, E. M. (2005). Prospective observational study of treatments for unexplained chronic fatigue. *Journal of Clinical Psychiatry, 66*(5), 625–632.

Benton, D., Griffiths, R., & Haller, J. (1997). Thiamine supplementation mood and cognitive functioning. *Psychopharmacology (Berlin), 129*(1), 66–71. (In German

Bereiter, D. A., Bereiter, D. F., & Ramos, M. (2002). Vagotomy prevents morphine-induced reduction in Fos-like immunoreactivity in trigeminal spinal nucleus produced after TMJ injury in a sex-dependent manner. *Pain, 96*(1–2), 205–213.

Beresford, S. A., Weiss, N. S., Voigt, L. F., & McKnight, B. (1997). Risk of endometrial cancer in relation to use of oestrogen combined with cyclic progestagen therapy in postmenopausal women. *Lancet, 349*(9050), 458–461.

Berga, S. L., & Loucks, T. L. (2006). Use of cognitive behavior therapy for functional hypothalamic amenorrhea. *Annals of the New York Academy of Sciences, 1092*, 114–129.

Berger, B. G., & Owen, D. R. (1992). Mood alteration with yoga and swimming: Aerobic exercise may not be necessary. *Perceptual Motor Skills, 75*(3 Pt 2), 1331–1343.

Berger, G. E., Smesny, S., & Amminger, G. P. (2006). Bioactive lipids in schizophrenia. *International Review of Psychiatry, 18*(2), 85–98.

Berger, R., & Nowak, H. (1987). A new medical approach to the treatment of osteoarthritis. Report of an open phase IV study with ademetionine (Gumbaral). *American Journal of Medicine, 83*(5A), 84–88.

Berk, M. (2007). *Australian Society for Biopolar Disorders Conference.* Retrieved October 20, 2007, from http://medicalmedia.upmc.com/webtraining/wpic/bipolar2007/berk060807245c/p-p-t4_1.gif.

Berlanga, C., Ortega-Soto, H. A., Ontiveros, M., & Senties, H. (1992). Efficacy of S-adenosyl-L-methionine in speeding the onset of action of imipramine. *Psychiatry Research, 44*(3), 257–262.

Berntson, G. G., Sarter, M., & Cacioppo, J. T. (2003). Ascending visceral regulation of cortical affective information processing. *European Journal of Neuroscience, 18*, 2103–2109.

Bersani, G., & Garavini, A. (2000). Melatonin add-on in manic patients with treatment resistant insomnia. *Progress in Neuropsychopharmacology and Biological Psychiatry, 24*(2), 185–191.

Betz, J. M., White, K. D., & der Marderosian, A. H. (1995). Gas chromatographic determination of yohimbine in commercial yohimbe products. *J AOAC Int, 78*(5), 1189–1194.

Bhalla, P., & Nehru, B. (2005). Modulatory effects of centrophenoxine on different regions of ageing rat brain. *Experimental Gerontology, 40*(10), 801–806.

Bhatia, M., Kumar, A., Kumar, N., Pandey, R. M., & Kochupillai, V. (2003). Electrophysiologic evaluation of Sudarshan Kriya: An EEG, BAER, P300 study. *Indian Journal of Physiology and Pharmacology, 47*(2), 157–163.

Bhattacharya, S. K. (1994). Nootropic effect of BR-16A (Mentat), a psychotropic herbal formulation, on cognitive deficits induced by prenatal undernutrition, postnatal environmental impoverishment and hypoxia in rats. *Indian Journal of Experimental Biology, 32*(1), 31–36.

Bianchetti, A., Rozzini, R., & Trabucchi, M. (2003). Effects of acetyl-L-carnitine in Alzheimer's disease patients unresponsive to acetylcholinesterase inhibitors. *Current Medical Research Opinion, 19*(4), 350–353.

Bikov, V. A., Zapesochnaya, G. G., & Kurkin, V. A. (1999). *Rhodiola rosea*: traditional and biotechnological aspects of obtaining medicinal and pharmacological compounds. *Pharmacology and Toxicology of Medicinal Plants*, 22–39.

Bilici, M., Yildirim, F., Kandil, S., Bekaroglu, M., Yildirmis, S., Deger, O. et al. (2004). Double-blind, placebo-controlled study of zinc sulfate in the treatment of attention-deficit hyperactivity disorder. *Progress Neuropsychopharmacology and Biological Psychiatry, 28*(1), 181–190.

Birch, E. E., Garfield, S., Hoffman, D. R., Uauy, R., & Birch, D. G. (2000). A randomized controlled trial of early dietary supply of long-chain polyunsaturated fatty acids and mental development in term infants. *Developmental Medicine and Child Neurology, 42*(3), 174–181.

Birks, J., & Grimley Evans, J. (2007). *Ginkgo biloba* for cognitive impairment and dementia. *Cochrane Database System Review,* (2), CD003120.

Bishnoi, M., Kumar, A., Chopra, K., & Kulkarni, S. K. (2007). Comparative neurochemical changes associated with chronic administration of typical and atypical neuroleptics: Implications in tardive dyskinesia. *Indian Journal of Experimental Biology, 45*(2), 175–179.

Bloch, M., Schmidt, P. J., Danaceau, M. A., Adams, L. F., & Rubinow, D. R. (1999). Dehydroepiandrosterone treatment of midlife dysthymia. *Biological Psychiatry, 45*(12), 1533–1541.

Blokland, A., Honig, W., Brouns, F., & Jolles, J. (1999). Cognition-enhancing properties of subchronic phosphatidylserine (PS) treatment in middle-aged rats: Comparison of bovine cortex PS with egg PS and soybean PS. *Nutrition, 15*(10), 778–83.

Blumenthal, J. A., Babyak, M. A., Moore, K. A., Craighead, W. E., Herman, S., Khatri, P. et al. (1999). Effects of exercise training on older patients with major depression. *Archives of Internal Medicine, 159*(19), 2349–2356.

Bocharova, O. A., Matveev, B. P., Baryshnikov, A. I. U., Figurin, K. M., Serebriakova, R. V., & Bodrova, N. B. (1995). The effect of a *Rhodiola rosea* extract on the incidence of recurrences of a superficial bladder cancer (experimental clinical research). *Urologiia I Nefrologiia (Moscow)*, (2), 46–47. (In Russian)

Bonne, O., Shemer, Y., Gorali, Y., Katz, M., & Shalev, A. Y. (2003). A randomized, double-blind, placebo-controlled study of classical homeopathy in generalized anxiety disorder. *Journal of Clinical Psychiatry*, 64(3), 282–287.

Bonoczk, P., Gulyas, B., Adam-Vizi, V., Nemes, A., Karpati, E., Kiss, B. et al. (2000). Role of sodium channel inhibition in neuroprotection: Effect of vinpocetine. *Brain Research Bulletin*, 53(3), 245–254.

Booth, N. L., Overk, C. R., Yao, P., Burdette, J. E., Nikolic, D., Chen, S. N. et al. (2006). The chemical and biologic profile of a red clover (*Trifolium pratense L.*) phase II clinical extract. *Journal of Alternative and Complementary Medicine*, 12(2), 133–139.

Bormann, J. E., Gifford, A. L., Shively, M., Smith, T. L., Redwine, L., Kelly, A., Becker, S., Gershwin, M., Bone, P., & Belding, W. (2006). Effects of spiritual mantram repetition on HIV outcomes: A randomized controlled trial. *Journal of Behavioral Medicine*, 29(4), 359–376.

Bormann, J. E., Oman, D., Kemppainen, J. K., Becker, S., Gershwin, M., & Kelly, A. (2006). Mantram repetition for stress management in veterans and employees: A critical incident study. *Journal of Advanced Nursing*, 53(5), 502–512.

Bosch, T. M., Meijerman, I., Beijnen, J. H., & Schellens, J. H. (2006). Genetic polymorphisms of drug-metabolising enzymes and drug transporters in the chemotherapeutic treatment of cancer. *Clinical Pharmacokinetics*, 45(3), 253–285.

Bottiglieri, T. (1996). Folate, vitamin B12, and neuropsychiatric disorders. *Nutrition Review*, 54(12), 382–390.

Bottiglieri, T. (2002). S-Adenosyl-L-methionine (SAMe): from the bench to the bedside—Molecular basis of a pleiotrophic molecule. *American Journal of Clinical Nutrition*, 76(5), 1151S–1157S.

Bottiglieri, T. (2005). Homocysteine and folate metabolism in depression. *Progress in Neuropsychopharmacology and Biological Psychiatry*, 29(7), 1103–1112.

Bourre, J. M. (2005a). Dietary omega-3 Fatty acids and psychiatry: Mood, behaviour, stress, depression, dementia and aging. *Journal of Nutrition and Healthy Aging*, 9(1), 31–38.

Bourre, J. M. (2005b). Effect of increasing the omega-3 fatty acid in the diets of animals on the animal products consumed by humans. *Medical Science (Paris)*, 21(8–9), 773–779. (In French)

Bourre, J. M. (2006). Effects of nutrients (in food) on the structure and function of the nervous system: Update on dietary requirements for brain. Part 1: Micronutrients. *Journal of Nutrition and Healthy Aging*, 10(5), 377–385.

Bourre, J. M. (2007). Dietary omega-3 fatty acids for women. *Biomedical Pharmacotherapy*, 61(2–3), 105–112.

Bourre, J. M., & Galea, F. (2006). An important source of omega-3 fatty acids, vitamins D and E, carotenoids, iodine and selenium: A new natural multi-enriched egg. *Journal of Nutrition and Healthy Aging, 10*(5), 371–376.

Bower, J. E., Woolery, A., Sternlieb, B., & Garet, D. (2005). Yoga for cancer patients and survivors. *Cancer Control, 12*(3), 165–171.

Bradley, J. D., Flusser, D., Katz, B. P., Schumacher, H. R. Jr, Brandt, K. D., Chambers, M. A. et al. (1994). A randomized, double blind, placebo controlled trial of intravenous loading with S-adenosylmethionine (SAM) followed by oral SAM therapy in patients with knee osteoarthritis. *Journal of Rheumatology, 21*(5), 905–911.

Brazier, A., Mulkins, A., & Verhoef, M. (2006). Evaluating a yogic breathing and meditation intervention for individuals living with HIV/AIDS. *American Journal of Health Promotion, 20*(3), 192–195.

Breckhman, I. I., & Dardymov, I. V. (1969). New substances of plant origin which increase nonspecific resistance. *Annual Review of Pharmacology, 9*, 419–430.

Brichenko, V. S., & Skorokhova, T. F. (1987). *Herbal adaptogens in rehabilitation of patients with depression, clinical and organisational aspects of early manifestations of nervous and mental diseases* (p. 15). Soviet Union: Barnaul. (In Russian)

Brooks, J. O. 3rd, Yesavage, J. A., Carta, A., & Bravi, D. (1998). Acetyl L-carnitine slows decline in younger patients with Alzheimer's disease: A reanalysis of a double-blind, placebo-controlled study using the trilinear approach. *International Psychogeriatrics, 10*(2), 193–203.

Brookins, C. C. (1996). Exploring psychosocial task resolution and self-concept among African-American adolescents. *Percept Mot Skills, 82*(3 Pt 1), 803–10.

Brown, D. (1996). Anti-anxiety effects of chamomile compounds. *Herbalgram, 39*, 19.

Brown, R. P., & Gerbarg, P. L. (2004). *The rhodiola revolution.* Emmaus, PA: Rodale.

Brown, R. P., & Gerbarg, P. L. (2005a). Sudarshan Kriya yogic breathing in the treatment of stress, anxiety, and depression: Part I: Neurophysiologic model. *Journal of Alternative and Complementary Medicine, 11*(1), 189–201.

Brown, R. P., & Gerbarg, P. L. (2005b). Sudarshan Kriya Yogic breathing in the treatment of stress, anxiety, and depression. Part II: Clinical applications and guidelines. *Journal of Alternative and Complementary Medicine, 11*(4), 711–717.

Brown, R. P., & Gerbarg, P. L. (in press). Yoga breathing, meditation, and longevity. *Annals of the New York Academy of Sciences.*

Brown, R. P., Gerbarg, P. L., & Bottiglieri, T. (2000). S-Adenosylmethionine (SAMe) in the clincial practice of psychiatry, neurology, and internal medicine. *Clinical Practice of Alternative Medicine, 1*(4), 230–241.

Brown, R. P., Gerbarg, P. L., & Bottiglieri, T. (2002). S-adenosylmethionine (SAMe) for depression: Biochemical and clinical evidence. *Psychiatric Annals, 32*(1), 29–44.

Brown, R. P., Gerbarg, P. L., & Muskin, P. R. (2003). Complementary and alternative treatments in psychiatry. In A. Tasman, J. Kay, & J. A. Lieberman (Eds.), *Psychiatry* (2nd ed., Vol. 2, pp. 2147–2183). London: Wiley.

Brown, R. P., Gerbarg, P. L., & Ramazanov, Z. (2002). A phythomedical review of *Rhodiola rosea. Herbalgram, 56,* 40–62.

Bruner, A. B., Joffe, A., Duggan, A. K., Casella, J. F., & Brandt, J. (1996). Randomised study of cognitive effects of iron supplementation in non-anaemic iron-deficient adolescent girls. *Lancet, 348*(9033), 992–996.

Brunstein, M. G., Ghisolfi, E. S., Ramos, F. L., & Lara, D. R. (2005). A clinical trial of adjuvant allopurinol therapy for moderately refractory schizophrenia. *Journal of Clinical Psychiatry, 66*(2), 213–219.

Bucci, K. K., Possidente, C. J., & Talbot, K. A. (2003). Strategies to improve medication adherence in patients with depression. *American Journal of Health Systems Pharmacology, 60*(24), 2601–2605.

Bucci, W. (2001). Pathways of emotional communication. *Psychoanalytic Inquiry, 20,* 40–70.

Bucci, W. (2003). Varieties of dissociative experiences: A multiple code account and a discussion of Bromberg's case of "William." *Psychoanalytic Psychology, 20*(3), 542–557.

Budeiri, D., Li Wan Po, A., & Dornan, J. C. (1996). Is evening primrose oil of value in the treatment of premenstrual syndrome? *Controlled Clinical Trials, 17*(1), 60–68.

Buscemi, N., Vandermeer, B., Hooton, N., Pandya, R., Tjosvold, L., Hartling, L., et al. (2005). The efficacy and safety of exogenous melatonin for primary sleep disorders. A meta-analysis. *Journal of General Internal Medicine, 20*(12), 1151–1158.

Buydens-Branchey, L., & Branchey, M. (2006). n-3 polyunsaturated fatty acids decrease anxiety feelings in a population of substance abusers. *Journal of Clinical Psychopharmacology, 26*(6), 661–665.

Caffarra, C., & Santamaria, V. (1987). The effects of phosphatidylserine in patients with mild cognitive decline: An open trial. *Clinical Trials Journal, 24,* 109–111.

Calabrese, P., Perrault, H., Dinh, T. P., Eberhard, A., & Benchetrit, G. (2000). Cardiorespiratory interactions during resistive load breathing. *American Journal of Physiology and Regulatory Integrated and Comparative Physiology, 279*(6), R2208–2213.

Calabrese, V., Scapagnini, G., Catalano, C., Dinotta, F., Bates, T. E., Calvani, M. et al. (2001). Effects of acetyl-L-carnitine on the formation of fatty acid ethyl esters in brain and peripheral organs after short-term ethanol administration in rat. *Neurochemical Research, 26*(2), 167–174.

Calabrese, V., Scapagnini, G., Latteri, S., Colombrita, C., Ravagna, A., Catalano, C. et al. (2002). Long-term ethanol administration enhances age-dependent modulation of redox state in different brain regions in the rat: Protection by acetyl carnitine. *International Journal of Tissue Reaction, 24*(3), 97–104.

Calatayud Maldonado, V., Calatayud Perez, J. B., & Aso Escario, J. (1991). Effects of

CDP-choline on the recovery of patients with head injury. *Journal of Neurological Science, 103* (Suppl.), S15–18.

Cameron, L. D., Booth, R. J., Schlatter, M., Ziginskas, D., & Harman, J. E. (2007). Changes in emotion regulation and psychological adjustment following use of a group psychosocial support program for women recently diagnosed with breast cancer. *Psychooncology, 16*(3), 171–180.

Cao, L. L., Du, G. H., & Wang, M. W. (2006). The effect of salidroside on cell damage induced by glutamate and intracellular free calcium in PC12 cells. *Journal of Asian Natural Products Research, 8*(1–2), 159–165.

Cao, Q., Mak, K. M., & Lieber, C. S. (2006). DLPC and SAMe prevent alpha1(I) collagen mRNA up-regulation in human hepatic stellate cells, whether caused by leptin or menadione. *Biochemical and Biophysical Research Communications, 350*(1), 50–55.

Cappo, B. M., & Holmes, D. S. (1984). The utility of prolonged respiratory exhalation for reducing physiological and psychological arousal in non-threatening and threatening situations. *Journal of Psychosomatic Research, 28*(4), 265–273.

Caraci, F., Chisari, M., Frasca, G., Canonico, P. L., Battaglia, A., Calafiore, M. et al. (2005). Nicergoline, a drug used for age-dependent cognitive impairment, protects cultured neurons against beta-amyloid toxicity. *Brain Research, 1047*(1), 30–37.

Carani, C., Salvioli, V., Scuteri, A., Borelli, A., Baldini, A., Granata, A. R. et al. (1991). Urological and sexual evaluation of treatment of benign prostatic disease using *Pygeum africanum* at high doses. *Archivio Italiano di Urologia, Nefrologia, Andrologia, 63*(3), 341–345.

Carlson, L. E., & Garland, S. N. (2005). Impact of mindfulness-based stress reduction (MBSR) on sleep, mood, stress and fatigue symptoms in cancer outpatients. *International Journal of Behavioral Medicine, 12*(4), 278–285.

Carlson, L. E., Speca, M., Patel, K. D., & Goodey, E. (2003). Mindfulness-based stress reduction in relation to quality of life, mood, symptoms of stress, and immune parameters in breast and prostate cancer outpatients. *Psychosomatic Medicine, 65*(4), 571–581.

Carney, M. W., & Ellis, P. F. (1988). Benzodiazepines in anxiety. *Lancet, 1*(8584), 537.

Carney, R. M., Saunders, R. D., Freedland, K. E., Stein, P., Rich, M. W., & Jaffe, A. S. (1995). Association of depression with reduced heart rate variability in coronary artery disease. *American Journal of Cardiology, 76*(8), 562–564.

Carrieri, P. B., Indaco, A., & Gentile, S. (1990). S-Adenosylmethionine treatment of depression in patients with Parkinson's disease: A double-blind crossover study versus placebo. *Current Therapeutic Research, 48*, 154–160.

Carter, J. J., & Byrne, G. G. (2004). A two year study of the use of yoga in a series of pilot studies as an adjunct to ordinary psychiatric treatment in a group of Vietnam War veterans suffering from posttraumatic stress disorder. www.Therapywithyoga.com, 1–11.

Carter, J. J., Byrne, G. G., Brown, R. P., Gerbarg, P. L., & Ware, R. (in process).

Sudarshan Kriya yoga reduces symptoms of PTSD in Vietnam Veterans: A randomized controlled trial.

Casini, M. L., Marelli, G., Papaleo, E., Ferrari, A., D'Ambrosio, F., & Unfer, V. (2006). Psychological assessment of the effects of treatment with phytoestrogens on postmenopausal women: A randomized, double-blind, crossover, placebo-controlled study. *Fertility and Sterility,* 85(4), 972–978.

Cavallini, G., Caracciolo, S., Vitali, G., Modenini, F., & Biagiotti, G. (2004). Carnitine versus androgen administration in the treatment of sexual dysfunction, depressed mood, and fatigue associated with male aging. *Urology,* 63(4), 641–6.

Cavallini, G., Modenini, F., Vitali, G., & Koverech, A. (2005). Acetyl-L-carnitine plus propionyl-L-carnitine improve efficacy of sildenafil in treatment of erectile dysfunction after bilateral nerve-sparing radical retropubic prostatectomy. *Urology,* 66(5), 1080–1085.

Cenacchi, T., Bertoldin, T., & Palin, E. (1987). Human tolerability of phosphatidyl serine assessed through laboratory examinations. *Clinical Trials Journal, 24,* 125–130.

Cerutti, R., Sichel, M. P., Perin, M., et al. (1993). Psychological distress during puerperium: A novel therapeutic approach using S-adenosylmethionine. *Current Therapeutic Research, 53,* 707–716.

Chacon, G. A. (1997). *La importancia de Lepidium peruvianum Chacon ("Maca") en la alimentacion y salud humano y animal 2,000 anos antes y despues de cristo y en el siglo XXI.* Unpublished doctoral dissertation, Universidad Nacional Mayor de San Marcos, Lima Peru. (In Spanish)

Chan, A., & Shea, T. B. (2007). Folate deprivation increases presenilin expression, gamma-secretase activity, and Abeta levels in murine brain: Potentiation by ApoE deficiency and alleviation by dietary S-adenosyl methionine. *Journal of Neurochemistry, 102(3),* 753–760.

Chan, E., Rappaport, L. A., & Kemper, K. J. (2003). Complementary and alternative therapies on childhood attention and hyperactivity problems. *Journal of Developmental and Behavioral Pediatrics,* 24(1), 4–8.

Chen, J., Wollman, Y., Chernichovsky, T., Iaina, A., Sofer, M., & Matzkin, H. (1999). Effect of oral administration of high-dose nitric oxide donor L-arginine in men with organic erectile dysfunction: Results of a double-blind, randomized, placebo-controlled study. *BJU International,* 83(3), 269–273.

Chen, K. W., Hassett, A. L., Hou, F., Staller, J., & Lichtbroun, A. S. (2006). A pilot study of external qigong therapy for patients with fibromyalgia. *Journal of Alternative and Complementary Medicine,* 12(9), 851–856.

Chen, R. W., Williams, A. J., Liao, Z., Yao, C., Tortella, F. C., & Dave, J. R. (2007). Broad spectrum neuroprotection profile of phosphodiesterase inhibitors as related to modulation of cell-cycle elements and caspase-3 activation. *Neuroscience Letters, 418(2),* 165–169.

Chengappa, K. N., Levine, J., Gershon, S., Mallinger, A. G., Hardan, A., Vagnucci, A. et al. (2000). Inositol as an add-on treatment for bipolar depression. *Bipolar Disorder,* 2(1), 47–55.

Choi, H. K., Seong, D. H., & Rha, K. H. (1995). Clinical efficacy of Korean red ginseng for erectile dysfunction. *International Journal of Impotence Research, 7*(3), 181–186.

Chong, O. T. (2006). An integrative approach to addressing clinical issues in complementary and alternative medicine in an outpatient oncology center. *Clinical Journal of Oncology Nursing, 10*(1), 83–88.

Chowdhuri, D. K., Parmar, D., Kakkar, P., Shukla, R., Seth, P. K., & Srimal, R. C. (2002). Antistress effects of bacosides of Bacopa monnieri: Modulation of Hsp70 expression, superoxide dismutase and cytochrome P450 activity in rat brain. *Phytotherapy Research, 16*(7), 639–645.

Cibin, M., Gentile, N., & Ferri, M. (1988). S-Adenosylmethionine (SAMe) is effective in reducing ethanol abuse in an outpatient program for alcoholics. In K. Kuriyama, A. Takada, & M. Ishii (Eds.), *Proceedings of the 4th congress of biomedical and social aspects of alcohol and alcoholism.* (pp. 357–360). Amsterdam: Elsevier Science Publishers.

Cicerchia, G., Santucci, R., & Palmieri, M. (1985). Use of piracetam in the treatment of cranial injuries. Observations on 903 cases. *Clinica Terapeutica, 114*(6), 481–487. (In Italian)

Cicero, A. F., Bandieri, E., & Arletti, R. (2001). *Lepidium meyenii Walp.* improves sexual behaviour in male rats independently from its action on spontaneous locomotor activity. *Journal of Ethnopharmacology, 75*(2–3), 225–229.

Clough, A. R., Bailie, R. S., & Currie, B. (2003). Liver function test abnormalities in users of aqueous kava extracts. *Journal of Clinical Toxicology, 41*(6), 821–829.

Cohen, A. J., & Bartlik, B. (1998). Ginkgo biloba for antidepressant-induced sexual dysfunction. *Journal of Sex and Marital Therapy, 24*(2), 139–143.

Cohen, H., Neumann, L., Alhosshle, A., Kotler, M., Abu-Shakra, M., & Buskila, D. (2001). Abnormal sympathovagal balance in men with fibromyalgia. *Journal of Rheumatology, 28*(3), 581–589.

Cohen, L., Warneke, C., Fouladi, R. T., Rodriguez, M. A., & Chaoul-Reich, A. (2004). Psychological adjustment and sleep quality in a randomized trial of the effects of a Tibetan yoga intervention in patients with lymphoma. *Cancer, 100*(10), 2253–2260.

Cohen, L. S., & Rosenbaum, J. F. (1998). Psychotropic drug use during pregnancy: Weighing the risks. *Journal of Clinical Psychiatry, 59* (Suppl. 2), 18–28.

Cohen, M. H., & Schouten, R. (2007). Legal, regulatory, and ethical issues. In J. Lake & D. Spiegel (Eds.), *Complementary and alternative treatments in mental health care* (pp. 21–33). Washington, DC: American Psychiatric Publishing.

Cohen-Mansfield, J., Garfinkel, D., & Lipson, S. (2000). Melatonin for treatment of sundowning in elderly persons with dementia—A preliminary study. *Archives of Gerontology and Geriatrics, 31*(1), 65–76.

Colditz, G. A., Hankinson, S. E., Hunter, D. J., Willett, W. C., Manson, J. E., Stampfer, M. J. et al. (1995). The use of estrogens and progestins and the risk of breast cancer in postmenopausal women. *New England Journal of Medicine, 332*(24), 1589–1593.

Colditz, G. A., Stampfer, M. J., Willett, W. C., Hennekens, C. H., Rosner, B., & Speizer, F. E. (1990). Prospective study of estrogen replacement therapy and risk of breast cancer in postmenopausal women. *Journal of the American Medical Association, 264*(20), 2648–2653.

Collins, A., Cerin, A., Coleman, G., & Landgren, B. M. (1993). Essential fatty acids in the treatment of premenstrual syndrome. *Obstetrics and Gynecology, 81*(1), 93–98.

Connor, K. M., Payne, V., & Davidson, J. R. (2006). Kava in generalized anxiety disorder: Three placebo-controlled trials. *International Clinical Psychopharmacology, 21*(5), 249–253.

Conquer, J. A., Tierney, M. C., Zecevic, J., Bettger, W. J., & Fisher, R. H. (2000). Fatty acid analysis of blood plasma of patients with Alzheimer's disease, other types of dementia, and cognitive impairment. *Lipids, 35*(12), 1305–1312.

Cooney, C. A., Wise, C. K., Poirier, L. A., & Ali, S. F. (1998). Methamphetamine treatment affects blood and liver S-adenosylmethionine (SAM) in mice. Correlation with dopamine depletion in the striatum. *Annals of the New York Academy of Sciences, 844*, 191–200.

Coppen, A., & Bailey, J. (2000). Enhancement of the antidepressant action of fluoxetine by folic acid: A randomised, placebo controlled trial. *Journal of Affective Disorders, 60*(2), 121–130.

Cott, J. M. (2002). Herb-drug interactions: Focus on pharmacokinetics. *CNS Spectrum, 6*(10), 827–832.

Cott, J. M., & Fugh-Berman, A. (1998). Is St. John's Wort (*Hypericum perforatum*) an effective antidepressant? *Journal of Nervous and Mental Disorders, 186*(8), 500–501.

Cozens, D. D., Barton, S. J., Clark, R., Gibson, W. A., Hughes, E. W., Masters, R. E. et al. (1988). Reproductive toxicity studies of ademetionine. *Arzneimittelforschung, 38*(11), 1625–1629.

Craft, L., & Landers, D. (1998). The effects of exercise on clinical depression and depression resulting from medical illness: A meta-analysis. *Journal of Sport and Exercise Psychology, 20*, 339–357.

Craig, A. D. (2003). Interoception: The sense of the physiological condition of the body. *Current Opinion in Neurobiology, 13*(4), 500–505.

Crawford, M. A. (1993). The role of essential fatty acids in neural development: Implications for perinatal nutrition. *American Journal of Clinical Nutrition, 57*(Suppl. 5), S703–S709. discussion 709S–710S.

Crellin, R., Bottiglieri, T., & Reynolds, E. H. (1993). Folates and psychiatric disorders. Clinical potential. *Drugs, 45*(5), 623–636.

Critchley, H. D. (2005). Neural mechanisms of autonomic, affective, and cognitive integration. *Journal of Comparative Neurology, 493*(1), 154–166.

Crook, T. H., Tinklenberg, J., Yesavage, J., Petrie, W., Nunzi, M. G., & Massari, D. C. (1991). Effects of phosphatidylserine in age-associated memory impairment. *Neurology, 41*(5), 644–449.

Culos-Reed, S. N., Shields, C., & Brawley, L. R. (2005). Breast cancer survivors involved in vigorous team physical activity: Psychosocial correlates of maintenance participation. *Psychooncology, 14*(7), 594–605.

Cutler, W. B., & Genovese, E. (2002). Pheromones, sexual attractiveness and quality of life in menopausal women. *Climacteric, 5*(2), 112–121.

Damasio, A. R. (1994). *Descartes' error: Emotion, reason and the human brain.* New York: Grosset/Putnam Books.

Damasio, A. R. (1999). *The feeling of what happens: Body and emotion in the making of consciousness.* New York: Harcourt Brace.

Darbinyan, V., Aslanyan, G., Embroyan, E., Gabrielyan, E., Malmstrom, C., & Panossian, A. 2007 Clinical trial of *Rhodiola rosea* L. extract SHR-5 in the treatment of mild to moderate depression. *Nordic Journal of Psychiatry, 61,* 343–348.

Darbinyan, V., Kteyan, A., Panossian, A., Gabrielian, E., Wikman, G., & Wagner, H. (2000). *Rhodiola rosea* in stress induced fatigue—A double blind cross-over study of a standardized extract SHR-5 with a repeated low-dose regimen on the mental performance of healthy physicians during night duty. *Phytomedicine, 7*(5), 365–371.

Das, P., Kemp, A. H., Liddell, B. J., Olivieri, G., Peduto, A., Gordon, E. et al. (2005). Pathways for fear perception: Modulation of amygdala activity by thalamocoritcal systems. *NeuroImage, 26,* 141–148.

Das, S. N., Kochupillai, V., Singh, D., Aggarwal, D., & Bhardwaj, N. (2002). Flowcytometric study of T-cell subset and natural killer cells in peripheral blood of art of living teachers, normal subjects and cancer patients. In *"Science of breath": International symposium on sudarshan kriya, pranayam and consciousness.* New Delhi: All India Institute of Medical Sciences.

Das, U. N. (2006). Fetal alcohol syndrome and essential fatty acids. *PLoS Medicine, 3*(5), e247. author reply e248.

Das, Y. T., Bagchi, M., Bagchi, D., & Preuss, H. G. (2004). Safety of 5-hydroxy-L-tryptophan. *Toxicology Letters, 150*(1), 111–122.

De Deyn, P. P., Reuck, J. D., Deberdt, W., Vlietinck, R., & Orgogozo, J. M., & Members of the Piracetam in Acute Stroke Study (PASS) Group. (1997). Treatment of acute ischemic stroke with piracetam. *Stroke, 28*(12), 2347–2352.

De La Cruz, J. P., Pavia, J., Gonzalez-Correa, J. A., Ortiz, P., & Sanchez de la Cuesta, F. (2000). Effects of chronic administration of S-adenosyl-L-methionine on brain oxidative stress in rats. *Naunyn Schmiedebergs Archives of Pharmacology, 361*(1), 47–52.

De Rosa, M., Boggia, B., Amalfi, B., Zarrilli, S., Vita, A., Colao, A., & Lombardi, G. (2005). Correlation between seminal carnitine and functional spermatozoal characteristics in men with semen dysfunction of various origins. *Drugs Research and Development, 6*(1), 1–9.

Dean, A. J., (2005) Natural and complementary therapies for substance use disorders. Current opinion in Psychiatry, 18(3), 271–276.

Deberdt, W. (1994). Interaction between psychological and pharmacological treatment in cognitive impairment. *Life Science 55*(25–26), 2057–2066.

Dement'eva, L. A., & Iaremenko, K. V. (1987). Effect of a *Rhodiola* extract on the tumor process in an experiment]. *Voprosy Onkologii, 33*(7), 57–60.

Denes, L., Szilagyi, G., Gal, A., Bori, Z., & Nagy, Z. (2006). Cytoprotective effect of two synthetic enhancer substances, (-)-BPAP and (-)-deprenyl, on human brain capillary endothelial cells and rat PC12 cells. *Life Sciences, 79*(11), 1034–1039.

Descilo, T. , Vedamurthachar, A., Gerbarg, P. G., Nagaraja, D., Gangadhar, R., Damodoran, R. et al. (2006). Comparison of a yoga breath-based program and a client-centered exposure therapy for relief of PTSD and depression in survivors of tsunami disaster. In *Proceedings World Conference Expanding Paradigms: Science Consciousness and Spirituality* (pp. 64–78). New Delhi, India: AIIMS.

Descilo, T. , Vedamurthachar, A., Gerbarg, P. G., Nagaraja, D., Gangadhar, R., Damodoran, R. et al. (2007, May 20–24). *Comparison of a yoga breath-based program and a client-centered exposure therapy for relief of PTSD and depression in survivors of tsunami disaster.* Paper presented at the American Psychiatric Association Annual Meeting. San Diego, CA,

Dhawan, K., Dhawan, S., & Chhabra, S. (2003). Attenuation of benzodiazepine dependence in mice by a tri-substituted benzoflavone moiety of Passiflora incarnata Linneaus: A non-habit forming anxiolytic. *J Pharmacology and Pharmaceutical Sciences, 6*(2), 215-222.

Di Donato, S., Frerman, F. E., Rimoldi, M., Rinaldo, P., Taroni, F., & Wiesmann, U. N. (1986). Systemic carnitine deficiency due to lack of electron transfer flavoprotein:ubiquinone oxidoreductase. *Neurology, 36*(7), 957–963.

Di Padova, C. (1987). S-adenosylmethionine in the treatment of osteoarthritis. Review of the clinical studies. *American Journal of Medicine, 83*(5A), 60–65.

Di Rocco, A., Rogers, J. D., Brown, R., Werner, P., & Bottiglieri, T. (2000). S-adenosyl-1-methionine improves depression in patients with Parkinson's disease in an open label clinical trial. *Journal of Movement Disorders, 15*(6), 1225–1229.

Diamond, B. J., Shiflett, S. C., Feiwel, N., Matheis, R. J., Noskin, O., Richards, J. A., & Schoenberger, N. E. (2000). Ginkgo biloba extract: Mechanisms and clinical indications. *Archives of Physical Medicine Rehabilitation, 81*(5), 668–678.

Dixon, C. E., Ma, X., & Marion, D. W. (1997). Effects of CDP-choline treatment on neurobehavioral deficits after TBI and on hippocampal and neocortical acetylcholine release. *Journal of Neurotrauma, 14*(3), 161–169.

Dodge, N. N., & Wilson, G. A. (2001). Melatonin for treatment of sleep disorders in children with developmental disabilities. *Journal of Child Neurology, 16*(8), 581–584.

Dodin, S., Lemay, A., Jacques, H., Legare, F., Forest, J. C., & Masse, B. (2005). The effects of flaxseed dietary supplement on lipid profile, bone mineral density, and symptoms in menopausal women: A randomized, double-blind, wheat germ placebo-controlled clinical trial. *Journal of Clinical Endocrinology and Metabolism, 90*(3), 1390–1397.

Dolberg, O. T., Hirschmann, S., & Grunhaus, L. (1998). Melatonin for the treatment of sleep disturbances in major depressive disorder. *American Journal of Psychiatry,* 155(8), 1119–1121.

Donath, F., Quispe, S., Diefenbach, K., Maurer, A., Fietze, I., & Roots, I. (2000). Critical evaluation of the effect of valerian extract on sleep structure and sleep quality. *Pharmacopsychiatry,* 33(2), 47–53.

Dorababu, M., Prabha, T., Priyambada, S., Agrawal, V. K., Aryya, N. C., & Goel, R. K. (2004). Effect of *Bacopa monniera* and *Azadirachta indica* on gastric ulceration and healing in experimental NIDDM rats. *Indian Journal of Experimental Biology,* 42(4), 389–397.

Dorofeev, B. F., & Kholodov, L. E. (1991). Pikamilon pharmacokinetics in animals. *Farmakologiia i Toksikologiia (Moscow),* 54(2), 66–69. (In Russian)

Dos Santos-Neto, L. L., de Vilhena Toledo, M. A., Medeiros-Souza, P., & de Souza, G. A. (2006). The use of herbal medicine in Alzheimer's disease-a systematic review. *Evidence Based Complementary and Alternative Medicine,* 3(4), 441–445.

Dowling, G. A., Mastick, J., Colling, E., Carter, J. H., Singer, C. M., & Aminoff, M. J. (2005). Melatonin for sleep disturbances in Parkinson's disease. *Sleep Medicine,* 6(5), 459–466.

Drieu, K., Vranckx, R., Benassayad, C., Haourigi, M., Hassid, J., Yoa, R. G. et al. (2000). Effect of the extract of *Ginkgo biloba* (EGb 761) on the circulating and cellular profiles of polyunsaturated fatty acids: Correlation with the antioxidant properties of the extract. *Prostaglandins Leukotrienes and Essential Fatty Acids,* 63(5), 293–300.

Dubichev, A. G., Kurkin, B. A., Zapesochnaya, G. G., & Vornotzov, E. D. (1991). Study of *Rhodiola rosea* root chemical composition using HPLC. *Chemico-Pharmaceutical Journal,* 2, 188–193.

du Bois, T. M., Deng, C., & Huang, X. F. (2005). Membrane phospholipid composition, alterations in neurotransmitter systems and schizophrenia. *Progress in Neuropsychopharmacologyand Biolological Psychiatry,* 29(6): 878–88.

Dumville, J. C., Miles, J. N., Porthouse, J., Cockayne, S., Saxon, L., & King, C. (2006). Can vitamin D supplementation prevent winter-time blues? A randomised trial among older women. *Journal of Nutrition and Healthy Aging,* 10(2), 151–153.

Dunnick, J. K., & Hailey, J. R. (1995). Experimental studies on the long-term effects of methylphenidate hydrochloride. *Toxicology,* 103(2), 77–84.

Duraiswamy, G., Thirthalli, J., Nagendra, H. R., & Gangadhar, B. N. (2007). Yoga therapy as an add-on treatment in the management of patients with schizophrenia—A randomized controlled trial. *Acta Psychiatrica Scandinavia,* 116(3), 226–232.

Dwivedi, C., Natarajan, K., & Matthees, D. P. (2005). Chemopreventive effects of dietary flaxseed oil on colon tumor development. *Nutrition and Cancer,* 51(1), 52–58.

Eagon, P. K., Elm, M. S., Gerberg, P. L., Brown, R. P., Check, J. J., Diorio, G. J., & Houghton, Jr. F. (2003). Evaluation of the medicinal botanical *Rhodiola rosea* for estrogenicity [Abstract]. American Association Cancer Research

Eastern Cooperative Oncology Group. (2007). Levocarnitine in treating fatigue in cancer patients. Study ID Numbers: CDR0000384087; ECOG-E4Z02.

Ebadi, M., Brown-Borg, H., Ren, J., Sharma, S., Shavali, S., El ReFaey, H. et al. (2006). Therapeutic efficacy of selegiline in neurodegenerative disorders and neurological diseases. *Current Drug Targets, 7*(11), 1513–1529.

Efrati, O., Barak, A., Modan-Moses, D., Augarten, A., Vilozni, D., Katznelson, D et al. (2003). Liver cirrhosis and portal hypertension in cystic fibrosis. *European Journal of Gastroenterology and Hepatology, 15*(10), 1073–1078.

Eisenberg, J., Ben-Daniel, N., Mei-Tal, G., & Wertman, E. (2004). An autonomic nervous system biofeedback modality for the treatment of attention-deficit hyperactivity disorder—An open pilot study. *Israel Journal of Psychiatry and Related Sciences, 41*(1), 45–53.

Elias, M. F., Robbins, M. A., Budge, M. M., Elias, P. K., Brennan, S. L., Johnston, C., Nagy, Z., & Bates, C. J. (2006). Homocysteine, folate, and vitamins B6 and B12 blood levels in relation to cognitive performance: The Maine-Syracuse study. *Psychosomatic Medicine, 68*(4), 547–554.

Elliott, S. , & Edmonson, D. (2005). *The new science of breath.* Allen, TX: Coherence Press.

Elliott S., & Edmonson, D. (2006). *The new science of breath* (2nd ed.). Allen, TX: Coherence Press.

Elsabagh, S., Hartley, D. E., & File, S. E. (2005). Limited cognitive benefits in Stage +2 postmenopausal women after 6 weeks of treatment with *Ginkgo biloba. Journal of Psychopharmacology, 19*(2), 173–181.

Emsley, R., Myburgh, C., Oosthuizen, P., & van Rensburg, S. J. (2002). Randomized, placebo-controlled study of ethyl-eicosapentaenoic acid as supplemental treatment in schizophrenia. *American Journal of Psychiatry, 159*(9), 1596–1598.

Enderby, P., Broeckx, J., Hospers, W., Schildermans, F., & Deberdt, W. (1994). Effect of piracetam on recovery and rehabilitation after stroke: A double-blind, placebo-controlled study. *Clinical Neuropharmacology, 17*(4), 320–331.

Engelmann, U., Walther, C., Bondarenko, B., Funk, P., & Schlafke, S. (2006). Efficacy and safety of a combination of sabal and urtica extract in lower urinary tract symptoms. A randomized, double-blind study versus tamsulosin. *Arzneimittelforschung, 56*(3), 222–229.

Epperson, C. N., Terman, M., Terman, J. S., Hanusa, B. H., Oren, D. A., Peindl, K. S. et al. (2004). Randomized clinical trial of bright light therapy for antepartum depression: Preliminary findings. *Journal of Clinical Psychiatry, 65*(3), 421–425.

Ernst, E. (Ed.). (2001). *The desktop guide to complementary and alternative medicine.* M. H. Pittler, C. Stevinson, & A. White (Eds.). New York: Mosby.

Ernst, E. (2003). Complementary medicine. *Current Opinion in Rheumatology, 15*(2), 151–155.

Ernst, E. (2004). Musculoskeletal conditions and complementary/alternative medicine. *Best Practice Research in Clinical Rheumatology, 18*(4), 539–556.

Ernst, E., & Pittler, M. H. (1998). Yohimbine for erectile dysfunction: A systematic review and meta- analysis of randomized clinical trials. *Journal of Urology,* 159(2), 433–436.

Facchinetti, F., Borella, P., Sances, G., Fioroni, L., Nappi, R. E., & Genazzani, A. R. (1991). Oral magnesium successfully relieves premenstrual mood changes. *Obstetrics and Gynecology,* 78(2), 177–181.

Facchinetti, F., Nappi, R. E., Sances, M. G., Neri, I., Grandinetti, G., & Genazzani, A. (1997). Effects of a yeast-based dietary supplementation on premenstrual syndrome. A double-blind placebo-controlled study. *Gynecology and Obstetrics Investigation,* 43(2), 120–124.

Fackleman, K. (1998). Medicine for menopause. *Science News,* 153, 392–393.

Faloon, M. (1999). BPH: The other side of the coin. *Life Extension Journal,* 12–17.

Fauteck, J. D., Schmidt, H., Lerchl, A. Kurleman, G. & Wittkowski, W. (1999). Melatonin in epilepsy: first results of replacement therapy and first clinical results. *Biological Signals and Receptors,* 8, 105–110.

Fava, M. (2006). Pharmacological approaches to the treatment of residual symptoms. *Journal of Psychopharmacology,* 20(Suppl. 3), 29–34.

Federation of State Medical Boards. (2002). *Federation of State Medical Boards: Model guidelines for physician use of complementary and alternative therapies in medical practice.*

Fehmi, L. G., & McKnight, J. T. (2001). Attention and neurofeedback synchrony training: Clinical results and their significance. *Journal of Neurotherapy,* 5(1/2), 45–61.

Fenton, W. S., Dickerson, F., Boronow, J., Hibbeln, J. R., & Knable, M. (2001). A placebo-controlled trial of omega-3 fatty acid (ethyl eicosapentaenoic acid) supplementation for residual symptoms and cognitive impairment in schizophrenia. *American Journal of Psychiatry,* 158(12), 2071–2074.

Ferrell, R. E., Salamatina, N. V., Dalakishvili, S. M., Bakuradze, N. A., & Chakraborty, R. (1985). A population genetic study in the Ochamchir region, Abkhazia, SSR. *American Journal of Physical Anthropology,* 66(1), 63–71.

Figley, C. R., & Nash, W. P. (2007). *Combat stress injury.* New York: Routledge.

Finasteride for benign prostatic hypertrophy. (1992). *Medical Letter on Drugs and Therapeutics,* 34(878), 83–84.

Fintelmann, V., & Gruenwald, J. (2007). Efficacy and tolerability of a *Rhodiola rosea* extract in adults with physical and cognitive deficiencies. *Advances in Therapy,* 24(4), 929–39.

Fioravanti, M., & Flicker, L. (2001). Efficacy of nicergoline in dementia and other age associated forms of cognitive impairment. *Cochrane Database System Review,* (4), CD003159.

Fioravanti, M., & Yanagi, M. (2005). Cytidinediphosphocholine (CDP-choline) for cognitive and behavioural disturbances associated with chronic cerebral disorders in the elderly. *Cochrane Database System Review,* (2), CD000269.

Fischer, H. D., Schmidt, J., & Wustmann, C. (1984). On some mechanisms of anti-hypoxic actions of nootropic drugs. *Biomedical and Biochemical Acta,* 43(4), 541–543.

Fish oil supplements. (2006). *Medical Letter on Drugs and Therapeutics, 48*(1239), 59–60.

Flicker, L., & Grimley Evans, G. (2001). Piracetam for dementia or cognitive impairment. *Cochrane Database System Review, 2,* CD001011.

Fontanari, D., Di Palma, C., Giorgetti, G. et al. (1994). Effects of S-adenosyl-L-methionine on cognitive and vigilance functions in the elderly. *Current Therapy Research, 55*(6), 682–689.

Foster, S. (1999). Black cohosh *Cimicifugae racemosa*: A literature review. *Herbalgram, 45,* 36–49.

Frangou, S., Lewis, M., & McCrone, P. (2006). Efficacy of ethyl-eicosapentaenoic acid in bipolar depression: Randomised double-blind placebo-controlled study. *British Journal of Psychiatry, 188,* 46–50.

Franzblau, S. H., Smith, M., Echevarria, S., & Van Cantford, T. E. (2006). Take a breath, break the silence: The effects of yogic breathing and testimony about battering on feelings of self-efficacy in battered women. *International Journal of Yoga Therapy, 16,* 49–57.

Freedman, R. R. (2005). Pathophysiology and treatment of menopausal hot flashes. *Seminars on Reproductive Medicine, 23*(2), 117–125.

Freedman, R. R., & Roehrs, T. A. (2006). Effects of REM sleep and ambient temperature on hot flash-induced sleep disturbance. *Menopause, 13*(4), 576–583.

Freedman, R. R., & Roehrs, T. A. (2007). Sleep disturbance in menopause. *Menopause, 14,* 826–829.

Freedman, R. R., & Woodward, S. (1992). Behavioral treatment of menopausal hot flushes: Evaluation by ambulatory monitoring. *American Journal of Obstetrics and Gynecology, 167*(2), 436–439.

Freeman, E. W., Stout, A. L., Endicott, J., & Spiers, P. (2002). Treatment of premenstrual syndrome with a carbohydrate-rich beverage. *International Journal of Gynaecology and Obstetrics (Limerick), 77*(3), 253–254.

Freeman, M. P., Hibbeln, J. R., Wisner, K. L., Brumbach, B. H., Watchman, M., & Gelenberg, A. J. (2006). Randomized dose-ranging pilot trial of omega-3 fatty acids for postpartum depression. *Acta Psychiatrica Scandinavica, 113*(1), 31–35.

Freeman, M. P., Hibbeln, J. R., Wisner, K. L., Davis, J. M., Mischoulon, D., Peet, M. et al. (2006). Omega-3 fatty acids: Evidence basis for treatment and future research in psychiatry. *Journal of Clinical Psychiatry, 67*(12), 1954–1967.

Freeman, M. P., Hibbeln, J. R., Wisner, K. L., & Watchman, M. G. A. J. (2006). An open trial of omega-3 fatty acids for depression in pregnancy. *Acta Neuropsychiatrica, 18*(1), 21–24.

Freud, S. (1930). Civilization and its discontents. In J. Strachey (Ed. & Trans.), *The standard edition of the complete psychological works of Sigmund Freud* (Vol. 21, pp. 72–73). London: Hogarth. (Original work published 1930)

Freudenstein, J., & Bodinet, C. (1999, January 15). *Influence of an isopropanolic aqueous extract of* Cimicifugae racemosa rhizoma *on the proliferation of MCF-7 cells.* Paper presented at the 23rd LOF-Symposium on Phytoestrogens, University of Ghent, Belgium.

Freund-Levi, Y., Eriksdotter-Jonhagen, M., Cederholm, T., Basun, H., Faxen-Irving, G., Garlind, A et al. (2006). Omega-3 fatty acid treatment in 174 patients with mild to moderate Alzheimer disease: OmegAD study: A randomized double-blind trial. *Archives of Neurology, 63*(10), 1402–1408.

Frezza, M., Centini, G., Cammareri, G., Le Grazie, C., & Di Padova, C. (1990). S-adenosylmethionine for the treatment of intrahepatic cholestasis of pregnancy. Results of a controlled clinical trial. *Hepatogastroenterology, 37* (Suppl. 2), 122–125.

Frezza, M., Surrenti, C., Manzillo, G., Fiaccadori, F., Bortolini, M., & Di Padova, C. (1990). Oral S-adenosylmethionine in the symptomatic treatment of intrahepatic cholestasis. A double-blind, placebo-controlled study. *Gastroenterology, 99*(1), 211–215.

Friedel, H. A., Goa, K. L., & Benfield, P. (1989). S-adenosyl-L-methionine. A review of its pharmacological properties and therapeutic potential in liver dysfunction and affective disorders in relation to its physiological role in cell metabolism. *Drugs, 38*(3), 389–416.

Friederich, H. C., Schellberg, D., Mueller, K., Bieber, C., Zipfel, S., & Eich, W. (2005). Stress and autonomic dysregulation in patients with fibromyalgia syndrome. *Schmerz, 19*(3), 185–194. (In German)

Fuchs, T., Birbaumer, N., Lutzenberger, W., Gruzelier, J. H., & Kaiser, J. (2003). Neurofeedback treatment for attention-deficit/hyperactivity disorder in children: A comparison with methylphenidate. *Applied Psychophysiology and Biofeedback, 28*(1), 1–12.

Fugh-Berman, A., & Kronenberg, F. (2003). Complementary and alternative medicine (CAM) in reproductive-age women: A review of randomized controlled trials. *Reproductive Toxicology, 17*(2), 137–152.

Furmanowa, M., Oledzka, H., Michalska, M., Sokolnicka, I., & Radomska, D. (1995). *Rhodiola rosea* L. (Roseroot): In vitro regeneration and the biological activity of roots. In Y. P. S. Bajaj (Ed.), *Biotechnology in agriculture and forestry: Vol. 33. Medicinal and aromatic plants 8* (pp. 412–426). Berlin & Heidelberg: Springer-Verlag.

Furmanowa, M., Skopinska-Rozewska, E., Rogala, E., & Malgorzata, H. (1998). *Rhodiola rosea* in vitro culture—Phytochemical analysis and antioxidant action. *Acta Societis Botanicorum Poloniae, 76*(1), 69–73.

Fux, M., Benjamin, J., & Nemets, B. (2004). A placebo-controlled cross-over trial of adjunctive EPA in OCD. *Journal of Psychiatric Research, 38*(3), 323–325.

Fux, M., Levine, J., Aviv, A., & Belmaker, R. H. (1996). Inositol treatment of obsessive-compulsive disorder. *American Journal of Psychiatry, 153*(9), 1219–1221.

Garno, J. L., Goldberg, J. F., Ramirez, P. M., & Ritzler, B. A. (2005). Bipolar disorder with comorbid cluster B personality disorder features: Impact on suicidality. *Journal of Clinical Psychiatry, 66*(3), 339–345.

Gastpar, M., Singer, A., & Zeller, K. (2005). Efficacy and tolerability of hypericum extract STW3 in long-term treatment with a once-daily dosage in comparison with sertraline. *Pharmacopsychiatry, 38*(2), 78–86.

Geehta, H., Chitra, H., Kubera, N. S., & Pranathi, M. (2006). Effect of Sudarshan Kriya on menopausal women. In *Proceedings World Conference Expanding Paradigms: Science, consciousness and spirituality*. New Delhi, India: All India Insitute of Medical Sciences.

Gerasimova, H. D. (1970). Effect of *Rhodiola rosea* extract on ovarian functional activity. In *Proceedings of the Scientific Conference on Endocrinology and Gynecology* (pp. 46–48). Sverdlovsk, Russia (In Russian)

Gerbarg, P. L. (2007). Yoga and neuro-psychoanalysis. In F. S. Anderson (Ed.), *Bodies in treatment: The unspoken dimension* (pp. 132–133). Hillsdale, NJ: Analytic Press.

Gerbarg, P. L. & Brown R. P. (2005). Yoga: A breath of relief for Hurricane Katrina refugees. *Current Psychiatry*, 4(10): 55–67.

Gerhard, I. I, Patek, A., Monga, B., Blank, A., & Gorkow, C. (1998). Mastodynon(R) bei weiblicher Sterilitat. *Forschende Komplementarmedizin*, 5(6), 272–278.

Germano, C., Ramazanov, Z., & Bernal Suarez, M. (1999). *Arctic Root (Rhodiola rosea): The powerful new ginseng alternative*. New York: Kensington.

Giacobini, E. (1998). Invited review: Cholinesterase inhibitors for Alzheimer's disease therapy: From tacrine to future applications. *Neurochemistry International*, 32(5–6), 413–419.

Gijsman, H. J., van Gerven, J. M., de Kam, M. L., Schoemaker, R. C., Pieters, M. S., Weemaes, M. et al. (2002). Placebo-controlled comparison of three dose-regimens of 5-hydroxytryptophan challenge test in healthy volunteers. *Journal of Clinical Psychopharmacology*, 22(2), 183–189.

Gillis, J. C., Benefield, P., & McTavish, D. (1994). Idebenone. A review of its pharmacodynamic and pharmacokinetic properties, and therapeutic use in age-related cognitive disorders. *Drugs and Aging*, 5(2), 133–152.

Glassman, A. H., Bigger, J. T., Gaffney, M., & Van Zyl, L. T. (2007). Heart rate variability in acute coronary syndrome patients with major depression: Influence of sertraline and mood improvement. *Archives of General Psychiatry*, 64(9), 1025–1931.

Glieck, J. (1988). *Chaos: The making of science*. New York: Penguin.

Gloth, F. M. 3rd, Alam, W., & Hollis, B. (1999). Vitamin D vs broad spectrum phototherapy in the treatment of seasonal affective disorder. *Journal of Nutrition, Health and Aging*, 3(1), 5–7.

Gomez-Ramirez, M., Higgins, B. A., Rycroft, J. A., Owen, G. N., Mahoney, J., Shpaner, M. et al. (2007). The deployment of intersensory selective attention: A high-density electrical mapping study of the effects of theanine. *Clinical Neuropharmacology*, 30(1), 25–38.

Gonzales, G. F., Cordova, A., Gonzales, C., Chung, A., Vega, K., & Villena, A. (2001). *Lepidium meyenii* (Maca) improved semen parameters in adult men. *Asian Journal of Andrology*, 3(4), 301–303.

Gonzales, G. F., Cordova, A., Vega, K., Chung, A., Villena, A., Gonez, C., & Castillo, S. (2002). Effect of *Lepidium meyenii* (MACA) on sexual desire and its absent relationship with serum testosterone levels in adult healthy men. *Andrologia*, 34(6), 367–372.

Gonzales, G. F., Gasco, M., Cordova, A., Chung, A., Rubio, J., & Villegas, L. (2004). Effect of *Lepidium meyenii* (Maca) on spermatogenesis in male rats acutely exposed to high altitude (4340 m). *Journal of Endocrinology, 180*(1), 87–95.

Gonzales, G. F., Nieto, J., Rubio, J., & Gasco, M. (2006). Effect of Black maca (*Lepidium meyenii*) on one spermatogenic cycle in rats. *Andrologia, 38*(5), 166–172.

Goodale, I. L., Domar, A. D., & Benson, H. (1990). Alleviation of premenstrual syndrome symptoms with the relaxation response. *Obstetrics and Gynecology, 75*(4), 649–655.

Gordon, J. S., Staples, J. K., Blyta, A., & Bytyqi, M. (2004). Treatment of posttraumatic stress disorder in postwar Kosovo high school students using mind-body skills groups: A pilot study. *Journal of Trauma and Stress, 17*(2), 143–147.

Gouliaev, A. H., & Senning, A. (1994). Piracetam and other structurally related nootropics. *Brain Research Review, 19*(2), 180–222.

Granath, J., Ingvarsson, S., von Thiele, U., & Lundberg, U. (2006). Stress management: A randomized study of cognitive behavioural therapy and yoga. *Cognitive Behavioral Therapy, 35*(1), 3–10.

Grassetto, M., & Varatto, A. (1994). Primary fibromyalgia is responsive to S-adenosyl-L-methionine. *Current Therapeutic Research, 55*, 797–806.

Graziano, F., Bisonni, R., Catalano, V., Silva, R., Rovidati, S., Mencarini et al. (2002). Potential role of levocarnitine supplementation for the treatment of chemotherapy-induced fatigue in non-anaemic cancer patients. *British Journal of Cancer, 86*(12), 1854–1857.

Green, P., Hermesh, H., Monselise, A., Marom, S., Presburger, G., & Weizman, A. (2006). Red cell membrane omega-3 fatty acids are decreased in nondepressed patients with social anxiety disorder. *European Neuropsychopharmacology, 16*(2), 107–113.

Grube, B., Walper, A., & Wheatley, D. (1999). St. John's Wort extract efficacy for menopausal symptoms of psychological origin. *Advances in Therapy, 16*(4), 177–186.

Guderian, S., & Duzel, E. (2005). Induced theta oscillations mediate large-scale synchrony with mediotemporal areas during recollection in humans. *Hippocampus, 15*(7), 901–912.

Gunther, R. T. (1968). *The Greek herbal of Dioscorides, book 4. 45. Rhodia radis, Sedum Rhodiola* (p. 438). London: Hafner.

Gurley, B. J., Gardner, S. F., Hubbard, M. A., Williams, D. K., Gentry, W. B., Cui, Y. et al. (2002). Cytochrome P450 phenotypic ratios for predicting herb-drug interactions in humans. *Clinical Pharmacology Therapy, 72*(3), 276–287.

Gurley, B. J., Gardner, S. F., Hubbard, M. A., Williams, D. K., Gentry, W. B., Khan, I. A. et al. (2005). In vivo effects of goldenseal, kava kava, black cohosh, and valerian on human cytochrome P450 1A2, 2D6, 2E1, and 3A4/5 phenotypes. *Clinical Pharmacology Therapy, 77*(5), 415–426.

Gurnell, E. M., & Chatterjee, V. K. (2001). Dehydroepiandrosterone replacement therapy. *European Journal of Endocrinology, 145*(2), 103–106.

Gutzmann, H., & Hadler, D. (1998). Sustained efficacy and safety of idebenone in the treatment of Alzheimer's disease: Update on a 2-year double-blind multicentre study. *Journal of Neural Transmitters* (Suppl. 54), 301–310.

Hackbert, L., & Heiman, J. R. (2002). Acute dehydroepiandrosterone (DHEA) effects on sexual arousal in postmenopausal women. *Journal of Women's Health and Gender Based Medicine, 11*(2), 155–162.

Haffner, J., Roos, J., Goldstein, N., Parzer, P., & Resch, F. (2006). The effectiveness of body-oriented methods of therapy in the treatment of attention-deficit hyperactivity disorder (ADHD): Results of a controlled pilot study. *Zeitschrift Kinder Jugendpsychiatr Psychother, 34*(1), 37–47. (In German)

Haimov, I., Lavie, P., Laudon, M., Herer, P., Vigder, C., & Zisapel, N. (1995). Melatonin replacement therapy of elderly insomniacs. *Sleep, 18*(7), 598–603.

Hakkarainen, H., & Hakamies, L. (1978). Piracetam in the treatment of postconcussional syndrome. A double-blind study. *European Neurology, 17*(1), 50–55.

Halil, M., Cankurtaran, M., Yavuz, B. B., Ozkayar, N., Ulger, Z., Dede, D. S., Shorbagi, A., Buyukasik, Y., Haznedaroglu, I. C., & Arogul, S. (2005). No alteration in the PFA-100 in vitro bleeding time induced by the Ginkgo biloba special extract, EGb 761, in elderly patients with mild cognitive impairment. *Blood Coagulation and Fibrinolysis, 16*(5): 349–53.

Hallahan, B., Hibbeln, J. R., Davis, J. M., & Garland, M. R. (2007). Omega-3 fatty acid supplementation in patients with recurrent self-harm. Single-centre double-blind randomised controlled trial. *British Journal of Psychiatry, 190*, 118–122.

Hansgen, K. D., Vesper, J., & Ploch, M. (1994). Multicenter double-blind study examining the antidepressant effectiveness of the hypericum extract LI 160. *Journal of Geriatric Psychiatry and Neurology, 7* (Suppl. 1), S15–S18.

Harris, D. S., Wolkowitz, O. M., & Reus, V. I. (2001). Movement disorder, memory, psychiatric symptoms and serum DHEA levels in schizophrenic and schizoaffective patients. *World Journal of Biology and Psychiatry, 2*(2), 99–102.

Hartley, D. E., Elsabagh, S., & File, S. E. (2004). Gincosan (a combination of *Ginkgo biloba* and *Panax ginseng*): The effects on mood and cognition of 6 and 12 weeks treatment in post-menopausal women. *Nutrition and Neuroscience, 7*(5–6), 325–333.

Harvey, B. H., Joubert, C., du Preez, J. L., & Berk, M. (2007). Effect of chronic n-acetyl cysteine administration on oxidative status in the presence and absence of induced oxidative stress in rat striatum. *Neurochemical Research*.

Hassett, A. L., Radvanski, D. C., Vaschillo, E. G., Vaschillo, B., Sigal, L. H., Karavidas, M. K., et al. (2007). A pilot study of the efficacy of heart rate variability (HRV) biofeedback in patients with fibromyalgia. *Applied Psychophysiology and Biofeedback, 32*(1), 1–10.

Hassing, L., Wahlin, A., Winblad, B., & Backman, L. (1999). Further evidence on the effects of vitamin B12 and folate levels on episodic memory functioning: A population-based study of healthy very old adults. *Biological Psychiatry, 45*(11), 1472–1480.

Hawkins, E. B. (2000, Sept 5). *Report on Houghton PJ: Leads to treatment of CNS disorders with plants, extracts and constituents*. Poster presentation, 48th Annual Meeting of the International Congress of the Society of Plant Research PL12. *Herbalgram, 50*, 71.

Helfgott, E., Rudel, R. G., & Kairam, R. (1986). The effect of piracetam on short- and long-term verbal retrieval in dyslexic boys. *International Journal of Psychophysiology, 4*(1), 53–61.

Helland, I. B., Smith, L., Saarem, K., Saugstad, O. D., & Drevon, C. A. (2003). Maternal supplementation with very-long-chain n-3 fatty acids during pregnancy and lactation augments children's IQ at 4 years of age. Pediatrics, 111(1), e39–44.

Helms, J. M. (1987). Acupuncture for the management of primary dysmenorrhea. *Obstetrics and Gynecology, 69*(1), 51–56.

Helyer, L. K., Chin, S., Chui, B. K., Fitzgerald, B., Verma, S., Rakovitch, E. et al. (2006). The use of complementary and alternative medicines among patients with locally advanced breast cancer—A descriptive study. *BMC Cancer, 6*, 39.

Henderson, M. C., Miranda, C. L., Stevens, J. F., Deinzer, M. L., & Buhler, D. R. (2000). In vitro inhibition of human P450 enzymes by prenylated flavonoids from hops, *Humulus lupulus*. *Xenobiotica, 30*(3), 235–251.

Herxheimer, A., & Petrie, K. J. (2001). Melatonin for preventing and treating jet lag. *Cochrane Database System Review*, (1), CD001520.

Hibbeln, J. R. (2002). Seafood consumption, the DHA content of mothers' milk and prevalence rates of postpartum depression: A cross-national, ecological analysis. *Journal of Affective Disorders, 69*(1–3), 15–29.

Hibbeln, J. R., & Salem, N. Jr. (1995). Dietary polyunsaturated fatty acids and depression: When cholesterol does not satisfy. *American Journal of Clinical Nutrition, 62*(1), 1–9.

Hill-House, B. J., Ming, D. S., French, C. J., & Towers, N. G. H. (2004). Acetylcholine esterase inhibitors in *Rhodiola rosea*. *Pharmaceutical Biology (Formerly International Journal of Pharmacognosy), 42*(1), 68–72.

Hiranita, T., Nawata, Y., Sakimura, K., Anggadiredja, K., & Yamamoto, T. (2006). Suppression of methamphetamine-seeking behavior by nicotinic agonists. *Proceedings of the National Academy of Sciences USA, 103*(22), 8523–8527.

Hirashima, F., Parow, A. M., Stoll, A. L., Demopulos, C. M., Damico, K. E., Rohan, M. L. et al. (2004). Omega-3 fatty acid treatment and T(2) whole brain relaxation times in bipolar disorder. *American Journal of Psychiatry, 161*(10), 1922–1924.

Hirata, J. D., Swiersz, L. M., Zell, Small, R., Ettinger, B. (1997). Does dong quai have estrogenic effects in postmenopausal women? A double-blind placebo controlled trial. *Fertility and Sterility, 68*, 981–986.

Hoge, C. W., Auchterlonie, J. L., & Milliken, C. S. (2006). Mental health problems, use of mental health services, and attrition from military service after returning from deployment to Iraq or Afghanistan. *Journal of the American Medical Association, 295*(9), 1023–1032.

Holdcraft, L. C., Assefi, N., & Buchwald, D. (2003). Complementary and alternative medicine in fibromyalgia and related syndromes. *Best Practice Research in Clinical Rheumatology, 17*(4), 667–683.

Hoppes, K. (2006). The application of mindfulness-based cognitive interventions in the treatment of co-occurring addictive and mood disorders. *CNS Spectrum, 11*(11), 829–851.

Horrobin, D. F. (1998). The membrane phospholipid hypothesis as a biochemical basis for the neurodevelopmental concept of schizophrenia. *Schizophrenia Research, 10*:30(3): 193–208.

Hote, P. T. , Sahoo, R., Jani, T. S., Ghare, S. S., Chen, T., Joshi-Barve, S. et al. (2007). Ethanol inhibits methionine adenosyltransferase II activity and S-adenosylmethionine biosynthesis and enhances caspase-3-dependent cell death in T lymphocytes: Relevance to alcohol-induced immunosuppression. *Journal of Nutrition and Biochemistry.*

Hudson, S., & Tabet, N. (2003). Acetyl-L-carnitine for dementia. *Cochrane Database System Review,* (2), CD003158.

Hummel, F., & Gerloff, C. (2005). Larger interregional synchrony is associated with greater behavioral success in a complex sensory integration task in humans. *Cerebral Cortex, 15*(5), 670–678.

Hung, T. M., Na, M., Min, B. S., Ngoc, T. M., Lee, I., Zhang, X., & Bae, K. (2007). Acetylcholinesterase inhibitory effect of lignans isolated from Schizandra chinensis. *Archives of Pharmacological Research, 30*(6), 685-690.

Huntley, A., & Ernst, E. (2003). A systematic review of the safety of black cohosh. *Menopause, 10*(1), 58–64.

Huong, N. T., Matsumoto, K., & Yamasaki, K. (1997). Majonoside-R2, a major constituent of Vietnamese ginseng, attenuates opioid-induced antinociception. *Pharmacology, Biochemistry and Behavior, 57*, 285–291.

Hurtado, O., Moro, M. A., Cardenas, A., Sanchez, V., Fernandez-Tome, P., Leza, J. C., Lorenzo, P., Secades, J. J., Lozano, R., Davalos, A., Castillo, J., & Lizasoain, I. (2005). Neuroprotection afforded by prior citicoline administration in experimental brain ischemia: Effects on glutamate transport. *Neurobiology of Disease, 18*(2), 336–345.

Hypericum Depression Trial Study Group. (2002). Effect of *Hypericum perforatum* (St John's Wort) in major depressive disorder: A randomized controlled trial. *Journal of the American Medical Association, 287*(14), 1807–1814

Ianiello, A., Ostuni, P. A., Sfriso, P. et al. (1994). S-adenosyl-L-methionine in Sjogren's syndrome and fibromyalgia. *Current Therapeutic Research, 55*, 699–705.

Ikeda, H. (1977). Effects of taurine on alcohol withdrawal. *Lancet, 2*(509).

Ingvar, M., Ambros-Ingerson, J., Davis, M., Granger, R., Kessler, M., Rogers, G. A., Schehr, R. S., & Lynch, G. (1997). Enhancement by an ampakine of memory encoding in humans. *Experimental Neurology, 146*(2), 553–559.

Innes, K. E., Bourguignon, C., & Taylor, A. G. (2005). Risk indices associated with the insulin resistance syndrome, cardiovascular disease, and possible protection with yoga: A systematic review. *Journal of the American Board of Family Practice, 18*(6), 491–519.

Itil, T. M. (2001). Uses and contraindications of *Ginkgo biloba* in psychiatry. *Psychiatric Times,* 47–48.

Itil, T. M., Menon, G. N., Songar, A., & Itil, K. Z. (1986). CNS pharmacology and clinical therapeutic effects of oxiracetam. *Clinical Neuropharmacology, 9* (Suppl. 3), S70–S72.

Ito, T. Y., Polan, M. L., Whipple, B., & Trant, A. S. (2006). The enhancement of female sexual function with ArginMax, a nutritional supplement, among women differing in menopausal status. *Journal of Sex and Marital Therapy, 32*(5), 369–378.

Ito, T. Y., Trant, A. S., & Polan, M. L. (2001). A double-blind placebo-controlled study of ArginMax, a nutritional supplement for enhancement of female sexual function. *Journal of Sex and Marital Therapy, 27*(5), 541–549.

Iwasaki, K., Satoh, Nakagawa, T., Maruyama, M., Monma, Y., Nemoto, M., Tomita, N., Tanji, H., Jujiwara, H., Seki, T., Fujii, M., Arai, H., & Sasaki, H. (2005). A randomized, observer-blind, controlled trial of the traditional Chines medicine Yi-Gan San for improvement of behavioral and psycological symptoms and activities of daily living in dementia patients. *Journal Clinical Psychiatry, 66*(2), 248–52.

Iyengar, B. K. S. (1966). *Light on yoga.* New York: Schocken Books.

Iyengar, B. K. S. (1988). *The tree of yoga.* Boston: Shambhala.

Jacobs, B. P., Bent, S., Tice, J. A., Blackwell, T., & Cummings, S. R. (2005). An internet-based randomized, placebo-controlled trial of kava and valerian for anxiety and insomnia. *Medicine (Baltimore), 84*(4), 197–207.

Jacobs, G. D. (2001). Clinical applications of the relaxation response and mind-body interventions. *Journal of Alternative and Complementary Medicine, 7*(Suppl. 1), S93–S101.

Jacobsen, F. M. (1992). Fluoxetine-induced sexual dysfunction and an open trial of yohimbine. *Journal of Clinical Psychiatry, 53*(4), 119–122.

Jacobsen, S., Danneskiold-Samsoe, B., & Andersen, R. B. (1991). Oral S-adenosylmethionine in primary fibromyalgia. Double-blind clinical evaluation. *Scandinavian Journal of Rheumatology, 20*(4), 294–302.

Jan, J. E., Espezel, H., & Appleton, R. E. (1994). The treatment of sleep disorders with melatonin. *Developmental Medicine and Child Neurology, 36*(2), 97–107.

Janakiramaiah, N., Gangadhar, B. N., Naga Venkatesha Murthy, P. J., Harish, M. G., Subbakrishna, D. K., & Vedamurthachar, A. (2000). Antidepressant efficacy of Sudarshan Kriya Yoga (SKY) in melancholia: A randomized comparison with electroconvulsive therapy (ECT) and imipramine. *Journal of Affective Disorders, 57*(1–3), 255–259.

Janakiramaiah, N., Gangadhar, B. N., Naga Venkatesha Murthy, P. J., Harish, M. G., Taranath Shetty, K., Subbakrishna, D. K. et al. (1998). Therapeutic efficacy of Sudarshan Kriya Yoga (SKY) in dysthymic disorder. *NIMHANS Journal*, 21–28.

Jang, M. H. , Shin, M. C., Kim, Y. J., Chung, J. H., Yim, S. V., Kim, E. H., Kim, Y., & Kim, C. J. (2001). Protective effects of puerariae flos against ethanol-induced apoptosis on human neuroblastoma cell line SK-N-MC. *Japanese Journal of Pharmacology*, 87(4), 338–342.

Jarry, H., Spengler, B., Porzel, A., Schmidt, J., Wuttke, W., & Christoffel, V. (2003). Evidence for estrogen receptor beta-selective activity of Vitex agnus-castus and isolated flavones. *Planta Medica*, 69(10), 945–947.

Jensen, C. L., Voigt, R. G., Prager, T. C., Zou, Y. L., Fraley, J. K., Rozelle, J. C., et al. (2005). Effects of maternal docosahexanoic acid intake on visual function and neurodevelopment in breastfed term infants. *American Journal of Clinical Nutrition*, 82(1),125–132.

Jensen, P. S., & Kenny, D. T. (2004). The effects of yoga on the attention and behavior of boys with attention-deficit/ hyperactivity disorder (ADHD). *Journal of Attention Disorders*, 7(4), 205–216.

Jin, P. (1989). Changes in heart rate, noradrenaline, cortisol and mood during Tai Chi. *Journal of Psychosomatic Research*, 33(2), 197–206.

Jorissen, B. L., Brouns, F., Van Boxtel, M. P., Ponds, R. W., Verhy, F. R., Jolles, J., & Riedel, W. J. (2001). The influence of soy-derived phosphatidylserine on cognition in age-associated memory impairment. *Nutr Neurosci*, 4(2), 121–34.

Jung, C. H., Jung, H., Shin, Y. C., Park, J. H., Jun, C. Y., Kim, H. M. et al. (2007). *Eleutherococcus senticosus* extract attenuates LPS-induced iNOS expression through the inhibition of Akt and JNK pathways in murine macrophage. *Journal of Ethnopharmacology*, 113(1), 183–187.

Jyoti, A., & Sharma, D. (2006). Neuroprotective role of *Bacopa monniera* extract against aluminium-induced oxidative stress in the hippocampus of rat brain. *Neurotoxicology*, 27(4), 451–457.

Kabat-Zinn, J. (1990). *Full catastrophe living: Using the wisdom of your body and mind to face stress, pain and illness.* New York: Delacourt.

Kabat-Zinn, J., Massion, A. O., Kristeller, J., Peterson, L. G., Fletcher, K. E., Pbert, L. et al. (1992). Effectiveness of a meditation-based stress reduction program in the treatment of anxiety disorders. *American Journal of Psychiatry*, 149(7), 936–943.

Kahn, E. (2004). *"Ha" breathe "Ou ka Leo O ka Pu" The voice of the shell sounds.* Hawaii: Zen Care.

Kang, S. Y., Kim, S. H., Schini, V. B., & Kim, N. D. (1995). Dietary ginsenosides improve endothelium-dependent relaxation in the thoracic aorta of hypercholesterolemic rabbit. *General Pharmacology*, 26(3), 483–487.

Kaplan, K. H., Goldenberg, D. L., & Galvin-Nadeau, M. (1993). The impact of a meditation-based stress reduction program on fibromyalgia. *General Hospital Psychiatry*, 15(5), 284–289.

Kasper, S. (1997). Treatment of seasonal affective disorder (SAD) with hypericum extract. *Pharmacopsychiatry*, 30 (Suppl. 2), 89–93.

Kasper, S., Anghelescu, I. G., Szegedi, A., Dienel, A., & Kieser, M. (2006). Superior efficacy of St John's wort extract WS 5570 compared to placebo in patients with major depression: A randomized, double-blind, placebo-controlled, multi-center trial. *BMC Medicine, 4,* 14.

Kataoka-Kato, A., Ukai, M., Sakai, M., Kudo, S., & Kameyama, T. (2005). Enhanced learning of normal adult rodents by repeated oral administration of soybean transphosphatidylated phosphatidylserine. *J Parmacol Sci, 9*(3), 307–14.

Kayumov, L., Brown, G., Jindal, R., Buttoo, K., & Shapiro, C. M. (2001). A randomized, double-blind, placebo-controlled crossover study of the effect of exogenous melatonin on delayed sleep phase syndrome. *Psychosomatic Medicine, 63*(1), 40–48.

Keck, P. E. Jr, Mintz, J., McElroy, S. L., Freeman, M. P., Suppes, T., Frye, M. A. et al. (2006). Double-blind, randomized, placebo-controlled trials of ethyl-eicosapentanoate in the treatment of bipolar depression and rapid cycling bipolar disorder. *Biological Psychiatry, 60*(9), 1020–1022.

Keinan-Boker, L., van Der Schouw, Y. T., Grobbee, D. E., & Peeters, P. H. (2004). Dietary phytoestrogens and breast cancer risk. *American Journal of Clinical Nutrition, 79*(2), 282–288.

Kelly, G. S. (2001). *Rhodiola rosea*: A possible plant adaptogen. *Alternive Medical Review, 6*(3), 293–302.

Kemppainen, J. K., Eller, L. S., Bunch, E., Hamilton, M. J., Dole, P., Holzemer, W. et al. (2006). Strategies for self-management of HIV-related anxiety. *AIDS Care, 18*(6), 597–607.

Kennedy, D. O., Little, W., & Scholey, A. B. (2004). Attenuation of laboratory-induced stress in humans after acute administration of *Melissa officinalis* (Lemon Balm). *Psychosomatic Medicine, 66*(4), 607–613.

Kennedy, D. O., Haskell, C. F., Mauri, P. L., & Scholey, A. B. (2007). Acute cognitive effects of standardised Ginkgo biloba extract complexed with phosphatidylserine. *Hum Psychopharmacol, 22*(4), 199–210.

Kennedy, D. O., Wake, G., Savelev, S., Tildesley, N. T., Perry, E. K., Wesnes, K. A., & Scholey, A. B. (2003). Modulation of mood and cognitive performance following acute administration of single doses of *Melissa officinalis* (Lemon balm) with human CNS nicotinic and muscarinic receptor-binding properties. *Neuropsychopharmacology, 28*(10), 1871–1881.

Kessler, J., Thiel, A., Karbe, H., & Heiss, W. D. (2000). Piracetam improves activated blood flow and facilitates rehabilitation of poststroke aphasic patients. *Stroke, 31*(9), 2112–2116.

Khalsa, S. B., & Cope, S. (2006). Effects of a yoga lifestyle intervention on performance-related characteristics of musicians: A preliminary study. *Medical Science Monitor, 12*(8), CR325–331.

Khalsa, S. S. K. (2007). Yoga therapy: Emotional aspects/ Yoga, meditation and the psychology of health recovery. Symposium on Yoga Therapy and Research SYTAR. January 20, 2007. Main Session 8. Retrieved October 8, 2007 from http://www.cmebyplaza.com/YOGA/registrants/SYTAR2007/SYTAR%202007%

20Course%20Companion%20Main%20Session%20PDF/MS%208%20Yoga%2
0Therapy%20Emotional%20Aspects-%20Khalsa.pdf. *Symposium on Yoga Therapy and Research SYTAR,* Los Angeles.

Khan, A., Khan, S. R., Walens, G., Kolts, R., & Giller, E. L. (2003). Frequency of positive studies among fixed and flexible dose antidepressant clinical trials: An analysis of the food and drug administration summary basis of approval reports. *Neuropsychopharmacology, 28*(3), 552–557.

Kharbanda, K. K., Rogers, D. D. 2nd, Mailliard, M. E., Siford, G. L., Barak, A. J., Beckenhauer, H. C. et al. (2005). A comparison of the effects of betaine and S-adenosylmethionine on ethanol-induced changes in methionine metabolism and steatosis in rat hepatocytes. *Journal of Nutrition, 135*(3), 519–524.

Khoo, S. K., Munro, C., & Battistutta, D. (1990). Evening primrose oil and treatment of premenstrual syndrome. *Medical Journal of Australia, 153*(4), 189–192.

Khumar, S. S., & Kaur, P. K. S. (1993). Effectiveness of Shavasana on depression in university students. *Indian Journal of Clinical Psychology, 20*(2), 82–87.

Kidd, P. M. (2000). Attention-deficit/hyperactivity disorder (ADHD) in children: Rationale for its integrative management. *Alternative Medicine Review, 5*(5), 402–428.

Kim, H. S., Kang, J. G., & Seong, Y. H. (1995). Blockade by ginseng total saponin of the development of cocaine induced reverse tolerance and dopamine receptor supersensitivity in mice. *Pharmacology, Biochemistry and Behavior, 50,* 23-27.

Kimura, H., Nagao, F., Tanaka, Y., Sakai, S., Ohnishi, S. T., & Okumura, K. (2005). Beneficial effects of the Nishino breathing method on immune activity and stress level. *Journal of Alternative and Complementary Medicine, 11*(2), 285–291.

Kimura, K., Ozeki, M., Juneja, L. R., & Ohira, H. (2007). L-Theanine reduces psychological and physiological stress responses. *Biological Psychology, 74*(1), 39–45.

Kitani, K., Minami, C., Maruyama, W., Kanai, S., Ivy, G. O., & Carrillo, M. C. (2000). Common properties for propargylamines of enhancing superoxide dismutase and catalase activities in the dopaminergic system in the rat: Implications for the life prolonging effect of (-)deprenyl. *Journal of Neural Transmission, 60* (Suppl.), 139–156.

Kjellgren, A., Bood, S.A., Axelsson, K., Norlander, T., & Saatcioglu, F. (2007). Wellness through a comprehensive Yogic breathing program: A controlled pilot trial. *BMC Complement Altern Med.* 7(1), 43.

Kleijnen, J., Ter Riet, G., & Knipschild, P. (1990). Vitamin B6 in the treatment of the premenstrual syndrome—A review. *British Journal of Obstetrics and Gynaecology, 97*(9), 847–852.

Klepser, T., & Nisly, N. (1999). Chaste tree berry for premenstrual syndrome. *Alternative Medicine Alert, 2*(6), 61–72.

Knoll, J. (2000). (-)Deprenyl (Selegiline): Past, present and future. *Neurobiology (Bp), 8*(2), 179–99.

Knoll, J. (2003). Enhancer regulation/endogenous and synthetic enhancer compounds: A neurochemical concept of the innate and acquired drives. *Neurochemical Research, 28*(8), 1275–1297.

Knuppel, L., & Linde, K. (2004). Adverse effects of St. John's Wort: A systematic review. *Journal of Clinical Psychiatry, 65*(11), 1470–1479.

Kobak, K. A., Taylor, L. V., Bystritsky, A., Kohlenberg, C. J., Greist, J. H., Tucker, P. et al. (2005). St John's wort versus placebo in obsessive-compulsive disorder: Results from a double-blind study. *International Clinical Psychopharmacology, 20*(6), 299–304.

Kobak, K. A., Taylor, L. V., Warner, G., & Futterer, R. (2005). St. John's Wort versus placebo in social phobia: Results from a placebo-controlled pilot study. *Journal of Clinical Psychopharmacology, 25*(1), 51–58.

Kochupillai, V., Kumar, P., Singh, D., Aggarwal, D., Bhardwaj, N., Bhutani, M., & Das, S. N. (2005). Effect of rhythmic breathing (Sudarshan Kriya and Pranayam) on immune functions and tobacco addiction. *Annals of the New York Academy of Sciences, 1056,* 242–252.

Kohama, T., Suzuki, N., Ohno, S., & Inoue, M. (2004). Analgesic efficacy of French maritime pine bark extract in dysmenorrhea: an open clinical trial. *Journal of Reproductive Medicine, 49*(10), 828–832.

Konig, H., Stahl, H., Sieper, J., & Wolf, K. J. (1995). Magnetic resonance tomography of finger polyarthritis: Morphology and cartilage signals after ademetionine therapy. *Aktuelle Radiologie, 5*(1), 36–40. (In German)

Konofal, E., Lecendreux, M., Arnulf, I., & Mouren, M. C. (2004). Iron deficiency in children with attention-deficit/hyperactivity disorder. *Archives of Pediatric and Adolescent Medicine, 158*(12), 1113–1115.

Kormosh, N., Laktionov, K., & Antoshechkina, M. (2006). Effect of a combination of extract from several plants on cell-mediated and humoral immunity of patients with advanced ovarian cancer. *Phytotherapy Research, 20*(5), 424–425.

Kraft, M., Spahn, T. W., Menzel, J., Senninger, N., Dietl, K. H., Herbst, H. et al. (2001). Fulminant liver failure after administration of the herbal antidepressant kava-kava. *Deutsche Medizin Wochenschrift, 126*(36), 970–972. (In German)

Krasnik, C., Montori, V. M., Guyatt, G. H., Heels-Ansdell, D., & Busse, J. W. (2005). The effect of bright light therapy on depression associated with premenstrual dysphoric disorder. *American Journal of Obstetrics and Gynecology, 193*(3 Pt 1), 658–661

Kraus, T., Hosl, K., Kiess, O., Schanze, A., Kornhuber, J., & Forster, C. (2007). BOLD fMRI deactivation of limbic and temporal brain structures and mood enhancing effect by transcutaneous vagus nerve stimulation. *Journal of Neural Transmission, 114,* 1485–1493.

Krisanaprakornkit, T., Krisanaprakornkit, W., Piyavhatkul, N., & Laopaiboon, M. (2006). Meditation therapy for anxiety disorders. *Cochrane Database System Review,* (1), CD004998.

Kruglikova, R. P. (1997). How and why Picamilon works. *Life Extension,* July, 34–39.

Krystal. A. D. , & Ressler, I. (2002). The use of valerian in neuropsychiatry. *CNS Spectrum, 6*(10), 841–847.

Krzeski, T., Kazon, M., Borkowski, A., Witeska, A., & Kuczera, J. (1993). Combined extracts of *Urtica dioica* and *Pygeum africanum* in the treatment of benign prostatic hyperplasia: Double-blind comparison of two doses. *Clinical Therapy, 15*(6), 1011–1020.

Kudolo, G. B. (2000). The effect of 3-month ingestion of *Ginkgo biloba* extract on pancreatic beta-cell function in response to glucose loading in normal glucose tolerant individuals. *Journal of Clinical Pharmacology, 40*(6), 647–654.

Kulkarni, S. K., & Ninan, I. (1997). Inhibition of morphine tolerance and dependence by *Withania somnifera* in mice. *Journal of Ethnopharmacology, 57*, 213–217.

Kumar, P. N. S., Andrade, C., Bhakta, S. G., & Singh, N. M. (2007). Melatonin in schizophrenic outpatients with insomnia: A double-blind, placebo-controlled study. *Journal of Clinical Psychiatry, 68*, 237–241.

Kunz, D., & Bes, F. (1997). Melatonin effects in a patient with severe REM sleep behavior disorder: Case report and theoretical considerations. *Neuropsychobiology, 36*(4), 211–214.

Kurkin V. A., Zapesochnaya G. G. (1986). Khimicheskiy sostav i farmakologicheskiye svoystva rasteniy roda Rhodiola. Obzor. (Chemical composition and pharmacological properties of *Rhodiola rosea.*) *Khim-Farm Zh (Chemical and Pharmaceutical Journal Moscow)*, 20:1231–1244.

Kuttner, L., Chambers, C. T., Hardial, J., Israel, D. M., Jacobson, K., & Evans, K. (2006). A randomized trial of yoga for adolescents with irritable bowel syndrome. *Pain Research Management, 11*(4), 217–223.

Kyle, D. J., & Arterburn, L. M. (1998). Single cell oil sources of docosahexaenoic acid: Clinical studies. *World Review of Nutrition and Diet, 83*, 116–131.

Lake, J. M. (2007). *Textbook of integrative treatments*. New York: Theime.

Lane, J. D., Seskevich, J. E., & Pieper, C. F. (2007). Brief meditation training can improve perceived stress and negative mood. *Alternative Therapy Health Medicine, 13*(1), 38–44.

Lange, H., Suryapranata, H., De Luca, G., Borner, C., Dille, J., Kallmayer, K., Pasalary, M. N., Scherer, E., & Dambrink, J. H. (2004). Folate therapy and instent restenosis after coronary stenting. *New England Journal of Medicine, 350*(26), 2673–81.

Lapane, K. L., Zierler, S., Lasater, T. M., Stein, M., Barbour, M. M., & Hume, A. L. (1995). Is a history of depressive symptoms associated with an increased risk of infertility in women? *Psychosomatic Medicine, 57*(6), 509–513. discussion 514–516.

Lara, D. R., Brunstein, M. G., Ghisolfi, E. S., Lobato, M. I., Belmonte-de-Abreu, P., & Souza, D. O. (2001). Allopurinol augmentation for poorly responsive schizophrenia. *International Clinical Psychopharmacology, 16*(4), 235–237.

LaRowe, S. D., Myrick, H., Hedden, S., Mardikian, P., Saladin, M., McRae, A. et al. (2007). Is cocaine desire reduced by N-acetylcysteine? *American Journal of Psychiatry, 164*(7), 1115–1117.

Larsen, S. (2006). *The healing power of neurofeedback: The revolutionary LENS technique for restoring optimal brain functioning.* Rochester, VT: Healing Arts Press.

Larsen, S., Yee, W., Gerbarg, P. L., Brown, R. P., Gunkelman, J., & Sherlin, L. (2006, February 24–25). Neurophysiolgocial markers of Sudarshan Kriya Yoga practices: A pilot study. In *Proceedings* the *World Conference Expanding Paradigms: Science, consciousness and spirituality* (pp. 36–48). Delhi, India. All India Institute of Medical Sciences.

Lavey, R., Sherman, T., Mueser, K. T., Osborne, D. D., Currier, M., & Wolfe, R. (2005). The effects of yoga on mood in psychiatric inpatients. *Psychiatric Rehabilitation Journal, 28*(4), 399–402.

Lazar, S. W., Kerr, C. E., Wasserman, R. H., Gray, J. R., Greve, D. N., Treadway, M. T. et al. (2005). Meditation experience is associated with increased cortical thickness. *Neuroreport, 16*(17), 1893–1897.

Le Bars, P. L., Velasco, F. M., Ferguson, J. M., Dessain, E. C., Kieser, M., & Hoerr, R. (2002). Influence of the severity of cognitive impairment on the effect of the *Ginkgo biloba* extract EGb 761 in Alzheimer's disease. *Neuropsychobiology, 45*(1), 19–26.

Lebret, T., Herve, J. M., Gorny, P., Worcel, M., & Botto, H. (2002). Efficacy and safety of a novel combination of L-arginine glutamate and yohimbine hydrochloride: A new oral therapy for erectile dysfunction. *European Urology, 41*(6), 608–613.

LeDoux, J. E. (2000). Emotion circuits in the brain. *Annual Review of Neuroscience, 23,* 155–184.

Lee, M. S., Huh, H. J., Jeong, S. M., Lee, H. S., Ryu, H., Park, J. H. et al. (2003). Effects of Qigong on immune cells. *American Journal of Chinese Medicine, 31*(2), 327–335.

Lee, M. S., Huh, H. J., Kim, B. G., Ryu, H., Lee, H. S., Kim, J. M., & Chung, H. T. (2002). Effects of Qi-training on heart rate variability. *American Journal of Chinese Medicine, 30*(4), 463–470.

Lehrer, P., Sasaki, Y., & Saito, Y. (1999). Zazen and cardiac variability. *Psychosomatic Medicine, 61*(6), 812–821.

Lerner, V., Bergman, J., Statsenko, N., & Miodownik, C. (2004). Vitamin B6 treatment in acute neuroleptic-induced akathisia: A randomized, double-blind, placebo-controlled study. *Journal of Clinical Psychiatry, 65*(11), 1550–1554.

Lerner, V., Miodownik, C., Kaptsan, A., Cohen, H., Matar, M., Loewenthal, U., & Kotler, M. (2001). Vitamin B(6) in the treatment of tardive dyskinesia: A double-blind, placebo-controlled, crossover study. *American Journal of Psychiatry, 158*(9), 1511–1514.

Leverich, G. S., & Post, R. M. (2006). Course of bipolar illness after history of childhood trauma. *Lancet, 367*(9516), 1040–1042.

Levin, H. S. (1991). Treatment of postconcussional symptoms with CDP-choline. *Journal of the Neurological Sciences, 103* (Suppl.), S39–S42.

Levine, J., Stahl, Z., Sela, B. A., Ruderman, V., Shumaico, O., Babushkin, I. et al. (2006). Homocysteine-reducing strategies improve symptoms in chronic schizophrenic patients with hyperhomocysteinemia. *Biological Psychiatry, 60*(3), 265–269.

Levy, S., Brizendine, L., & Nachtigall, R. (2006). How to treat depression, stress associated with infertility Tx. *Current Psychiatry, 5*(10), 65–74.

Li, F., Fisher, K. J., Harmer, P., Irbe, D., Tearse, R. G., & Weimer, C. (2004). Tai chi and self-rated quality of sleep and daytime sleepiness in older adults: A randomized controlled trial. *Journal of the American Geriatric Society, 52*(6), 892–900.

Li, M., Chen, K., & Mo, Z. (2002). Use of qigong therapy in the detoxification of heroin addicts. *Alternative Therapy and Health Medicine, 8*(1), 50–59.

Liao, Y., Wang, R., & Tang, X. C. (2004). Centrophenoxine improves chronic cerebral ischemia induced cognitive deficit and neuronal degeneration in rats. *Acta Pharmacologica Sinica, 25*(12), 1590–1596.

Lichius, J. J., & Muth, C. (1997). The inhibiting effects of *Urtica dioica* root extracts on experimentally induced prostatic hyperplasia in the mouse. *Planta Medica, 63*(4), 307–310.

Lieber, C. S. (1999). Role of S-adenosyl-L-methionine in the treatment of liver diseases. *Journal of Hepatology, 30*(6), 1155–1159.

Lieber, C. S. (2001). Liver diseases by alcohol and hepatitis C: Early detection and new insights in pathogenesis lead to improved treatment. *American Journal of Addiction, 10* (Suppl.), 29–50.

Lieber, C. S. (2002). S-adenosyl-L-methionine: Its role in the treatment of liver disorders. *American Journal of Clinical Nutrition, 76*(5), S1183–S1187.

Lieber, C. S. (2005). Pathogenesis and treatment of alcoholic liver disease: Progress over the last 50 years. *Roczniki Akademii Medycznej w Bialymstoku (Bialystok), 50*, 7–20. (In Polish)

Lieberman, S. (1998). A review of the effectiveness of *Cimicifuga racemosa* (black cohosh) for the symptoms of menopause. *Journal of Women's Health, 7*(5), 525–529.

Linde, K., Ramirez, G., Mulrow, C. D., Pauls, A., Weidenhammer, W., & Melchart, D. (1996). St John's wort for depression—An overview and meta-analysis of randomised clinical trials. *BMJ, 313*(7052), 253–258.

Linden, M., Habib, T., & Radojevic, V. (1996). A controlled study of the effects of EEG biofeedback on cognition and behavior of children with attention-deficit disorder and learning disabilities. *Biofeedback Self Regulation, 21*(1), 35–49.

Linehan, M. M., Dimeff, L. A., Reynolds, S. K., Comtois, K. A., Welch, S. S., Heagerty, P. et al. (2002). Dialectical behavior therapy versus comprehensive validation therapy plus 12-step for the treatment of opioid dependent women meeting criteria for borderline personality disorder. *Drug and Alcohol Dependency, 67*(1), 13–26.

Ling, D. S., & Benardo, L. S. (2005). Nootropic agents enhance the recruitment of fast GABAA inhibition in rat neocortex. *Cerebral Cortex, 15*(7), 921–928.

Loizzo, M. R., Tundis, R., Menichini, F., & Menichini, F. (2008). Natural products and their derivatives as cholinesterase inhibitors in the treatment of neurodegenerative disorders: An update. *Current Medicinal Chemistry, 15*(12): 1209–28.

Lolic, M. M., Fiskum, G., & Rosenthal, R. E. (1997). Neuroprotective effects of acetyl-L-carnitine after stroke in rats. *Annals of Emergency Medicine, 29*(6), 758–765.

Lopatkin, N., Sivkov, A., Walther, C., Schlafke, S., Medvedev, A., Avdeichuk, J. et al. (2005). Long-term efficacy and safety of a combination of sabal and urtica extract for lower urinary tract symptoms—A placebo-controlled, double-blind, multicenter trial. *World Journal of Urology, 23*(2), 139–146.

Lozano, R. (1991). CDP-choline in the treatment of cranio-encephalic traumata. *Journal of the Neurological Sciences, 103* (Suppl.), S43–S47.

Lu, K., Gray, M. A., Oliver, C., Liley, D. T., Harrison, B. J., Bartholomeusz et al. (2004). The acute effects of L-theanine in comparison with alprazolam on anticipatory anxiety in humans. *Human Psychopharmacology, 19*(7), 457–465.

Lubar, J. F., & Bahler, W. W. (1976). Behavioral management of epileptic seizures following EEG biofeedback training of the sensorimotor rhythm. *Biofeedback and Self Regulation, 1* (1), 77–104.

Lubar, J. O., & Lubar, J. F. (1984). Electroencephalographic biofeedback of SMR and beta for treatment of attention-deficit disorders in a clinical setting. *Biofeedback and Self Regulation, 9*(1), 1–23.

Lukas, S. E., Penetar, D., Berko, J., Vicens, L., Palmer, C., Mallya, G., Macklin, E. A., & Lee, D. Y. (2005). An extract of the Chinese herbal root kudzu reduces alcohol drinking by heavy drinkers in a naturalistic setting. *Alcoholism, Clinical and Experimental Research, 29*(5), 756–762.

Luo, Y., Chen, D., Ren, L., Zhao, X., & Qin, J. (2006). Solid lipid nanoparticles for enhancing vinpocetine's oral bioavailability. *Journal of Controlled Release, 114*(1), 53–59.

Lutz, A., Greischar, L. L., Rawlings, N. B., Ricard, M., & Davidson, R. J. (2004). Long-term meditators self-induce high-amplitude gamma synchrony during mental practice. *Proceedings of the National Academy of Sciences USA, 101*(46), 16369–16373.

Lyon, M. R., Cline, J. C., Totosy de Zepetnek, J., Shan, J. J., Pang, P., & Benishin, C. (2001). Effect of the herbal extract combination *Panax quinquefolium* and *Ginkgo biloba* on attention-deficit hyperactivity disorder: a pilot study. *Journal of Psychiatry and Neuroscience, 26*(3), 221–228.

MacNeil, J. S. (2006). Consider pregnancy risks in bipolar women. *Clinical Psychiatry News, 34*(8), 20.

Malathi, A., & Damodaran, A. (1999). Stress due to exams in medical students—Role of yoga. *Indian Journal of Physiology and Pharmacology, 43*(2), 218–224.

Mangano, N. G., Clementi, G., Costantino, G., Calvani, M., & Matera, M. (2000). Effect of acetyl-L-carnitine on ethanol consumption and alcohol abstinence syndrome in rats. *Drugs under Experimental and Clinical Research, 26*(1), 7–12.

Mangoni, A., Grassi, M. P., Frattola, L., Piolti, R., Bassi, S., Motta, A. et al. (1991). Effects of a MAO-B inhibitor in the treatment of Alzheimer disease. *European Neurology, 31*(2), 100–107.

Manheimer, E., Anderson, B. J., & Stein, M. D. (2003). Use and assessment of complementary and alternative therapies by intravenous drug users. *American Journal of Drug and Alcohol Abuse, 29*(2), 401–413.

Manjunath, N. K., & Telles, S. (2005). Influence of Yoga and Ayurveda on self-rated sleep in a geriatric population. *Indian Journal of Medical Research, 121*(5), 683–690.

Mardikian, P. N., LaRowe, S. D., Hedden, S., Kalivas, P. W., & Malcolm, R. J. (2007). An open-label trial of N-acetylcysteine for the treatment of cocaine dependence: A pilot study. *Progress in Neuropsychopharmacology and Biological Psychiatry, 31*(2), 389–394.

Martinez-Lavin, M., Hermosillo, A. G., Rosas, M., & Soto, M. E. (1998). Circadian studies of autonomic nervous balance in patients with fibromyalgia: A heart rate variability analysis. *Arthritis and Rheumatism, 41*(11), 1966–1971.

Maruyama, W., & Naoi, M. (1999). Neuroprotection by (-)-deprenyl and related compounds. *Mechanics of Ageing and Development, 111*(2–3), 189–200.

Maslova, L. V., Kondrat'ev, B. I. U., Maslov, L. N., & Lishmanov, I. u. B. (1994). The cardioprotective and antiadrenergic activity of an extract of *Rhodiola rosea* in stress. *Eksp Klin Farmakol, 57*(6), 61–63. (In Russian)

Mathews, J. D., Riley, M. D., Fejo, L., Munoz, E., Milns, N. R., Gardner, I. D. et al. (1988). Effects of the heavy usage of kava on physical health: Summary of a pilot survey in an aboriginal community. *Medical Journal of Australia, 148*(11), 548–555.

Mathews, J. M., Etheridge, A. S., & Black, S. R. (2002). Inhibition of human cytochrome P450 activities by kava extract and kavalactones. *Drug Metabolism and Disposition: The Biological Fate of Chemicals, 30*(11), 1153–1157.

Mathie, R. T., & Robinson, T. W. (2006). Outcomes from homeopathic prescribing in medical practice: A prospective, research-targeted, pilot study. *Homeopathy, 95*(4), 199–205.

Mato, J. M., Camara, J., Fernandez de Paz, J., Caballeria, L., Coll, S., Caballero, A. et al. (1999). S-adenosylmethionine in alcoholic liver cirrhosis: A randomized, placebo-controlled, double-blind, multicenter clinical trial. *Journal of Hepatology, 30*(6), 1081–1089.

Matsumoto, S., Mori, N., Tsuchihashi, N., Ogata, T., Lin, Y., Yokoyama, H., & Ishida, S. (1998). Enhancement of nitroxide-reducing activity in rats after chronic administration of vitamin E, vitamin C, and idebenone examined by an in vivo electron spin resonance technique. *Magnetic Resonance Medicine, 40*(2), 330–333.

Mattarello, M. J., Benedini, S., Fiore, C., Camozzi, V., Sartorato, P., Luisetto, G., & Armanini, D. (2006). Effect of licorice on PTH levels in healthy women. *Steroids, 71*(5), 403–408.

Mayo, J. L. (1997). A natural approach to menopause. *Clinical Nutritional Insights, 5*(6), 1–8.

McCabe, S. E., Teter, C. J., & Boyd, C. J. (2004). The use, misuse and diversion of prescription stimulants among middle and high school students. *Substance Use and Misuse, 39*(7), 1095–1116.

McCaleb, R. (1995). *Vitex agnus-castus.* Golden, CO: Herb Research Foundation.

McCormick, M. A. P. (2002). Yoga therapy and post traumatic stress disorder. Retrieved September 20, 2007 from http://www.iayt.org/site/publications/studies.htm?ProfileNumber=&UStatus=&AutoID=&LS=&AM=&Ds=&CI=&AT=&Return=. *Yoga Studies*.

McDaniel, M. A., Maier, S. F., & Einstein, G. O. (2003). "Brain-specific" nutrients: A memory cure? *Nutrition, 19*(11–12), 957–975.

McNamara, R. K., Hahn, C. G., Jandacek, R., Rider, T., Tso, P., Stanford, K. E. et al. (2007). Selective deficits in the omega-3 fatty acid docosahexaenoic acid in the postmortem orbitofrontal cortex of patients with major depressive disorder. *Biological Psychiatry, 62*(1), 17–24.

Melatonin. (1995). *Medical Letter on Drugs and Therapeutics, 37*(962), 111–112.

Mellor, J. E., Laugharne, J. D., & Peet, M. (1995). Schizophrenic symptoms and dietary intake of n-3 fatty acids. *Schizophrenia Research, 18*(1), 85–86.

Meseguer, E., Taboada, R., Sanchez, V., Mena, M. A., Campos, V., & Garcia De Yebenes, J. (2002). Life-threatening parkinsonism induced by kava-kava. *Movement Disorders, 17*(1), 195–196.

Meuret, A. E., Ritz, T., Wilhelm, F. H., & Roth, W. T. (2005). Voluntary hyperventilation in the treatment of panic disorder—functions of hyperventilation, their implications for breathing training, and recommendations for standardization. *Clinical Psychology Review, 25*(3), 285–306.

Mezzacappa, E., Tremblay, R. E., Kindlon, D., Saul, J. P., Arseneault, L., Seguin, J., Pihl, R. O., & Earls, F. (1997). Anxiety, antisocial behavior, and heart rate regulation in adolescent males. *Journal of Child Psychology and Psychiatry, 38*(4), 457–469.

Michalsen, A., Grossman, P., Acil, A., Langhorst, J., Ludtke, R., Esch, T. et al. (2005). Rapid stress reduction and anxiolysis among distressed women as a consequence of a three-month intensive yoga program. *Medical Science Monitor, 11*(12), CR555–561.

Miller, J. J., Fletcher, K., & Kabat-Zinn, J. (1995). Three-year follow-up and clinical implications of a mindfulness meditation-based stress reduction intervention in the treatment of anxiety disorders. *General Hospital Psychiatry, 17*(3), 192–200.

Millichap, J. G., Yee, M. M., & Davidson, S. I. (2006). Serum ferritin in children with attention-deficit hyperactivity disorder. *Pediatric Neurology, 34*(3), 200–203.

Ming, D. S., Hillhouse, B. J., Guns, E. S., Eberding, A., Xie, S., Vimalanathan, S., & Towers, G. H. (2005). Bioactive compounds from *Rhodiola rosea* (Crassulaceae). *Phytotherapy Research, 19*(9), 740–743.

Mirzoian, R. S., Gan'shina, T. S., Kosoi, M. I., Aleksandrin, V. V., & Aleksandrin, P. N. (1989). Effect of pikamilon on the cortical blood supply and microcirculation in the pial arteriole system. *Biulleten Eksperimentalnoi Biologii I Meditsiny (Moscow), 107*(5), 581–582. (In Russian)

Mitka, M. (2002). News about neuroprotectants for the treatment of stroke. *Journal of the American Medical Association, 287*(10), 1253–1254.

Mittal, C. M., Wig, N., Mishra, S., & Deepak, K. K. (2004). Heart rate variability in human immunodeficiency virus-positive individuals. *International Journal of Cardiology, 94*(1), 1–6.

Mizuhara, H., Wang, L. O., Kobayashi, K., & Yamaguchi, Y. (2005). Long-range EEG phase synchronization during an arithmetic task indexes a coherent cortical network simultaneously measured by fMRI. *Neuroimage, 27*(3), 553–563.

Mizuno, T., Kuno, R., Nitta, A., Nabeshima, T., Zhang, G., Kawanokuchi, J. et al. (2005). Protective effects of nicergoline against neuronal cell death induced by activated microglia and astrocytes. *Brain Research, 1066*(1–2), 78–85.

Moadel, A. B., Shah, C., Wylie-Rosett, J., Harris, M. S., Patel, S. R., Hall, C. B., & Sparano, J. A. (2007). Randomized controlled trial of yoga among a multiethnic sample of breast cancer patients: Effects on quality of life. *Journal of Clinical Oncology, 25*(28), 4387–4395.

Monaco, P., Pastore, L., Rizzo, S., et al. (1996). *Safety and tolerability of ademetionine (ADE) SD for inpatients with stroke: A pilot randomized double-blind, placebo-controlled study* [abstract]. Paper presented at the Third World Stroke Conference and Fifth European Stroke Conference.

Monastra, V. J., Monastra, D. M., & George, S. (2002). The effects of stimulant therapy, EEG biofeedback, and parenting style on the primary symptoms of attention-deficit/hyperactivity disorder. *Applied Psychophysiology and Biofeedback, 27*(4), 231–249.

Montgomery, S. A., Thal, L. J., & Amrein, R. (2003). Meta-analysis of double blind randomized controlled clinical trials of acetyl-L-carnitine versus placebo in the treatment of mild cognitive impairment and mild Alzheimer's disease. *International Clinical Psychopharmacology, 18*(2), 61–71.

Mood, M. A. (2007). Returning vets mental health worsens over time. *Clinical Psychiatry News, 35*(12), 8.

Morales, A., Condra, M., Owen, J. A., Surridge, D. H., Fenemore, J., & Harris, C. (1987). Is yohimbine effective in the treatment of organic impotence? Results of a controlled trial. *Journal of Urology, 137*(6), 1168–1172.

Mordente, A., Martorana, G. E., Minotti, G., & Giardina, B. (1998). Antioxidant properties of 2,3-dimethoxy-5-methyl-6-(10-hydroxydecyl)-1,4-benzoquinone (idebenone). *Chemical Research in Toxicology, 11*(1), 54–63.

Morin, C. M., Koetter, U., Bastien, C., Ware, J. C., & Wooten, V. (2005). Valerian-hops combination and diphenhydramine for treating insomnia: A randomized placebo-controlled clinical trial. *Sleep, 28*(11), 1465–1471.

Morris, M. C., Evans, D. A., Bienias, J. L., Tangney, C. C., Bennett, D. A., Aggarwal, N., Schneider, J., & Wilson, R. S. (2003). Dietary fats and the risk of incident Alzheimer disease. *Archives of Neurology, 60*(2), 194–200.

Mowrey, D. B. (1996). *Muira-puama* (Liriosma ovata), *in herbal tonic therapies.* Avenel, NJ: Wings Books.

Mueller, S. C., Uehleke, B., Woehling, H., Petzsch, M., Majcher-Peszynska, J., Hehl, E. M. et al. (2004). Effect of St John's Wort dose and preparations on the pharmacokinetics of digoxin. *Clinical Pharmacology and Therapeutics, 75*(6), 546–557.

Muller, S. F., & Klement, S. (2006). A combination of valerian and lemon balm is effective in the treatment of restlessness and dyssomnia in children. *Phytomedicine, 13*(6), 383–387.

Muller, T., Mannel, M., Murck, H., & Rahlfs, V. W. (2004). Treatment of somatoform disorders with St. John's Wort: A randomized, double-blind and placebo-controlled trial. *Psychosomatic Medicine, 66*(4), 538–547.

Murck, H., Spitznagel, H., Ploch, M., Seibel, K., & Schaffler, K. (2006). Hypericum extract reverses S-ketamine-induced changes in auditory evoked potentials in humans—Possible implications for the treatment of schizophrenia. *Biological Psychiatry, 59*(5), 440–445.

Murphy, M. P., & Smith, R. A. (2007). Targeting antioxidants to mitochondria by conjugation to lipophilic cations. *Annual Review of Pharmacology and Toxicology, 47*, 629–656.

Naga Venkatesha Murthy, P. J., Janakiramaiah, N., Gangadhar, B. N., & Subbakrishna, D. K. (1998). P300 amplitude and antidepressant response to Sudarshan Kriya Yoga (SKY). *Journal of Affective Disorders, 50*(1), 45–4-8.

Najm, W. I., Reinsch, S., Hoehler, F., Tobis, J. S., & Harvey, P. W. (2004). S-adenosyl methionine (SAMe) versus celecoxib for the treatment of osteoarthritis symptoms: A double-blind cross-over trial. *BMC Musculoskeletal Disorders, 5*, 6.

Nandy, K. (1978). Centrophenoxine: Effects on aging mammalian brain. *Journal of the American Geriatric Society, 26*(2), 74–81.

Narahashi, T., Moriguchi, S., Zhao, X., Marszalec, W., & Yeh, J. Z. (2004). Mechanisms of action of cognitive enhancers on neuroreceptors. *Biology and Pharmacology Bulletin, 27*(11), 1701–1706.

Nash, J. K. (2000). Treatment of attention-deficit hyperactivity disorder with neurotherapy. *Clinical Electroencephalography, 31*(1), 30–37.

Nathan, P. J., Clarke, J., Lloyd, J., Hutchison, C. W., Downey, L., & Stough, C. (2001). The acute effects of an extract of *Bacopa monniera* (Brahmi) on cognitive function in healthy normal subjects. *Human Psychopharmacology, 16*(4), 345–351.

Neese, S., La Grange, L., Trujillo, E., & Romero, D. (2004). The effects of ethanol and silymarin treatment during gestation on spatial working memory. *BMC Complementary and Alternative Medicine, 4*, 4.

Negi, K. S. , Singh, Y. D., Kushwaha, K. P., et al. (2000). Clinical evaluation of memory enhancing properties of Memory Plus in children with attention-deficit hyperactivity disorder. [Abstract]. *Indian Journal of Psychiatry, 42.*

Nemets, B., Stahl, Z., & Belmaker, R. H. (2002). Addition of omega-3 fatty acid to maintenance medication treatment for recurrent unipolar depressive disorder. *American Journal of Psychiatry, 159*(3), 477–47-9.

Nespor, K. (2000). Yoga for treatment of substance abuse [Electronic Version]. Retrieved from http://www.yogamag.net/archives/2000/6nov00/yogadds.shtml. n.p.

Newton, K. M., Reed, S. D., LaCroix, A. Z., Grothaus, L. C., Ehrlich, K., & Guiltinan, J. (2006). Treatment of vasomotor symptoms of menopause with black cohosh, multibotanicals, soy, hormone therapy, or placebo: A randomized trial. *Annals of Internal Medicine, 145*(12), 869–879.

Nidecker, A. (1997). Probing genes, drugs, and fatty acids in dementia. *Clinical Psychiatry News,* December, 4.

Nidich, S. I., Morehead, P., Nidich, R. J., Sands, D., & Sharma, H. (1993). The effect of the Maharishi Student Rasayana food supplement on non-verbal intelligence. *Personality and Individual Differences, 15*(5), 599–602.

Nierenberg, A. A., Ostacher, M. J., Calabrese, J. R., Ketter, T. A., Marangell, L. B., Miklowitz, D. J. et al. (2006). Treatment-resistant bipolar depression: A STEP-BD equipoise randomized effectiveness trial of antidepressant augmentation with lamotrigine, inositol, or risperidone. *American Journal of Psychiatry, 163*(2), 210–216.

Nishio, T., Sunohara, N., Furukawa, S., Akiguchi, I., & Kudo, Y. (1998). Repeated injections of nicergoline increase the nerve growth factor level in the aged rat brain. *Japan Journal of Pharmacology, 76*(3), 321–323. (In Japanese)

Noaghiul, S., & Hibbeln, J. R. (2003). Cross-national comparisons of seafood consumption and rates of bipolar disorders. *American Journal of Psychiatry, 160*(12), 2222–2227.

Noorbala, A. A., Akhondzadeh, S., Davari-Ashtiani, R., & Amini-Nooshabadi, H. (1999). Piracetam in the treatment of schizophrenia: implications for the glutamate hypothesis of schizophrenia. *Journal of Clinical Pharmacy and Therapeutics, 24*(5), 369–374.

Occhiuto, F., Pasquale, R. D., Guglielmo, G., Palumbo, D. R., Zangla, G., Samperi, S., Renzo, A., & Circosta, C. (2007). Effects of phytoestrogenic isoflavones from red clover (*Trifolium pratense L.*) on experimental osteoporosis. *Phytotherapy Research, 21*(2), 130–134.

Ochs, L. (2006). Low energy neurofeedback system (LENS): Theory, background, and introduction. *Journal of Neurotherapy, 10*(2/3), 5–39.

Ochs, L. (1994). EEG-driven stimulation and heterogeneous head injured patients: Extended findings. A peer-reviewed abstract from the 1994 Berrol Head Injury Conference, Las Vegas, NV [web page, cited December 7, 2001]. Available from: http://www.flexyx.com/contents/pubs/Extended. htm.

Oh, K. W., Kim, H. S., & Wagner, G. C. (1997). Ginseng total saponin inhibits the dopaminergic depletions induced by methamphetamine. *Planta Medica, 63,* 80–81.

Okuyama, S., & Aihara, H. (1988). Action of nootropic drugs on transcallosal responses in rats. *Neuropharmacology, 27*(1), 67–72.

Olin, J., Schneider, L., Novit, A., & Luczak, S. (2001). Hydergine for dementia. *Cochrane Database System Review,* (2), CD000359.

Oren, D. A., Wisner, K. L., Spinelli, M., Epperson, C. N., Peindl, K. S., Terman, J. S., & Terman, M. (2002). An open trial of morning light therapy for treatment of antepartum depression. *American Journal of Psychiatry, 159*(4), 666-9.

Osher, Y., Bersudsky, Y., & Belmaker, R. H. (2005). Omega-3 eicosapentaenoic acid in bipolar depression: Report of a small open-label study. *Journal of Clinical Psychiatry, 66*(6), 726–729.

Otto, M. W., Church, T. S., Craft, L. L., Greer, T. L., Smits, J. A., & Trivedi, M. H. (2007). Exercise for mood and anxiety disorders. *Journal of Clinical Psychiatry, 68*(5), 669–676.

Overk, C. R., Yao, P., Chadwick, L. R., Nikolic, D., Sun, Y., Cuendet, M. A., Deng, Y. et al. (2005). Comparison of the in vitro estrogenic activities of compounds from hops (*Humulus lupulus*) and red clover (*Trifolium pratense*). *Journal of Agricultural and Food Chemistry, 53*(16), 6246–6253.

Overstreet, D. H., Rezvani, A. H., Cowen, M., Chen, F., & Lawrence, A. J. (2006). Modulation of high alcohol drinking in the inbred Fawn-Hooded (FH/Wjd) rat strain: Implications for treatment. *Addictive Biology, 11*(3–4), 356–373.

Owen, D. J., & Fang, M. L. (2003). Information-seeking behavior in complementary and alternative medicine (CAM): An online survey of faculty at a health sciences campus. *Journal of the Medical Library Association, 91*(3), 311–321.

Oz, M. (2004). Emerging role of integrative medicine in cardiovascular disease. *Cardiology Review, 12*(2), 120–123.

Packer, L., & Colman, C. (1999). *The antioxidant miracle.* New York: Wiley.

Pampallona, S., Bollini, P., Tibaldi, G., Kupelnick, B., & Munizza, C. (2004). Combined pharmacotherapy and psychological treatment for depression: A systematic review. *Archives of General Psychiatry, 61*(7), 714–719.

Pan, N. L., Brown, R. P., Gerbarg, P. L., Liao, F.-F. L. H.-P., Jiang, M.-J., & Huang A-M. (in process). Modulation of serum brain-derived neurotrophic factor and indices of depression after the Sudarshan Kriya Yoga courses and practices.

Pan, N.-L., Liao, F.-F., Jiang, M.-J., Wang, C.-L., & Huang, A.-M. (2006, February 22–24). Serum levels of brain-derived neurotrophic factor before and after the practice of pranayam and Sudarshan Kriya. In *Proceedings World Conference Expanding Paradigms: Science, consciousness and spirituality.* (pp. 156–168). New Delhi: All India Institute of Medical Sciences.

Pandi-Perumal, S. R., Zisapel, N., Srinivasan, V., & Cardinali, D. P. (2005). Melatonin and sleep in aging population. *Experimental Gerontology, 40*(12), 911–925.

Panjwani, U., Selvamurthy, W., Singh, S. H., Gupta, H. L., Thakur, L., & Rai, U. C. (1996). Effect of Sahaja yoga practice on seizure control & EEG changes in patients of epilepsy. *Indian Journal of Medical Research, 103*, 165–172.

Panossian, A., & Wagner, H. (2005). Stimulating effect of adaptogens: An overview with particular reference to their efficacy following single dose administration. *Phytotherapy Research, 19*(10), 819–838.

Pantoni, L. (2004). Treatment of vascular dementia: Evidence from trials with non-cholinergic drugs. *Journal of Neurological Science, 226*(1–2), 67–70.

Paparrigopoulos, T. J. (2005). REM sleep behaviour disorder: Clinical profiles and pathophysiology. *International Review of Psychiatry, 17*(4), 293–300.

Parker, G., Gibson, N. A., Brotchie, H., Heruc, G., Rees, A. M., & Hadzi-Pavlovic, D. (2006). Omega-3 fatty acids and mood disorders. *American Journal of Psychiatry, 163*(6), 969–978.

Parnetti, L., Mignini, F., Tomassoni, D., Traini, E., & Amenta, F. (2007). Cholinergic precursors in the treatment of cognitive impairment of vascular origin: Ineffective approaches or need for re-evaluation? *Journal of Neurological Science,* 257(1–2), 264–269.

Parry, B. L., Hauger, R., Lin, E., Le Veau, B., Mostofi, N., Clopton, P. L., & Gillin, J. C. (1994). Neuroendocrine effects of light therapy in late luteal phase dysphoric disorder. *Biological Psychiatry,* 36(6), 356–364.

Parry, B. L., Mahan, A. M., Mostofi, N., Klauber, M. R., Lew, G. S., & Gillin, J. C. (1993). Light therapy of late luteal phase dysphoric disorder: An extended study. *American Journal of Psychiatry,* 150(9), 1417–1419.

Patrick, L. R. (2007). Restless legs syndrome: Pathophysiology and the role of iron and folate. *Alternative Medicine Review.*

Paul, M. A., Brown, G., Buguet, A., Gray, G., Pigeau, R. A., Weinberg, H., & Radomski, M. (2001). Melatonin and zopiclone as pharmacologic aids to facilitate crew rest. *Aviation Space and Environmental Medicine,* 72(11), 974–984.

Pavia, J., Martos, F., Gonzalez-Correa, J. A., Garcia, A. J., Rius, F., Laukkonen, S. et al. (1997). Effect of S-adenosyl methionine on muscarinic receptors in young rats. *Life Sciences,* 60(11), 825–832.

Peet, M., Brind, J., Ramchand, C. N., Shah, S., & Vankar, G. K. (2001). Two double-blind placebo-controlled pilot studies of eicosapentaenoic acid in the treatment of schizophrenia. *Schizophrenia Research,* 49(3), 243–251.

Peet, M., & Horrobin, D. F. (2002). A dose-ranging exploratory study of the effects of ethyl-eicosapentaenoate in patients with persistent schizophrenic symptoms. *Journal of Psychiatic Research,* 36(1), 7–18.

Pek, G., Fulop, T., & Zs-Nagy, I. (1989). Gerontopsychological studies using NAI ("Nurnberger Alters-Inventar") on patients with organic psychosyndrome (DSM III, Category 1) treated with centrophenoxine in a double blind, comparative, randomized clinical trial. *Archives of Gerontology and Geriatrics,* 9(1), 17–30.

Peled, A. (2005). Plasticity imbalance in mental disorders the neuroscience of psychiatry: Implications for diagnosis and research. *Medical Hypotheses,* 65(5), 947–952.

Pelka, R. B., & Leuchtgens, H. (1995). Pre-Alzheimer study: Action of a herbal yeast preparation (Bio-Strath) in a randomised double-blind trial. *Ars Neducu,* 85(1).

Peniston, E. G., & Kulkosky, P. J. (1989). Alpha-theta brainwave training and beta-endorphin levels in alcoholics. *Alcoholism, Clinical and Experimental Research,* 13(2), 271–279.

Pepeu, G., Pepeu, I. M., & Amaducci, L. (1996). A review of phosphatidylserine pharmacological and clinical effects. Is phosphatidylserine a drug for the ageing brain? *Pharmacology Research,* 33(2), 73–80.

Petersen, T. J. (2006). Enhancing the efficacy of antidepressants with psychotherapy. *Journal of Psychopharmacology,* 20(Suppl. 3), 19–28.

Petkov, V. D., Yonkov, D., Mosharoff, A., Kambourova, T., Alova, L., Petkov, V. V. et al. (1986). Effects of alcohol aqueous extract from *Rhodiola rosea L.* roots on learning and memory. *Acta Physiologica et Pharmacologica Bulgarica, 12*(1), 3–16. (In Bulgarian)

Pettegrew, J. W., Levine, J., & McClure, R. J. (2000). Acetyl-L-carnitine physical-chemical, metabolic, and therapeutic properties: Relevance for its mode of action in Alzheimer's disease and geriatric depression. *Molecular Psychiatry, 5*(6), 616–632.

Pezzoli, C., Galli-Kienle, M., & Stramentinoli, G. (1987). Lack of mutagenic activity of ademetionine in vitro and in vivo. *Arzneimittelforschung, 37*(7), 826–829.

Philipp, M., Kohnen, R., & Hiller, K. O. (1999). Hypericum extract versus imipramine or placebo in patients with moderate depression: Randomised multicentre study of treatment for eight weeks. *BMJ, 319*(7224), 1534–1538.

Philippot, P., Gaetane, C., & Blairy, S. (2002). Respiratory feedback in the generation of emotion. *Cognition and Emotion, 16*(5), 605–607.

Piersen, C. E. (2003). Phytoestrogens in botanical dietary supplements: Implications for cancer. *Integrated Cancer Therapy, 2*(2), 120–138.

Pilkington, K., Kirkwood, G., Rampes, H., Fisher, P., & Richardson, J. (2005). Homeopathy for depression: A systematic review of the research evidence. *Homeopathy, 94*(3), 153–163.

Pilkington, K., Kirkwood, G., Rampes, H., & Richardson, J. (2005). Yoga for depression: The research evidence. *Journal of Affective Disorders, 89*(1–3), 13–24.

Pilkington, K., Kirkwood, G., Rampes, H., Fisher, P., & Richardson, J. (2006). Homeopathy for anxiety and anxiety disorders: a systematic review of the research. *Homeopathy, 95*(3), 151–162.

Pittler, M. H., & Ernst, E. (2000). Efficacy of kava extract for treating anxiety: Systematic review and meta-analysis. *Journal of Clinical Psychopharmacology, 20*(1), 84–89.

Polan, M. L., Hochberg, R. B., Trant, A. S., & Wuh, H. C. (2004). Estrogen bioassay of ginseng extract and ArginMax, a nutritional supplement for the enhancement of female sexual function. *Journal of Women's Health (Larchmont), 13*(4), 427–430.

Polyakov, V. V. (1966). The use of a new phytoadaptogen under conditions of space flight. (Abstract) presented at symposium, Adaptogens: A New group of Pharmacogicially Active Substances which Increase the Nonspecific Resistance of the organism, Gothenberg, Sweden, Nov 4–5, 1966.

Porges, S. W. (2001). The polyvagal theory: Phylogenetic substrates of a social nervous system. *International Journal of Psychophysiology, 42*(2), 123–146.

Praschak-Rieder, N., Willeit, M., Neumeister, A., Hilger, E., Stastny, J., Thierry, N. et al. (2001). Prevalence of premenstrual dysphoric disorder in female patients with seasonal affective disorder. *Journal of Affective Disorders, 63*(1–3), 239–242.

Prathikanti, S. (2007). Ayurvedic treatments. In J. Lake & D. Spiegel (Eds.), *Complementary and alternative treatments* (pp. 225–272). Washington, DC: American Psychiatric Publishing.

Procter, A. (1991). Enhancement of recovery from psychiatric illness by methylfolate. *British Journal of Psychiatry, 159*, 271–272.

Pynoos, R. S., Frederick, C., Nader, K., Arroyo, W., Steinberg, A., Eth, S., Nonez, F.,

& Fairbanks, L. (1987). Life threat and posttraumatic stress in school-age children. *Arch Gen Psychiatry, 44*(12), 1057–63.

Quiros, C. F., & Cardenas, R. A. (1997). Maca (*Lepidium meyenii Walp*). In M. Herman & J. Heller (Eds.), *Promoting the conservation and use of underutilized and neglected crops: Vol. 21. Andean roots and tubers: Ahipa, arricacha, maco, yacon* (pp. 184–185). Rome, Italy: Institute of Plant Genetics and Crop Plant Research, Gatersleben/ International Plant Resources Institute.

Rabkin, J. G., McElhiney, M. C., Rabkin, R., McGrath, P. J., & Ferrando, S. J. (2006). Placebo-controlled trial of dehydroepiandrosterone (DHEA) for treatment of nonmajor depression in patients with HIV/AIDS. *American Journal of Psychiatry, 163*(1), 59–66.

Radad, K., Gille, G., Liu, L., & Rausch, W. D. (2006). Use of ginseng in medicine with emphasis on neurodegenerative disorders. *Journal of Pharmacological Science, 100*(3), 175–186.

Raghuraj, P., Ramakrishnan, A. G., Nagendra, H. R., & Telles, S. (1998). Effect of two selected yogic breathing techniques of heart rate variability. *Indian Journal of Physiology and Pharmacology, 42*(4), 467–472.

Rai, D., Bhatia, G., Palit, G., Pal, R., Singh, S., & Singh, H. K. (2003). Adaptogenic effect of *Bacopa monniera* (Brahmi). *Pharmacology and Biochemistry of Behavior, 75*(4), 823–830.

Ramarao, P. , Rao, K. T., Srivastava, R. S., & Ghosal, S. (1995). Effects of glycowithanolides from Withania somnifera on morphine-induced inhibition of intestinal motility and tolerance to analgesia in mice. *Phytotherapy Research, 9,* 66–68.

Ramaratnam, S., & Sridharan, K. (2000). Yoga for epilepsy. *Cochrane Database System Review,* (3), CD001524.

Ramassamy, C. (2006). Emerging role of polyphenolic compounds in the treatment of neurodegenerative diseases: a review of their intracellular targets. *European Journal of Pharmacology, 545*(1), 51–64.

Ramirez, P. M., Desantis, D., & Opler, L. A. (2001). EEG biofeedback treatment of ADD. A viable alternative to traditional medical intervention? *Annals of New York Academy of Sciences, 931,* 342–358.

Rao, A. M., Hatcher, J. F., & Dempsey, R. J. (1999). CDP-choline: Neuroprotection in transient forebrain ischemia of gerbils. *Journal of Neuroscience Research, 58*(5), 697–705.

Raskin, M., Bali, L. R., & Peeke, H. V. (1980). Muscle biofeedback and transcendental meditation. A controlled evaluation of efficacy in the treatment of chronic anxiety. *Archives of General Psychiatry, 37*(1), 93–97.

Raskind, M. A., Burke, B. L., Crites, N. J., Tapp, A. M., & Rasmussen, D. D. (2007). Olanzapine-induced weight gain and increased visceral adiposity is blocked by melatonin replacement therapy in rats. *Neuropsychopharmacology, 32*(2), 284–288.

Raskind, M. A., Peskind, E. R., Wessel, T., & Yuan, W. (2000). Galantamine in AD: A 6-month randomized, placebo-controlled trial with a 6-month extension. The Galantamine USA-1 Study Group. *Neurology, 54*(12), 2261–2268.

Rasmusson, A. M., Vasek, J., Lipschitz, D. S., Vojvoda, D., Mustone, M. E., Shi, Q. et al. (2004). An increased capacity for adrenal DHEA release is associated with decreased avoidance and negative mood symptoms in women with PTSD. *Neuropsychopharmacology,* 29(8), 1546–1557.

Raus, K., Brucker, C., Gorkow, C., & Wuttke, W. (2006). First-time proof of endometrial safety of the special black cohosh extract (*Actaea* or *Cimicifuga racemosa* extract) CR BNO 1055. *Menopause, 13*(4), 678–691.

Razina, T. G., Zueva, E. P., Amosova, E. N., & Krylova, S. G. (2000). Medicinal plant preparations used as adjuvant therapeutics in experimental oncology. *Eksp Klin Farmakol, 63*(5), 59–61. (In Russian)

Reay, J. L., Kennedy, D. O., & Scholey, A. B. (2006). Effects of Panax ginseng, consumed with and without glucose, on blood glucose levels and cognitive performance during sustained "mentally demanding" tasks. *Journal of Psychopharmacology, 20*(6), 771–781.

Rego, A. C., Santos, M. S., & Oliveira, C. R. (1999). Influence of the antioxidants vitamin E and idebenone on retinal cell injury mediated by chemical ischemia, hypoglycemia, or oxidative stress. *Free Radical Biological Medicine, 26*(11–12), 1405–1417.

Reiter, W. J., Schatzl, G., Mark, I., Zeiner, A., Pycha, A., & Marberger, M. (2001). Dehydroepiandrosterone in the treatment of erectile dysfunction in patients with different organic etiologies. *Urology Research, 29*(4), 278–281.

Richardson, A. J. (2006). Omega-3 fatty acids in ADHD and related neurodevelopmental disorders. *International Review Psychiatry, 18*(2), 155–172.

Ridenour, T., Ferrer-Wreder, L., & Gottschall, A. Exploratory factor analysis of the ALEXSA: A measure for evidence based prevention in school. (In review).

Robbers, J. E., & Tyler, V. E. (1999). *Tyler's herbs of choice: The therapeutic use of herbal medicinals.* New York: Hawthorne Herbal Press.

Robbins, J. (2000). *A symphony in the brain: The evolution of the new brain wave biofeedback.* New York: Atlantic Monthly Press.

Roemheld-Hamm, B. (2005). Chasteberry. *American Family Physician, 72*(5), 821–824.

Rohdewald, P. (2002). A review of the French maritime pine bark extract (Pycnogenol), a herbal medication with a diverse clinical pharmacology. *International Journal of Clinical Pharmacological Therapy, 40*(4), 158–168.

Roodenrys, S., Booth, D., Bulzomi, S., Phipps, A., Micallef, C., & Smoker, J. (2002). Chronic effects of Brahmi (*Bacopa monnieri*) on human memory. *Neuropsychopharmacology, 27*(2), 279–281.

Rosadini, G., Marenco, S., Nobili, F., Novellone, G., & Rodriguez, G. (1990). Acute effects of acetyl-L-carnitine on regional cerebral blood flow in patients with brain ischaemia. *International Journal of Clinical Pharmacological Research, 10*(1–2), 123–128.

Roseff, S. J. (2002). Improvement in sperm quality and function with French maritime pine tree bark extract. *Journal of Reproductive Medicine, 47*(10), 821–824.

Rosenberg, M., Schooler, C., & Schoenbach, C. (1989). Self-esteem and adolescent problems: Modeling reciprocal effects. *American Sociological Review*, 54(6), 1004–1018.

Rosenthal, D. A., Gurney, R. M., & Moore, S. M. (1981). From trust on intimacy: A new inventory for examining Erikson's stages of psychosocial development. *Journal of Youth and Adolescence, 10*(6), 525–537.

Rowland, D. L., & Tai, W. (2003). A review of plant-derived and herbal approaches to the treatment of sexual dysfunctions. *Journal of Sex and Marital Therapy, 29*(3), 185–205.

Ruiz-Luna, A. C., Salazar, S., Aspajo, N. J., Rubio, J., Gasco, M., & Gonzales, G. F. (2005). *Lepidium meyenii* (Maca) increases litter size in normal adult female mice. *Reproductive Bioliological Endocrinology, 3*, 16.

Russello, D., Randazzo, G., Favetta, A., Cristaldi, C., Petino, A. G., Carnazzo, S. A., & Latteri, F. (1990). Oxiracetam treatment of exogenous post-concussion syndrome. Statistical evaluation of results. *Minerva Chirurgica, 45*(20), 1309–1314.

Safarinejad, M. R. (2005). *Urtica dioica* for treatment of benign prostatic hyperplasia: A prospective, randomized, double-blind, placebo-controlled, crossover study. *Journal of Herb Pharmacotherapy, 5*(4), 1–11.

Sageman, S. (2002). Women with PTSD: The psychodynamic aspects of psychopharmacologic and "hands-on" psychiatric management. *Journal of the American Academy of Psychoanalysis, 30*(3), 415–427.

Sageman, S. (2004). Breaking through the despair: Spiritually oriented group therapy as a means of healing women with severe mental illness. *Journal of the American Academy of Psychoanalysis and Dynamic Psychiatry, 32*(1), 125–141.

Sageman, S., & Brown, R. P. (2006a). 3-acetyl-7-oxo-dehydroepiandrosterone for healing treatment-resistant posttraumatic stress disorder in women: 5 case reports. *Journal of Clinical Psychiatry, 67*(3), 493–496.

Sageman, S., & Brown, R. P. (2006b). Free at last: Natural and conventional treatment of a patient with multiple comorbid psychiatric disorders. In R. L. Spitzer, M. B. First, & B. W. Williams (Eds.), *DSM-IV-TR casebook* (Vol. 2, pp. 109–121). Washington, DC: American Psychiatric Publishing.

Sakai, M., Yamatoya, H., & Kudo, S. (1996). Pharmacological effects of phosphatidylserine enzymatically synthesized from soybean lecithin on brain functions in rodents. *J Nutr Sci Vitaminol (Tokyo), 42*(1), 47–54.

Salem, N., Jr. (1989). Omega-3-fatty acids: molecular and chemical aspects. In G. A. Spiller, & L. Scala (Eds.), *New roles for selective nutrients* (pp. 109–228). New York: Alan R. Liss.

Salem, N. Jr. , Kim, N. Y., & Yergey, J. A. (1986). Docosohexanoic acid: Membrane function and metabolism. In A. Simopoulos, R. R. Kifer, & R. Martin (Eds.), *Health effects of polyunsaturated seafoods* (Vol. 15, pp. 263–317). New York: Academic Press.

Saletu, B., Grunberger, J., Linzmayer, L., & Anderer, P. (1990). Brain protection of nicergoline against hypoxia: EEG brain mapping and psychometry. *Journal of Neural Transmission. Parkinson's Disease and Dementia Section (Vienna), 2*(4), 305–325. (In German)

Sano, M. (2003). Noncholinergic treatment options for Alzheimer's disease. *Journal of Clinical Psychiatry, 64* (Suppl. 9), 23–28.

Saratikov, A. S., & Krasnov, E. A. (1987a). Stimulative properties of *Rhodiola rosea*. In A. S. Saratikov & E. A. Krasnov (Eds.), *Rhodiola rosea is a valuable medicinal plant (golden root)* (pp. 69–90). Tomsk, Russia: Tomsk State University. (In Russian)

Saratikov, A. S., & Krasnov, E. A. (1987b). The influence of *Rhodiola* on endocrine glands and the liver. In A. S. Saratikov & E. A. Krasnov (Eds.), *Rhodiola rosea is a valuable medicinal plant (golden root)* (pp. 180–193). Tomsk, Russia: Tomsk State University. (In Russian)

Saratikov, A. S., & Krasnov, E. A. (1987c). Clinical studies of *Rhodiola rosea*. In A. S. Saratikov & E. A. Krasnov (Eds.), *Rhodiola rosea is a valuable medicinal plant (golden root)* (pp. 216–227). Tomsk, Russia: Tomsk State University.

Satyanarayana, M., Rajeswari, K. R., Rani, N. J., Krishna, C. S., & Rao, P. V. (1992). Effect of Santhi Kriya on certain psychophysiological parameters: A preliminary study. *Indian Journal of Physiology and Pharmacology, 36*(2), 88–92.

Saxon, D. W., & Hopkins, D. A. (2006). Ultrastructure and synaptology of the paratrigeminal nucleus in the rat: primary pharyngeal and laryngeal afferent projections. *Synapse, 59*(4), 220–234.

Sayegh, R., Schiff, I., Wurtman, J., Spiers, P., McDermott, J., & Wurtman, R. (1995). The effect of a carbohydrate-rich beverage on mood, appetite, and cognitive function in women with premenstrual syndrome. *Obstetrics and Gynecology, 86*(4 Pt 1), 520–528.

Scarmeas, N., Stern, Y., Tang, M. X., Mayeux, R., & Luchsinger, J. A. (2006). Mediterranean diet and risk for Alzheimer's disease. *Annals of Neurology, 59*(6), 912–921.

Schaenfield, D. (in process). Youth empowerment seminar: Effects on students from three high schools. Manuscript in preparation.

Schaller, J. L., Thomas, J., & Bazzan, A. J. (2004). SAMe use in children and adolescents. *European Child and Adolescent Psychiatry, 13*(5), 332–334.

Schellenberg, R. (2001). Treatment for the premenstrual syndrome with agnus castus fruit extract: Prospective, randomised, placebo controlled study. *BMJ, 322*(7279), 134–347.

Schenck, C. H., Bundlie, S. R., Ettinger, M. G., & Mahowald, M. W. (1986). Chronic behavioral disorders of human REM sleep: A new category of parasomnia. *Sleep, 9*(2), 293–308.

Schiff, B. B., & Rump, S. A. (1995). Asymmetrical hemispheric activation and emotion: The effects of unilateral forced nostril breathing. *Brain and Cognition, 29*(3), 217–231.

Schmidt, P. J., Daly, R. C., Bloch, M., Smith, M. J., Danaceau, M. A., St. Clair, L. S. et al. (2005). Dehydroepiandrosterone monotherapy in midlife-onset major and minor depression. *Archives of General Psychiatry, 62*(2), 154–162.

Schneider, F., Popa, R., Mihalas, G., Stefaniga, P., Mihalas, I. G., Maties, R et al.

(1994). Superiority of antagonic-stress composition versus nicergoline in gerontopsychiatry. *Annals of the New York Academy of Sciences, 717,* 332–342.

Schoenberger, N. E., Shif, S. C., Esty, M. L., Ochs, L., & Matheis, R. J. (2001). Flexyx neurotherapy system in the treatment of traumatic brain injury: An initial evaluation. *Journal of Head Trauma Rehabilitation, 16*(3), 260–274.

Schoenthaler, S. J., & Bier, I. D. (1999). Vitamin-mineral intake and intelligence: A macrolevel analysis of randomized controlled trials. *Journal of Alternative and Complementary Medicine, 5*(2), 125–134.

Schouten, J. W. (2007). Neuroprotection in traumatic brain injury: A complex struggle against the biology of nature. *Current Opinion in Critical Care, 13*(2), 134–142.

Schrader, E. (2000). Equivalence of St John's wort extract (Ze 117) and fluoxetine: A randomized, controlled study in mild-moderate depression. *International Clinical Psychopharmacology, 15*(2), 61–68.

Schumacher, K., Schneider, B., Reich, G., Stiefel, T., Stoll, G., Bock, P. R. et al. (2003). Influence of postoperative complementary treatment with lectin-standardized mistletoe extract on breast cancer patients. A controlled epidemiological multicentric retrolective cohort study. *Anticancer Research, 23*(6D), 5081–5087.

Schwarzenbach, F. H., & Brunner, K. W. (1996). Effects of a herbal yeast preparation in convalescent patients. *Schweizerische Zeitschrift Ganzheits Medizin,* 226–273. (In German)

Scott, J. (1997). Yoga and schizophrenia. *Yoga Magazine.* http://yogamagazine.net/archives/1997/3Sep97/shrm/. Updated Sept 1997. Accessed Aug 2007.

Scott, R., MacPherson, A., Yates, R. W., Hussain, B., & Dixon, J. (1998). The effect of oral selenium supplementation on human sperm motility. *British Journal of Urology, 82*(1), 76–80.

Scripnikov, A., Khomenko, A., & Napryeyenko, O. (2007). Effects of *Ginkgo biloba* extract EGb 761 on neuropsychiatric symptoms of dementia: Findings from a randomised controlled trial. *Wien Medizin Wochenschrift, 157*(13–14), 295–300. (In German)

Shaffer, H. J., LaSalvia, T. A., & Stein, J. P. (1997). Comparing Hatha yoga with dynamic group psychotherapy for enhancing methadone maintenance treatment: A randomized clinical trial. *Alternative Therapeutic Health Medicine, 3*(4), 57–66.

Shamir, E., Barak, Y., Shalman, I., Laudon, M., Zisapel, N., Tarrasch, R. et al. (2001). Melatonin treatment for tardive dyskinesia: A double-blind, placebo-controlled, crossover study. *Archives of General Psychiatry, 58*(11), 1049–1052.

Shamir, E., Laudon, M., Barak, Y., Anis, Y., Rotenberg, V., Elizur, A., & Zisapel, N. (2000). Melatonin improves sleep quality of patients with chronic schizophrenia. *Journal of Clinical Psychiatry, 61*(5), 373–377.

Shannahoff-Khalsa, D. S. (2003). Kundalini yoga meditation techniques for the treatment of obsessive-compulsive and OC spectrum disorders. *Grief Treatment and Crisis Intervention, 3*(3), 369–382.

Shannahoff-Khalsa, D. S. (2006a). A perspective on the emergence of meditation techniques for medical disorders. *Journal of Alternative and Complementary Medicine, 12*(8), 709–713.

Shannahoff-Khalsa, D. S. (2006b). *Kundalini yoga meditation.* New York: W. W. Norton.

Shannahoff-Khalsa, D. S. (2007). Selective unilateral autonomic activation: Implications for psychiatry. *CNS Spectrum, 12*(8), 625–634.

Shannahoff-Khalsa, D. S., Ray, L. E., Levine, S. et al. (1999). Randomized controlled trial of yogic meditation techniques for patients with obsessive-compulsive disorder. *CNS Spectrums, 4*(12), 34–47.

Shapiro, D., Cook, I. A., Davydov, D. M., Ottaviani, C., Leuchter, A. F., & Abrams, M. (2007) *Yoga as a complementary treatment of depression: Effects of traits and moods on treatment outcome.* Oxford: Oxford University Press.

Sharma, H., Aggarwal, D., Sen, S., Singh, A., Kochupillai, V., & Singh, N. (2002). Effects of Sudarshan Kriya on antioxidant status and blood lactate level. In *"Science of breath": International symposium on sudarshan kriya, pranayam and consciousness .* New Delhi: All India Institute of Medical Sciences.

Sharma, R., Chaturvedi, C., & Tewari, P. V. (1987). Efficacy of Bacopa monnieri in revitalizing intellectual functions in children. *Journal of Research Education in Indian Medicine,* (1–12).

Sharma, H. M,. Hanna, A. N., Kauffman, E. M., Newman, H. A. (1995). Effect of herbal mixture student Rasayana on lipoxygenase activity and lipid peroxidation. *Free Radic Biolology and Medicine, 18*(4): 687–97.

Shebek, J., & Rindone, J. P. (2000). A pilot study exploring the effect of kudzu root on the drinking habits of patients with chronic alcoholism. *Journal of Alternative and Complementary Medicine, 6*(1), 45–48.

Shekim, W. O., Antun, F., Hanna, G. L., McCracken, J. T., & Hess, E. B. (1990). S-adenosyl-L-methionine (SAM) in adults with ADHD, residual state: Preliminary results from an open trial. *Psychopharmacology Bulletin, 26*(2), 249–253.

Shelton, R. C., Keller, M. B., Gelenberg, A., Dunner, D. L., Hirschfeld, R., Thase, M. E., et al. (2001). Effectiveness of St John's Wort in major depression: A randomized controlled trial. *Journal of the American Medical Association, 285*(15), 1978–1986.

Shen, Y. C., & Wang, Y. F. (1984). Urinary 3-methoxy-4-hydroxyphenylglycol sulfate excretion in seventy-three schoolchildren with minimal brain dysfunction syndrome. *Biological Psychiatry, 19*(6), 861–870.

Shevtsov, V. A., Zholus, B. I., Shervarly, V. I., Vol'skij, V. B., Korovin, Y. P., Khristich, M. P. et al. (2003). A randomized trial of two different doses of a SHR-5 *Rhodiola rosea* extract versus placebo and control of capacity for mental work. *Phytomedicine, 10*(2-3), 95–105.

Shippy, A. (2004). HIV and aging. *Positive Aware, 15*(5), 38–41.

Shippy, R. A., Mendez, D., Jones, K., Cergnul, I., & Karpiak, S. E. (2004). S-adenosylmethionine (SAMe) for the treatment of depression in people living with HIV/AIDS. *BMC Psychiatry, 4,* 38.

Shnayder, N. A., Agarkova, N. O., Liouliakina, E. G., Naumova, E. B., & Shnayer, V. A.

(2006). *The biolelectrical brain activity in humans who practiced Sudarshan Kriya.* Presented at the World Conference Expanding Paradigms: Science, consciousness & spirituality. New Delhi, India: All India Insitute of Medical Sciences.

Silver, J. M., McAllistar, T. W., & Yudofsky, S. C. (2005). Psychopharmacology. In J. M. Silver, D. B. Arciniegas, & S. C. Yudofsky (Eds.), *Textbook of traumatic brain injury* (pp. 624–626). Washington, DC: American Psychiatric Press.

Simone, N. L., Simone, V., & Simone, C. B. (2007a). Antioxidants and other nutrients do not interfere with chemotherapy or radiation therapy and can increase kill and increase survival, Part 1. *Alternative Therapies in Health and Medicine, 13*(1): 22–8.

Simone, N. L., Simone, V., & Simone, C. B. (2007b). Antioxidants and other nutrients do not interfere with chemotherapy or radiation therapy and can increase kill and increase survival, Part 2. *Alternative Therapies in Health and Medicine, 13*(2): 40–7.

Simons, A. J., Dawson, I. K., & Duguma, B. (1998). Passing problems, prostate and prunus. *Herbalgram, 43,* 49–53.

Singh, Y. N., & Blumenthal, M. (1996). Kava: an overview. *Herbalgram, Special Review, 39,* 33–55.

Sitges, M., Chiu, L. M., Guarneros, A., & Nekrassov, V. (2007). Effects of carbamazepine, phenytoin, lamotrigine, oxcarbazepine, topiramate and vinpocetine on Na+ channel-mediated release of. *Neuropharmacology, 52*(2), 598–605.

Sivrioglu, E. Y., Kirli, S., Sipahioglu, D., Gursoy, B., & Sarandol, E. (2007). The impact of omega-3 fatty acids, vitamins E and C supplementation on treatment outcome and side effects in schizophrenia patients treated with haloperidol: An open-label pilot study. *Progress in Neuropsychopharmacology and Biological Psychiatry, 31*(7), 1493–1499.

Smits, M. G., Nagtegaal, E. E., van der Heijden, J., Coenen, A. M., & Kerkhof, G. A. (2001). Melatonin for chronic sleep onset insomnia in children: A randomized placebo-controlled trial. *Journal of Child Neurology, 16*(2), 86–92.

Soderberg, M., Edlund, C., Kristensson, K., & Dallner, G. (1991). Fatty acid composition of brain phospholipids in Soffa, V. M. (1996). Alternatives to hormone replacement. *Alternative Therapies, 2*(2), 34–39.

Sohn, M., & Sikora, R. (1991). *Ginkgo biloba* extract in the therapy of erectile dysfunction. *Journal of Sex Education Therapy, 17,* 53–61.

Sokeland, J., & Albrecht, J. (1997). Combination of *Sabal* and *Urtica* extract vs. finasteride in benign prostatic hyperplasia (Aiken stages I to II). Comparison of therapeutic effectiveness in a one year double-blind study. *Urologe Ausgabe A, 36*(4), 327–333.

Song, H. S., & Lehrer, P. M. (2003). The effects of specific respiratory rates on heart rate and heart rate variability. *Applied Psychophysiology and Biofeedback, 28*(1), 13–23.

Sood, A., Barton, D. L., Bauer, B. A., & Loprinzi, C. L. (2007). A critical review of complementary therapies for cancer-related fatigue. *Integrated Cancer Therapy, 6*(1), 8–13.

Sorensen, H., & Sonne, J. (1996). A double-masked study of the effects of ginseng on cognitive functions. *Current Therapy Research, 57*(12), 959–968.

Sota, M., Allegri, C., Cortesi, M., Barale, F., Politi, P., & Fusar-Poli, P. (2007). Targeting the effects of omega-3 and omega-6 fatty acid supplementation on schizophrenic spectrum disorders: Role of neuroimaging. *Medical Hypotheses, 69*(2): 466–7.

Sotaniemi, E. A., Haapakoski, E., & Rautio, A. (1995). Ginseng therapy in non-insulin-dependent diabetic patients. *Diabetes Care, 18*(10), 1373–1375.

Spasov, A. A., Mandrikov, V. B., & Mironova, I. A. (2000). The effect of the preparation rodakson on the psychophysiological and physical adaptation of students to an academic load. *Eksp Klin Farmakol, 63*(1), 76–78. (In Russian)

Spasov, A. A., Wikman, G. K., Mandrikov, V. B., Mironova, I. A., & Neumoin, V. V. (2000). A double-blind, placebo-controlled pilot study of the stimulating and adaptogenic effect of *Rhodiola rosea* SHR-5 extract on the fatigue of students caused by stress during an examination period with a repeated low-dose regimen. *Phytomedicine, 7*(2), 85–89.

Speca, M., Carlson, L. E., Goodey, E., & Angen, M. (2000). A randomized, wait-list controlled clinical trial: The effect of a mindfulness meditation-based stress reduction program on mood and symptoms of stress in cancer outpatients. *Psychosomatic Medicine, 62*(5), 613–622.

Spiegel, A. D. (1988). Temporary insanity and premenstrual syndrome: Medical testimony in an 1865 murder trial. *New York State Journal of Medicine, 88*(9), 482–492.

Srinivasan, V., Pandi-Perumal, S., Cardinali, D., Poeggeler, B., & Hardeland, R. (2006). Melatonin in Alzheimer's disease and other neurodegenerative disorders. *Behavior and Brain Function, 2*(1), 15.

Srinivasan, V., Pandi-Perumal, S. R., Maestroni, G. J., Esquifino, A. I., Hardeland, R., & Cardinali, D. P. (2005). Role of melatonin in neurodegenerative diseases. *Neurotoxicology Research, 7*(4), 293–318.

Stancheva, S. L., & Mosharrof, A. (1987). Effect of the extract of *rhodiola rosea L.* on the content of the brain biogenic monoamines. *Medecine Physiologie Comptes Rendus De L'Academie Bulgare Des Sciences, 40*(6), 85–87.

Stanislavov, R., & Nikolova, V. (2003). Treatment of erectile dysfunction with pycnogenol and L-arginine. *Journal of Sex and Marital Therapy, 29*(3), 207–213.

Stein, E., & Hunter, C. (2004). To exercise or not to exercise in chronic fatigue syndrome? *Medical Journal of Australia, 181*(10), 579. author reply 579-80.

Steinberg, S., Annable, L., Young, S. N., & Liyanage, N. (1999). A placebo-controlled clinical trial of L-tryptophan in premenstrual dysphoria. *Biological Psychiatry, 45*(3), 313–320.

Sterman, M. B., & Macdonald, L. R. (1978). Effects of central cortical EEG feedback training on incidence of poorly controlled seizures. *Epilepsia, 19*(3), 207–222.

Stevinson, C., & Ernst, E. (1999). Hypericum for depression. An update of the clinical evidence. *European Neuropsychopharmacology, 9*(6), 501–505.

Stevinson, C., & Ernst, E. (2000). Valerian for insomnia: A systematic review of randomized clinical trials. *Sleep Medicine, 1*(2), 91–99.

Stoddard, J. L., Dent, C. W., Shames, L., & Bernstein, L. (2007). Exercise training effects on premenstrual distress and ovarian steroid hormones. *European Journal of Applied Physiology, 99*(1), 27–37.

Stoll, A. L., Sachs, G. S., Cohen, B. M., Lafer, B., Christensen, J. D., & Renshaw, P. F. (1996). Choline in the treatment of rapid-cycling bipolar disorder: Clinical and neurochemical findings in lithium-treated patients. *Biological Psychiatry, 40*(5), 382–388.

Stoll, A. L., Severus, W. E., Freeman, M. P., Rueter, S., Zboyan, H. A., Diamond, E. et al. (1999). Omega 3 fatty acids in bipolar disorder: A preliminary double-blind, placebo-controlled trial. *Archives of General Psychiatry, 56*(5), 407–412.

Stough, C., Lloyd, J., Clarke, J., Downey, L. A., Hutchison, C. W., Rodgers, T., & Nathan, P. J. (2001). The chronic effects of an extract of *Bacopa monniera* (Brahmi) on cognitive function in healthy human subjects. *Psychopharmacology (Berlin), 156*(4), 481–484. (In German)

Strous, R. D. (2005). Dehydroepiandrosterone (DHEA) augmentation in the management of schizophrenia symptomatology. *Essential Psychopharmacology, 6*(3), 141–147.

Strous, R. D., Maayan, R., Kotler, M., & Weizman, A. (2005). Hormonal profile effects following dehydroepiandrosterone (DHEA) administration to schizophrenic patients. *Clinical Neuropharmacology, 28*(6), 265–269.

Strous, R. D., Maayan, R., Lapidus, R., Stryjer, R., Lustig, M., Kotler, M. et al.(2003). Dehydroepiandrosterone augmentation in the management of negative, depressive, and anxiety symptoms in schizophrenia. *Archives of General Psychiatry, 60*(2), 133–141.

Strous, R. D., Stryjer, R., Maayan, R., Gal, G., Viglin, D., Katz, E. et al. (2007). Analysis of clinical symptomatology, extrapyramidal symptoms and neurocognitive dysfunction following dehydroepiandrosterone (DHEA) administration in olanzapine treated schizophrenia patients: A randomized, double-blind placebo controlled trial. *Psychoneuroendocrinology, 32*(2), 96–105.

Stukin, S. (2001). Health, Hope and HIV yoga journal [Electronic version]. Retrieved on September 20, 2007 from www.iayt.org/site/publications/ aids.pdf. n.p.

Su, K. P., Huang, S. Y., Chiu, C. C., & Shen, W. W. (2003). Omega-3 fatty acids in major depressive disorder. A preliminary double-blind, placebo-controlled trial. *European Neuropsychopharmacology, 13*(4), 267–271.

Sublette, M. E., Hibbeln, J. R., Galfalvy, H., Oquendo, M. A., & Mann, J. J. (2006). Omega-3 polyunsaturated essential fatty acid status as a predictor of future suicide risk. *American Journal of Psychiatry, 163*(6), 1100–1102.

Suhner, A., Schlagenhauf, P., Johnson, R., Tschopp, A., & Steffen, R. (1998). Comparative study to determine the optimal melatonin dosage form for the alleviation of jet lag. *Chronobiology International, 15*(6), 655–666.

Sun, Y., Wang, Y., Qu, X., Wang, J., Fang, J., & Zhang, L. (1994). Clinical observation and treatment of hyperkinesia in children by traditional Chinese medicine. *Journal of Traditional Chinese Medicine, 14*(2), 105–109.

Surtees, R., & Hyland, K. (1989). A method for the measurement of S-adenosylmethionine in small volume samples of cerebrospinal fluid or brain using high-performance liquid chromatography-electrochemistry. *Annals of Biochemistry, 181*(2), 331–335.

Suzuki, S., Furushiro, M., Takahashi, M., Sakai, M., & Kudo, S. (1999). Oral administration of osybean lecithin transphosphatidylated phosphatidylserine (SB-tPS) reduces ischemic damage in the gerbil hippocampus. *Japanese Journal of Pharmacology, 81*(2), 237–9.

Suzuki, S., Kataoka, A., & Furushiro, M. (2000). Effect of intracerebroventricular administration of soybean lecithin transphosphatidylated phosphatidylserine on scopolamine-induced amnesic mice. *Japanese Journal of Pharmacology, 84*(1), 86–8.

Suzuki, S., Yamatoya, H., Sakai, M., Kataoka, A., Furushiro, M., & Kudo, S. (2001). Oral administration of soybean lecithin transphosphatidylated phosphatidylserine improves memory impairment in aged rats. *Journal of Nutrition, 131*(11), 2951–6.

Szalma, I., Kiss, A., Kardos, L., Horvath, G., Nyitrai, E., Tordai, Z., & Csiba, L. (2006). Piracetam prevents cognitive decline in coronary artery bypass: A randomized trial versus placebo. *Annals of Thoracic Surgery, 82*(4), 1430–1435.

Szegedi, A., Kohnen, R., Dienel, A., & Kieser, M. (2005). Acute treatment of moderate to severe depression with *hypericum* extract WS 5570 (St John's Wort): Randomised controlled double blind non-inferiority trial versus paroxetine. *BMJ, 330*(7490), 503.

Tai chi gives immune system a boost. (2007). *Harvard Health Letter, 32*(8), 7.

Takahashi, J., Nishino, H., & Ono, T. (1986). Effect of S-adenosyl-L-methionine (SAMe) on disturbances in hand movement and delayed response tasks after lesion of motor or prefrontal cortex in the monkey. *Nippon Yakurigaku Zasshi, 87*(5), 507–519.

Takahashi, J., Nishino, H., & Ono, T. (1987). S-adenosyl-L-methionine facilitates recovery from deficits in delayed response and hand movement tasks following brain lesions in monkeys. *Experimental Neurology, 98*(3), 459–471.

Tallal, P., Chase, C., Russell, G., & Schmitt, R. L. (1986). Evaluation of the efficacy of *piracetam* in treating information processing, reading and writing disorders in dyslexic children. *International Journal of Psychophysiology, 4*(1), 41–52.

Tamsulosin for benign prostatic hyperplasia. (1997). *Medical Letter on Drugs and Therapeutics, 39*(1011), 96.

Taneja, I., Deepak, K. K., Poojary, G., Acharya, I. N., Pandey, R. M., & Sharma, M. P. (2004). Yogic versus conventional treatment in diarrhea-predominant irritable bowel syndrome: A randomized control study. *Applied Psychophysiology and Biofeedback, 29*(1), 19–33.

Tang, X. C. (1996). Huperzine A (shuangyiping): A promising drug for Alzheimer's disease. *Zhongguo Yao Li Xue Bao, 17*(6), 481–484. (In Chinese)

Tariot, P. N., Solomon, P. R., Morris, J. C., Kershaw, P., Lilienfeld, S., & Ding, C. (2000). A 5-month, randomized, placebo-controlled trial of galantamine in AD. The Galantamine USA-10 Study Group. *Neurology*, 54(12), 2269–2276.

Tavoni, A., Jeracitano, G., & Cirigliano, G. (1998). Evaluation of S-adenosylmethionine in secondary fibromyalgia: a double-blind study. *Clinical and Experimental Rheumatology*, 16(1), 106–107.

Tavoni, A., Vitali, C., Bombardieri, S., & Pasero, G. (1987). Evaluation of S-adenosylmethionine in primary fibromyalgia. A double-blind crossover study. *American Journal of Medicine*, 83(5A), 107–110.

Telles, S., & Desiraju, T. (1992). Heart rate alterations in different types of pranayams. *Indian Journal of Physiology and Pharmacology*, 36(4), 287–288.

Temkin, N. R., Anderson, G. D., Winn, H. R., Ellenbogen, R. G., Britz, G. W., Schuster et al. (2007). Magnesium sulfate for neuroprotection after traumatic brain injury: a randomised controlled trial. *Lancet Neurology*, 6(1), 29–38.

Tempesta, E., Troncon, R., Janiri, L., Colusso, L., Riscica, P., Saraceni, G. et al. (1990). Role of acetyl-L-carnitine in the treatment of cognitive deficit in chronic alcoholism. *International Journal of Clinical Pharmacology Research*, 10(1–2), 101–107.

Teter, C. J., McCabe, S. E., Cranford, J. A., Boyd, C. J., & Guthrie, S. K. (2005). Prevalence and motives for illicit use of prescription stimulants in an undergraduate student sample. *Journal of American College Health*, 53(6), 253–262.

Thal, L. J., Grundman, M., Berg, J., Ernstrom, K., Margolin, R., Pfeiffer, E., Weiner, M. F., Zamrini, E., & Thomas, R. G. (2003). Idebenone treatment fails to slow cognitive decline in Alzheimer's disease. *Neurology*, 61(11), 1498–14502.

Thase, M. E. (2003). Evaluating antidepressant therapies: Remission as the optimal outcome. *Journal of Clinical Psychiatry*, 64(Suppl. 13), 18–25.

Thayer, J. F., & Brosschot, J. F. (2005). Psychosomatics and psychopathology: Looking up and down from the brain. *Psychoneuroendocrinology*, 30(10), 1050–1058.

Thomas, J. D., Garcia, G. G., Dominguez, H. D., & Riley, E. P. (2004). Administration of eliprodil during ethanol withdrawal in the neonatal rat attenuates ethanol-induced learning deficits. *Psychopharmacology (Berlin)*, 175(2), 189–195.

Thommessen, B., & Laake, K. (1996). No identifiable effect of ginseng (Gericomplex) as an adjuvant in the treatment of geriatric patients. *Aging (Milano)*, 8(6), 417–420.

Thys-Jacobs, S., McMahon, D., & Bilezikian, J. P. (2007). Cyclical changes in calcium metabolism across the menstrual cycle in women with premenstrual dysphoric disorder (PMDD). *Journal of Clinical Endocrinology and Metabolism*, 92(8), 2952–2959.

Thys-Jacobs, S., Starkey, P., Bernstein, D., & Tian, J. (1998). Calcium carbonate and the premenstrual syndrome: effects on premenstrual and menstrual symptoms. Premenstrual Syndrome Study Group. *American Journal of Obstetrics and Gynecology*, 179(2), 444–452.

Tice, J. A., Ettinger, B., Ensrud, K., Wallace, R., Blackwell, T., & Cummings, S. R. (2003). Phytoestrogen supplements for the treatment of hot flashes: The Isoflavone Clover Extract (ICE) Study: A randomized controlled trial. *Journal of the American Medical Association, 290*(2), 207–214.

Tildesley, N. T., Kennedy, D. O., Perry, E. K., Ballard, C. G., Wesnes, K. A., & Scholey, A. B. (2005). Positive modulation of mood and cognitive performance following administration of acute doses of Salvia lavandulaefolia essential oil to healthy young volunteers. *Physiology and Behavior, 83*(5), 699–709.

Timonen, M., Horrobin, D., Jokelainen, J., Laitinen, J., Herva, A., & Rasanen, P. (2004). Fish consumption and depression: The Northern Finland 1966 birth cohort study. *Journal of Affective Disorders, 82*(3), 447–452.

Toffano, G., Leon, A., Benvegnu, D., Boarato, E., & Azzone, G. F. (1976). Effect of brain cortex phospholipids on catechol-amine content of mouse brain. *Pharmacology Research Communications, 8*(6), 581–590.

Toneatto, T., & Nguyen, L. (2007). Does mindfulness meditation improve anxiety and mood symptoms? A review of the controlled research. *Canadian Journal Psychiatry, 52*(4), 260–266.

Torrioli, M. G., Vernacotola, S., Mariotti, P., Bianchi, E., Calvani, M., De Gaetano, A. et al. (1999). Double-blind, placebo-controlled study of L-acetylcarnitine for the treatment of hyperactive behavior in fragile X syndrome. *American Journal of Medical Genetics, 87*(4), 366–368.

Torta, R., Zanalda, F., Rocca, P. et al. (1988). Inhibitory activity of S-adenosyl-L-methionine on serum gamma-glutamyl-transpeptidase increase induced by psychodrugs and anticonvulsants. *Current Therapeutic Research, 44*, 144–159.

Trebaticka, J., Kopasova, S., Hradecna, Z., Cinovsky, K., Skodacek, I., Suba, J. et al. (2006). Treatment of ADHD with French maritime pine bark extract, Pycnogenol. *European Child and Adolescent Psychiatry, 15*(6), 329–335.

Trivedi, B. T. (1999). A clinical trial on Mentat. *Probe, 38*(4), 226.

Trivedi, M. H., Rush, A. J., Wisniewski, S. R., Nierenberg, A. A., Warden, D., Ritz, L. et al. (2006). Evaluation of outcomes with citalopram for depression using measurement-based care in STAR*D: Implications for clinical practice. *American Journal of Psychiatry, 163*(1), 28–40

Trock, B. J., Hilakivi-Clarke, L., & Clarke, R. (2006). Meta-analysis of soy intake and breast cancer risk. *Journal of the National Cancer Institute, 98*(7), 459–471.

Tsang, H. W., Fung, K. M., Chan, A. S., Lee, G., & Chan, F. (2006). Effect of a qigong exercise programme on elderly with depression. *International Journal of Geriatric Psychiatry, 21*(9), 890–297.

Tucker, M. (2007). Antioxidants studied for bipolar disorder, schizophrenia. *Psychiatry News, 35*(7), 3.

Turner, E. H., Loftis, J. M., & Blackwell, A. D. (2006). Serotonin a la carte: Supplementation with the serotonin precursor 5-hydroxytryptophan. *Pharmacology andl Therapeutics, 109*(3), 325–338.

Udintsev, S. N., & Shakhov, V. P. (1989). Decrease in the growth rate of Ehrlich's tumor and Pliss' lymphosarcoma with partial hepatectomy. *Voprosy Onkolologii*, 35(9), 1072–1075.

Udintsev, S. N., & Shakhov, V. P. (1990). Changes in clonogenic properties of bone marrow and transplantable mice tumor cells during combined use of cyclophosphane and biological response modifiers of adaptogenic origin. *Eksp Onkol*, 12(6), 55–56. (In Russian)

Udintsev, S. N., & Schakhov, V. P. (1991). Decrease of cyclophosphamide haematotoxicity by *Rhodiola rosea* root extract in mice with Ehrlich and Lewis transplantable tumors. *European Journal of Cancer*, 27(9), 1182.

Udintsev, S. N., Fomina, T. I., & Razina, T. G. (1992). An experimental model of metastatic liver involvement by using Ehrlich's ascitic cancer. *Voprosy Onkologii*, 38(6), 723–726. (In Russian)

U.S. Department of Health and Human Services, Agency for Healthcare Research and Quality (2002a). *Hormone replacement therapy and osteoporosis in HSTAT: Guide to clinical preventive services* (3rd ed.). Recommendations and Systematic Evidence Reviews, Guide to Community Preventive Services, Preventive Services Task Force Evidence Syntheses. Health Services/Technology Assessment Text.

U.S. Department of Health and Human Services, Agency for Healthcare Research and Quality (AHRQ). (2002b). S-adenosyl-L-metionine for treatment of depression, osteoarthritis, and liver disease. Summary, Evidence Report/Technology Assessment: Number 64. AHRQ Publication No. 02-E033. August 2002. Retrieved October 8, 2007 from www.ahrq.gov/clinic/epcsums/samesum .htm.

U.S. Food and Drug Administration Center for Safety and Applied Nutrition. (2002, March). Letter to health care professionals: FDA issues consumer advisory that Kava products may be associated with severe liver injury. www.cfsanifda .gov/ndms/addskava.html

Vairetti, M., Ferrigno, A., Canonico, P. L., Battaglia, A., Berte, F., & Richelmi, P. (2004). Nicergoline reverts haloperidol-induced loss of detoxifying-enzyme activity. *European Journal of Pharmacology*, 505(1–3), 121–125.

Valentova, K., Buckiova, D., Kren, V., Peknicova, J., Ulrichova, J., & Simanek, V. (2006). The in vitro biological activity of *Lepidium meyenii* extracts. *Cell Biology and Toxicology*, 22(2), 91–99 .

van Niekerk, J. K., Huppert, F. A., & Herbert, J. (2001). Salivary cortisol and DHEA: Association with measures of cognition and well-being in normal older men, and effects of three months of DHEA supplementation. *Psychoneuroendocrinology*, 26(6), 591–612.

Vaschillo, E. G., Vaschillo, B., & Lehrer, P. M. (2006). Characteristics of resonance in heart rate variability stimulated by biofeedback. *Applied Psychophysiology and Biofeedback*, 31(2), 129–142.

Vastag, B. (2007). Warming to a cold war herb. *Science News*, 172(12), 184–189.

Vedamurthachar, A., Janakiramaiah, N., Hegde, J. M., Shetty, T. K., Subbakrishna, D. K., Sureshbabu, S. V. et al. (2006). Antidepressant efficacy and hormonal effects of Sudarshana Kriya Yoga (SKY) in alcohol dependent individuals. *Journal of Affective Disorders, 94*(1–3), 249–253.

Vellas, B., Andrieu, S., Ousset, P. J., Ouzid, M., & Mathiex-Fortunet, H. (2006). The GuidAge study: methodological issues. A 5-year double-blind randomized trial of the efficacy of EGb 761 for prevention of Alzheimer disease in patients over 70 with a memory complaint. *Neurology, 67*(9 Suppl. 3), S6–S11.

Vermeulen, R. C., & Scholte, H. R. (2004). Exploratory open label, randomized study of acetyl- and propionylcarnitine in chronic fatigue syndrome. *Psychosomatic Medicine, 66*(2), 276–282.

Vernon, M. W., & Sorkin, E. M. (1991). Piracetam. An overview of its pharmacological properties and a review of its therapeutic use in senile cognitive disorders. *Drugs and Aging, 1*(1), 17–35.

Vickers, A. (2004). Alternative cancer cures: "unproven" or "disproven"? *CA: A Cancer Journal for Clinicians, 54*(2), 110–118.

Volkmann, H., Norregaard, J., Jacobsen, S., Danneskiold-Samsoe, B., Knoke, G., & Nehrdich, D. (1997). Double-blind, placebo-controlled cross-over study of intravenous S-adenosyl-L-methionine in patients with fibromyalgia. *Scandinavian Journal of Rheumatology, 26*(3), 206–211.

Volkow, N. D., Chang, L., Wang, G. J., Fowler, J. S., Leonido-Yee, M., Franceschi, D. et al. (2001). Association of dopamine transporter reduction with psychomotor impairment in methamphetamine abusers. *American Journal of Psychiatry, 158*(3), 377–382.

Volz, H. P., Murck, H., Kasper, S., & Moller, H. J. (2002). St John's wort extract (LI 160) in somatoform disorders: results of a placebo-controlled trial. *Psychopharmacology (Berlin), 164*(3), 294–300.

von Weiss, D. (2002). Use of mindfulness meditation for fibromyalgia. *American Family Physician, 65*(3), 380–384.

Vorbach, E. U., Arnoldt, K. H., & Hubner, W. D. (1997). Efficacy and tolerability of St. John's wort extract LI 160 versus imipramine in patients with severe depressive episodes according to ICD-10. *Pharmacopsychiatry, 30*(Suppl. 2), 81–85.

Wan, F. J., Lin, H. C., Kang, B. H., Tseng, C. J., & Tung, C. S. (1999). D-amphetamine-induced depletion of energy and dopamine in the rat striatum is attenuated by nicotinamide pretreatment. *Brain Research Bulletin, 50*(3), 167–171.

Wang, L. H., Li, C. S., & Li, G. Z. (1995). Clinical and experimental studies on tiaoshen liquor for infantile hyperkinetic syndrome. *Zhongguo Zhong Xi Yi Jie He Za Zhi, 15*(6), 337–340. (In Chinese)

Wang, R., Yan, H., & Tang, X. C. (2006). Progress in studies of huperzine A, a natural cholinesterase inhibitor from Chinese herbal medicine. *Acta Pharmacology Sinica (Beijin), 27*(1), 1–26. (In Chinese)

Warner, A. (2006, February 24–26). The psycho-spiritual benefits of Sudarshan KriyaYoga (SKY) for women diagnosed with breast cancer. In *Proceedings World Conference Expanding Paradigms: Science consciousness and spirituality* (pp. 124–136). New Delhi, India: All India Institute of Medical Sciences.

Watanabe, A., Hobara, N., & Nagashima, H. (1985). Lowering of liver acetaldehyde but not ethanol concentrations by pretreatment with taurine in ethanol-loaded rats. *Experientia, 41*, 1421–1422.

Watson, C. G., Tuorila, J. R., Vickers, K. S., Gearhart, L. P., & Mendez, C. M. (1997). The efficacies of three relaxation regimens in the treatment of PTSD in Vietnam War veterans. *Journal of Clinical Psychology, 53*(8), 917–923.

Waynberg, J. (1990, June 5–9). *Aphrodisiacs: Contribution to the clinical validation of traditional use of Ptychopetalum guyanna.* Paper presented at the First International Congress on Ethnopharmacology. Strasbourg, France.

Waynberg, J., & Brewer, S. (2000). Effects of Herbal vX on libido and sexual activity in premenopausal and postmenopausal women. *Advances in Therapy, 17*(5), 255–262.

Wdowiak, A., Wdowiak, L., & Wiktor, H. (2007). Evaluation of the effect of using mobile phones on male fertility. *Annals of Agricultural and Environmental Medicine, 14*(1), 169–172.

Weintraub, A. (2004). *Yoga for depression.* New York: Broadway Books.

Werntz, D. A., Bickford, R. G., & Shannahoff-Khalsa, D. (1987). Selective hemispheric stimulation by unilateral forced nostril breathing. *Human Neurobiology, 6*(3), 165–171.

Wesnes, K. A., Faleni, R. A., Hefting, N. R., Hoogsteen, G., Houben, J. J., Jenkins, E. et al. (1997). The cognitive, subjective, and physical effects of a ginkgo biloba/panax ginseng combination in healthy volunteers with neurasthenic complaints. *Psychopharmacology Bulletin, 33*(4), 677–683.

Westphal, L. M., Polan, M. L., & Trant, A. S. (2006). Double-blind, placebo-controlled study of Fertilityblend: A nutritional supplement for improving fertility in women. *Clinical and Experimental Obstetrics and Gynecology, 33*(4), 205–208.

Weydert, J. A., Shapiro, D. E., Acra, S. A., Monheim, C. J., Chambers, A. S., & Ball, T. M. (2006). Evaluation of guided imagery as treatment for recurrent abdominal pain in children: A randomized controlled trial. Bio Med Central *Pediatrics, 6*, 29.

Wheatley, D. (1999). Hypericum in seasonal affective disorder (SAD). *Current Medical Research Opinion, 15*(1), 33–37.

Widodo, N., Kaur, K., Shrestha, B. G., Takagi, Y., Ishii, T., Wadhwa, R. et al. (2007). Selective killing of cancer cells by leaf extract of Ashwagandha: Identification of a tumor-inhibitory factor and the first molecular insights to its effect. *Clinical Cancer Research, 13*(7), 2298–2306.

Willatts, P., Forsyth, J. S., DiModugno, M. K., Varma, S., & Colvin, M. (1998). Effect of long-chain polyunsaturated fatty acids in infant formula on problem solving at 10 months of age. *Lancet, 352*(9129), 688–691.

Williams, K. E., Marsh, W. K., & Rasgon, N. L. (2007). Mood disorders and fertility in women: A critical review of the literature and implications for future research. *Human Reproduction Update, 13*, 607–616.

Wilsher, C. R., Bennett, D., Chase, C. H., Conners, C. K., DiIanni, M., Feagans, L.

et al. (1987). Piracetam and dyslexia: effects on reading tests. *Journal of Clinical Psychopharmacology, 7*(4), 230–237.

Winman, A. (2004). Do perfume additives termed human pheromones warrant being termed pheromones? *Physiology and Behavior, 82*(4), 697–701.

Winn, H. R., Temkin, N. R., Anderson, G. D., & Dikmen, S. S. (2007). Magnesium for neuroprotection after traumatic brain injury. *Lancet Neurology, 6*(6), 478–479.

Withania somnifera. (2004). Monograph. *Alternative Medicine Review, 9*(2), 211–114.

Woelk, H., Arnoldt, K. H., Kieser, M., & Hoerr, R. (2007). *Ginkgo biloba* special extract EGb 761 in generalized anxiety disorder and adjustment disorder with anxious mood: A randomized, double-blind, placebo-controlled trial. *Journal of Psychiatric Research, 41*(6), 472–480.

Wolkowitz, O. M., Reus, V. I., Keebler, A., Nelson, N., Friedland, M., Brizendine, L. et al. (1999). Double-blind treatment of major depression with dehydroepiandrosterone. *American Journal of Psychiatry, 156*(4), 646–649.

Wong, A. H., Smith, M., & Boon, H. S. (1998). Herbal remedies in psychiatric practice. *Archives of General Psychiatry, 55*(11), 1033–1044.

Wong, W. Y., Merkus, H. M., Thomas, C. M., Menkveld, R., Zielhuis, G. A., & Steegers-Theunissen, R. P. (2002). Effects of folic acid and zinc sulfate on male factor subfertility: A double-blind, randomized, placebo-controlled trial. *Fertility and Sterility, 77* (3), 491–498.

Wood, C. (1993). Mood change and perceptions of vitality: A comparison of the effects of relaxation, visualization and yoga. *Journal of the Royal Society of Medicine, 86*(5), 254–258.

Woolery, A., Myers, H., Sternlieb, B., & Zeltzer, L. (2004). A yoga intervention for young adults with elevated symptoms of depression. *Alternative Therapy and Health Medicine, 10*(2), 60–63.

Wozniak, J., Biederman, J., Mick, E., Waxmonsky, J., Hantsoo, L., Best, C., Cluette-Brown, J. E., & Laposata, M. (2007). Omega-3 fatty acid monotherapy for pediatric bipolar disorder: A prospective open-label trial. *European Neuropsychopharmacology, 17*(6–7), 440–447.

Wu, X., Zhu, D., Jiang, X., Okagaki, P., Mearow, K., Zhu, G., McCall, S., Banaudha, K., Lipsky, R. H., & Marini, A. M. (2004). AMPA protects cultured neurons against glutamate excitotoxity through a phosphatidylinositol 3-kinase-dependent activation in extracellular signal-regulated kinase to upregulate BDNF gene expression. *Journal of Neurochemistry, 90*(4), 807–818.

Wuttke, W., Jarry, H., Christoffel, V., Spengler, B., & Seidlova-Wuttke, D. (2003). Chaste tree (*Vitex agnus-castus*)—Pharmacology and clinical indications. *Phytomedicine, 10*(4), 348–357.

Xu, R., Zhao, W., Xu, J., Shao, B., & Qin, G. (1996). Studies on bioactive saponins from Chinese medicinal plants. *Advances in Experimental Medicine and Biology, 404*, 371–382.

Yadav, S., Dhawan, A., Sethi, H., & Chopra, A. (2006, February 24–25). *Effect of*

AOL breathing process on heroin users. In *Proceedings World Conference Expanding Paradigms: Science, consciousness and spirituality* (pp. 169–177). New Delhi: All India Institutes of Medical Sciences.

Yamada, T., Terashima, T., Okubo, T., Juneja, L. R., & Yokogoshi, H. (2005). Effects of theanine, r-glutamylethylamide, on neurotransmitter release and its relationship with glutamic acid neurotransmission. *Nutrition and Neuroscience, 8*(4), 219–226.

Yehuda, S., Rabinovitz, S., & Mostofsky, D. I. (2005). Mixture of essential fatty acids lowers test anxiety. *Nutrition and Neuroscience, 8*(4), 265–267.

Yen, M. H., Weng, T. C., Liu, S. Y., Chai, C. Y., & Lin, C. C. (2005). The hepatoprotective effect of Bupleurum kaoi, an endemic plant to Taiwan, against dimethylnitrosamine-induced hepatic fibrosis in rats. *Biological and Pharmaceutical Bulletin, 28*(3), 442–448.

Yen, S. S. (2001). Dehydroepiandrosterone sulfate and longevity: New clues for an old friend. *Proceedings of the National Academy of Sciences USA, 98*(15), 8167–8169.

Youdim, K. A., Martin, A., & Joseph, J. A. (2000). Essential fatty acids and the brain: Possible health implications. *International Journal of Developmental Neuroscience, 18*(4–5), 383–399.

Youle, M., & Osio, M. (2007). A double-blind, parallel-group, placebo-controlled, multicentre study of acetyl L-carnitine in the symptomatic treatment of anti-retroviral toxic neuropathy in patients with HIV-1 infection. *HIV Medicine, 8*(4), 241–250.

Younus, J., Simpson, I., Collins, A., & Wang, X. (2003). Mind control of menopause. *Women's Health Issues, 13*(2), 74–78.

Yu, J. (2005). Airway mechanosensors. *Respiration Physiology and Neurobiology, 148*(3), 217–243.

Zanarini, M. C., & Frankenburg, F. R. (2003). Omega-3 Fatty acid treatment of women with borderline personality disorder:A double-blind, placebo-controlled pilot study. *American Journal of Psychiatry, 160*(1), 167–169.

Zandi, P. P., Anthony, J. C., Khachaturian, A. S., Stone, S. V., Gustafson, D., Tschanz, J. T. et al. (2004). Reduced risk of Alzheimer disease in users of antioxidant vitamin supplements: The Cache County Study. *Archives of Neurology, 61*(1), 82–88.

Zhang, H., & Huang, J. (1990). Preliminary study of traditional Chinese medicine treatment of minimal brain dysfunction: analysis of 100 cases. *Zhong Xi Yi Jie He Za Zhi, 10*(5), 278–279, 260. (In Chinese)

Zhang, X. Y., Zhou, D. F., Zhang, P. Y., Wu, G. Y., Su, J. M., & Cao, L. Y. (2001). A double-blind, placebo-controlled trial of extract of Ginkgo biloba added to haloperidol in treatment-resistant patients with schizophrenia. *Journal of Clinical Psychiatry, 62*(11), 878–883.

Zhdanova, I. V., Wurtman, R. J., Regan, M. M., Taylor, J. A., Shi, J. P., & Leclair, O. U. (2001). Melatonin treatment for age-related insomnia. *Journal of Clinical Endocrinology and Metabolism, 86*(10), 4727–4730.

Zheng, B. L., He, K., Kim, C. H., Rogers, L., Shao, Y., Huang, Z. Y., Lu, Y., Yan, S. J., Qien, L. C., & Zheng, Q. Y. (2000). Effect of a lipidic extract from lepidium meyenii on sexual behavior in mice and rats. *Urology,* 55(4), 598–602.

Zhu, J., Hamm, R. J., Reeves, T. M., Povlishock, J. T., & Phillips, L. L. (2000). Postinjury administration of L-deprenyl improves cognitive function and enhances neuroplasticity after traumatic brain injury. *Experimental Neurology,* 166(1), 136–152.

Zimatkin, S. M., & Zimatkina, T. I. (1996). Thiamine deficiency as predisposition to, and consequence of, increased alcohol consumption. *Alcohol and Alcoholism,* 31(4), 421–427.

Zs-Nagy, I. (1994). A survey of the available data on a new nootropic drug, BCE-001. *Annals of the New York Academy of Sciences, 717,* 102–214.

Zs-Nagy, I. (2002). Pharmacological interventions against aging through the cell plasma membrane: A review of the experimental results obtained in animals and humans. *Annals of the New York Academy of Sciences, 959,* 308–320.

Index

Note: Figures and tables are indicated by *f* or *t*, respectively, following the page number.

aging, 141–42
AIDS. *See* HIV/AIDS
akathisia, 341
Alcar. *See* acetyl-1 -carnitine
alcohol abuse. *See* substance abuse
allopurinol, 279–80
alpha-adrenergic blockers, 258
alpha-lipoic acid (ALA), 181
alternate nostril breathing, 97
Alzheimer's disease, 154–58
amantadine (Symmetrel), 338
American ginseng, 204, 216t
American Psychiatric Association
    (APA), 220
amino acids, attention-deficit disor-
    der and, 202
Amrit Kalash, 292, 315t, 340, 345
amygdala, 77
Anapanasati Sutta, 91
aniracetam
    attention-deficit disorder, 207
    cognition/memory disorders, 179
anorgasmia, 343
antidepressants
    augmentation of, 34, 43
    prescription, 15–17, 24–25
    SAMe, 18–30
antioxidants, cancer and, 286–87
anxiety disorders, 71–139
    case studies, 61–67, 81–83, 95–97,
        102–6, 123–24
    herbs and nutrients for, 125–35
    homeopathy, 136
    hormones for, 116–24
    medications, 74
    mind-body practices, 78–116
    post-traumatic stress disorder,
        97–104
    precautions and contraindications,
        110
    SAMe and, 21
    stress response systems and, 71–78
    treatment guidelines, 137–39t

apathy, 169–70
Arctic root. *See* Rhodiola rosea
arginine, 249, 256–57, 263t
ArginMax, 249, 256–57, 266t
ART-Excel, 208
Art of Living Foundation, 208
arthritis, 25, 301–2
ashwaganda
    cancer, 292
    cognition/memory disorders, 166
    treatment guidelines, 191t, 216t,
        313t
Asian ginseng. *See* Panax ginseng
asthenia, 336
astragalus, 344
attention, 93–94
attention-deficit disorder (ADD),
        195–206
    biofeedback for, 205–6
    case studies, 83, 197–99, 209–11
    causes, 195
    dietary treatments, 199–203
    herbs for, 203–5
    integrative approach, 209–15
    mind-body practices, 207–9
    neurotherapy for, 205–6
    pharmacological interventions,
        195–97
    treatment guidelines, 216–17t
AUM chant, 85
autism, 119
avoidance, 83
Ayurvedic medicine
    cancer, 291–92
    defined, 50
    mood disorders, 50–51
    theory of, 291

B vitamins
    akathisia treatment, 341
    cognition/memory disorders, 147
    hair loss treatment, 345
    mood disorders, 38–41